Be a Leader in Nursing

Be a Leader in Nursing

A Practical Guide for Nursing Students

HEATHER HENRY RN, BSC HONS NURSING, MBA, QUEEN'S NURSE

Honorary Senior Lecturer
University of Salford,
Greater Manchester, UK
Founder, BreathChamps CIC
Trustee, Being There

ELSEVIER

Notices

Practitioners and researchers must always rely on their own experience and knowledge in evaluating and using any information, methods, compounds or experiments described herein. Because of rapid advances in the medical sciences, in particular, independent verification of diagnoses and drug dosages should be made. To the fullest extent of the law, no responsibility is assumed by Elsevier, authors, editors or contributors for any injury and/or damage to persons or property as a matter of products liability, negligence or otherwise, or from any use or operation of any methods, products, instructions, or ideas contained in the material herein.

ISBN: 978-0-7020-8439-3

Content Strategist: Robert Edwards
Content Project Manager: Shravan Kumar
Design: Amy Buxton
Marketing Manager: Samantha Page

Printed in Poland

Last digit is the print number: 9   8   7   6   5   4   3   2   1

Working together
to grow libraries in
developing countries

www.elsevier.com • www.bookaid.org

CONTENTS

Nurses' Leadership Experiences Videos (available online on EVOLVE)

by Dr Katerina Kolyva

The literature of leadership in health care has steadily grown over the last decades to include a now very long list of theories and practices of leadership. From system to professional leadership, we have seen ideas and practices growing vigorously including the role of users, patients, and carers alongside the experts of developing and delivering systems of health care. In a parallel context, higher education also has seen a shift to its leadership theory, embracing the concept of student leadership and recognising the contribution of students as co-creators of education systems.

Leadership development is particularly relevant to health care students as these are students educated in a theoretical academic setting while they also learn in practice. Advances in academic theory, science and technology have led health care students to be exposed to different forms and types of leadership, whether these take place face to face in the classroom and in a practice learning setting or online via many forms of media, social media, augmented reality, artificial intelligence, robotics, etc. The list of opportunities for students to get exposed to leadership, to learn from role models and to practise their own leadership are now vast and extremely diverse.

Heather Henry's book is relevant and timely. In a post pandemic context, students have learned to adapt to different forms of learning and engagement with leadership. In demonstrating their leadership, students have taken ownership of their own learning, have networked with others in ways they have not done before, have promoted health care careers to newcomers and have raised awareness of issues affecting health care education and practice. In becoming proactive, students have demonstrated that leadership is not about hierarchy but rather about behaviour and the ability to inspire others.

I became involved in the concept of student leadership in health care five years ago. When we set up in 2017 the @150Leaders Student Leadership Programme at the Council of Deans of Health in partnership with the Burdett Trust for Nursing, we never expected it to grow to what it has become today. What started as a pilot to support students to learn about leadership and to debate with universities on teaching leadership in a more engaging way, has now become a movement. Over 300 students will have completed the programme in 2022 with more joining every year as the programme grows. What this initiative has taught me is that offering students leadership opportunities at a very early stage in their careers not only strengthens their confidence but helps us as a system to engage more directly with the future workforce. We can then better understand students' needs and develop policies and education curricula accordingly. Every single one of the 300 students that were exposed to leadership through this programme will have made a contribution to health care education, research and policy. I am proud of all their achievements.

Heather's book brings home all the key aspects of student leadership. From discussing and offering good critique of leadership theories, Heather focuses on what I would call the 'core' of student leadership: emotional intelligence, role modelling, networking, feedback, and reflection, coaching and mentoring. In each and every one of the chapters in this book, students will learn about an aspect of leadership theory and practice, but they will also learn from others. The examples and case studies from students, academics and practitioners are an excellent addition to the academic and policy context that Heather provides in each of the themes of her book. The specific tips and resources add value as students can tap into so many examples and material outside this book without necessarily always having to read more, as some of the resources include videos and social media material. References to the regulator's code of conduct and practice and the standards that relate to each of the themes discussed are helpful. Students can understand how leadership links to professionalism and feel confident that what they are learning in practical terms links to the learning outcomes expected of them as future newly qualified professionals.

The case studies used in the chapters are from real life examples and many come from students themselves including several from the @150Leaders programme. It is excellent to role model students in this publication, inspiring their fellow colleagues to pick up where others left or to develop totally new ventures and initiatives.

Storytelling is a strong component of this book, which is easy to read either from start to finish or in a more agile way by picking a chapter as they can be read independently. The structure of the book is easy to follow too: every chapter has a clear leadership theme, linked to the regulatory standards and the Nursing and Midwifery Council code, followed by case studies, tips and further resources.

I commend Heather for bringing together so many aspects of leadership in one place and yet managed to adapt them all to a student leadership context. I hope you enjoy reading this book as much as I did. For those of you who are students in the beginning of your leadership journey, I advise you to jump to every opportunity that offers engagement in leadership debate and action.

Dr Katerina Kolyva
CEO Council of Deans of Health
January 2022

by Craig Davidson

When the fantastic nurse leader Heather Henry first reached out and asked me to write a foreword to her book "Being a Leader in Nursing", I was flattered. My first thought was, I am so lucky to be one of the first to read her book. And I have been; you are in for a stellar treat. So, strap in, grab a notebook and get ready to begin your leadership journey. However, my next thought, as I am sure is true of nearly every nurse and student out there, was here comes the inevitable imposter syndrome – a topic I am delighted is covered in detail in this book. I had never written a foreword before, and although I am thirty-six, I only started nursing in 2016. What did I possibly have to say? But that is what Heather does so well both in practice and throughout this book. She encourages us to realise, celebrate and maximise our potential.

Heather is personable and honest throughout and gives insight into how she is also developing and learning as a leader. It is like having a friendly voice in your ear while reading the book, cheering you on. She talks throughout about "listening with fascination", but I am sure you will be reading with fascination like I was. This book is an invaluable tool for all nursing students, helping you realise your leadership potential. However, it is also an excellent refresher and resource guide for nurses at any stage of their career. As I was reading, I could not help but wish this resource was available when I started my leadership development. And from now on, I will be utilising both the teachings and the additional resources suggested. Because that is what this book does so brilliantly, it not only gives a robust introduction to various leadership behaviours, theories, models and styles, but also suggests further reading you can undertake and resources you can use to develop leadership potential the way you want, making it unique to you.

I particularly love the links to the Nursing and Midwifery Council (NMC) Code at the start of each chapter, illustrating how leadership should be a part of all our nurse development. Also, the top tips boxes and timeouts for reflection are so helpful. Heather discusses the importance of role-modelling while giving excellent lived examples of nursing students and registered nurse role models, demonstrating leadership in action. Reading the case studies and hearing the inspirational contributions from nursing students and other professionals is insightful, giving each of us something to aspire towards.

Heather reminds us that the days of traditional hierarchal leadership and followership are becoming a thing of the past. Modern leadership, as described throughout, can and should be a core part of everyday nursing. I have been extremely fortunate, both as a nursing student and now as an early-career nurse, to have held various formal and informal leadership positions. As a student, I was a departmental representative at Glasgow Caledonian University. I was also delighted to be elected as one of the two Scottish representatives on the Royal College of Nursing's (RCN) Students' Committee, becoming committee chair in the second year of my term. These student leadership opportunities enabled me to build my network and find allies, mentors and coaches who helped shape my leadership journey. Heather discusses how important building these relationships is in developing our leadership potential. Through networking and forging these alliances, I was invited to become a member of the Scottish Government's country-specific working group for the Year of the Nurse and Midwife in 2020 and sit on the working group for the NHS Scotland Pride badge initiative. So as students, you truly can make a difference – and more importantly, professionals at all levels realise your potential and want to hear your contribution and understand your unique perspective.

Embracing these opportunities as a student has given me the confidence to continue to pursue my leadership development as an early-career nurse. I now sit on the steering committee members of the RCN Nurses in Management and Leadership Forum and I am honoured to be co-chair of the Nursing Now Challenge's European regional hub. I get to work with other nurses pushing for real change at all stages of their careers. I also discover and discuss other nurses' passions and career progression as co-host of the award-winning podcast series, "Retaining the Passion: Journeys through Nursing", with my fellow early-career nurse Clare Manley.

As Heather and the other contributors of this book do, I encourage you to acknowledge your transferable leadership skills. Just because you are starting your nursing career, it does not mean you are beginning your leadership development from scratch. Too often in leadership and life, we focus on our weaknesses, the elements we perceive as holding us back. That is not to say we should not acknowledge and address these; as Heather identifies, we should "recognise [our] blind spots and be willing to learn." But our strengths make us unique; they are our assets. And we should look to them when creating our leadership blueprint, as Heather and the contributors of the book encourage us to do. So, as you read this book and develop your leadership potential, remember what your strengths are. Celebrate what you are good at; use your strengths as your guide. My final piece of advice, which Heather and the contributors echo throughout, is get to know your authentic self and be led by your ethics, morals, and values. Be bold, brave and courageous in your nursing leadership. Most importantly, believe you can be a leader; because you can.

Craig Davidson RN BSc (Hons)
Senior Nurse
Asylum Health Bridging Team
Glasgow City Health and Social Care Partnership

I came to this book thinking that I'd share a few leadership models and theories that I'd always found helpful and enjoyed with student nurses, but it has turned out to be much more than this.

By collaborating with nursing, midwifery and allied health professional students to write this book I entered their world, which is so incredibly different to my own student experience that started when I was 18 years old. I was so inexperienced in life that I didn't even know how to talk to people properly. I didn't have the worries of financing my studies or caring for family members. I lived in the nurse's home for the first 2 years and I was paid a (tiny) salary. My student life was a very sheltered experience.

I recognised that although students today come from diverse backgrounds, with many having had careers and/or families before entering nurse training, there are some major hurdles to overcome if they are to exercise their leadership muscles, such as that students are not often seen as assets.

> 'That is the student nurse experience: of being at the very starting rung, whether or not you have a wealth of life experience, that's not necessarily recognised.'
> AALIJAH BUTTIMER, DUAL MENTAL HEALTH/ADULTS NURSE PROGRAMME

I didn't write a word until I had given the student nursing community what my mentor would call 'a good listening to'. I discovered insecurity and inspiration in equal measure. All were driven by their values and passion.

Strange things happened when I listened: the students started praising my abilities as a coach, not as a writer, yet all I was doing was listening and asking questions. I was giving them my full attention and the space to hear themselves think out loud—something I would urge you to do as a leader.

I have been hugely impressed by the students that I have met and I hope that some of them may become lifelong colleagues. They walk a tightrope where, when they look ahead, they walk with expertise, but when they look down or around they wobble. These feelings are all natural. The trick is to believe and trust in yourself, and fake it till you make it. For us who are more senior in nursing it is our responsibility to nurture their talent and support them.

My own nurse training at Manchester Royal Infirmary was blissfully lacking in leadership knowledge: I was told what to do and exactly how to do it by sister-tutors, nursing officers and ward sisters. On my second ward the staff nurse told me that I was 'bolshy' and not cut out for nursing. My job was to replicate what they taught me and nothing more. I remember that one of my assessments in my third year was to manage the ward for a shift and I was frankly terrified. My first action was to break a bottle of orange squash and then have the ward clerk slip on the residue and fall. I lost my right-hand woman in the first 10 minutes.

When I became a newly registered nurse I became this ball of unstoppable ambition to be a ward sister, or ward manager as it is now, in my chosen specialism of cardiothoracic nursing. I thought, at that stage, that a sister was somebody who was very good at nursing rather than very good at managing and leading, so it was a good job that I didn't get promoted to be a sister.

I first learnt about leadership by role modelling: I watched other nurses whom I admired and basically followed them around and copied what worked and tried hard to avoid the things that didn't. In those days the support for those transitioning to registered nurse consisted of a short 'first-line management' course, that somehow I missed.

What I learnt much later was that you can be a leader and influencer at any level in an organisation, and that was the path for me. Those hierarchical leadership positions within the system that I strove for—and achieved—just made me more uncomfortable. It took me a long time to realise what my particular talents were and to employ them to the best of my ability, rather than try to be something I wasn't. I did what was expected of me, which was to climb the slippery slope of management. This will suit some of you; others will want to lead from where you are; others will work in research or education and lead from there; and others will volunteer like I did with the NHS Alliance—these are all valid leadership choices.

My family were extremely proud of me, but my social life was a mess because I worked such long hours and I worried a lot about my leadership challenges. I don't really thrive with constant pressure. I like to reflect on what is happening around me and be creative and inventive. Sometimes I was promoted for this, but sometimes I was seen as a threat. I got into trouble for being a dreamer, voicing my opinions and having too many ideas above my station. Seeing people like me as assets, at that time, was rare, but things have changed now and diversity of thought is embraced.

By the time I reached the level of an NHS director I was totally miserable. I was on a 6-month leadership course at the King's Fund in London called the Top Manager's Programme, which still operates today, as preparation for me to become a chief executive. It was a fantastic immersive experience, where I joined a temporary learning community and got to participate in various experiential leadership activities, focusing on emotional intelligence. I became much more able to recognise my own emotions and those of others. This experience very much reminds me of the #150Leaders programme that many of the students quoted in this book have been exposed to. But the more the King's Fund faculty members spoke about the role of the CEO, the more I became convinced that it wasn't for me. I felt trapped.

And then I was made compulsorily redundant, which forced me to rethink what I really wanted to do, and my career pivoted in another direction. I met a retired health visitor called Hazel Stuteley OBE of C2 Connecting Communities. Hazel's team partners with communities to enable them to change their own lives and address the deep disadvantages they face. What she said and did resonated with things that I'd thought and done with a community partnership that I'd worked with in Stretford, Greater Manchester.

Hazel was everything that I wanted to be, and so I apprenticed myself to her for a couple of years to 'learn the trade' of asset-based community development. Then I started working with a social enterprise in Salford called Unlimited Potential, whose CEO, Chris Dabbs, is one of the premier social entrepreneurs in the land. Being an anthropologist, he taught me much about societies and cultures, so I began to understand what was going on around me. I got to do some of the most enthralling social innovation projects with him that began to be noticed nationally.

I joined the NHS Alliance (now called The Health Creation Alliance CIC), a membership organisation that influences the health system. They encouraged me to write and speak about my experiences of working alongside communities to address inequality. As soon as I joined, their senior executives (mostly GPs) became my role models, showed me how to disrupt and influence the system, and invited me to do the same. My capacity to challenge, cajole and inspire people was encouraged. It turns out that my particular leadership talent is to be a positive irritant for change. The NHS embraces this talent now, and there are programmes to help 'radicals' to work within the system. I have written about this because several students that I interviewed have a strong drive to change the world. I'd say, go for it.

I ended up, to my utter surprise, being the first nurse—and first female—elected as chairman of the NHS Alliance. I had this huge opportunity, without any formal authority, to talk to government, policy-makers, academics, thought leaders and many more about those thoughts and dreams that used to get me into trouble: how things could be different for communities experiencing deep disadvantage. There I would be on some national platform, usually with a citizen leader, speaking truth to power about tackling health inequalities based on what I'd seen, read about and reflected on—a far cry from my student dream of being a ward sister. I knew myself and I'd found my voice. I no longer equated leadership with hierarchy and I felt valued for my strengths. I even got a Christmas card from the Secretary of State for Health.

A year ago, I launched my second social enterprise, BreathChamps CIC, which helps children, families and communities to learn about breathing problems in fun ways. My 18-year-old self is still a little shocked about this, because having uncontrolled asthma as a child and a right upper and middle lobectomy unexpectedly at just 21 rather shatters your confidence. Ian Unitt, a learning disability nurse whom I interviewed for this book, said it perfectly—if you work outside your comfort zone, then your comfort zone gets bigger.

The Alliance, Chris and Hazel taught me how to work right across the system, connecting with citizen leaders, housing, criminal justice, fire and rescue, faith, education and much more. Getting out of my silo, understanding how complex systems work and getting to know the role of others and how their organisations contribute to health and wellbeing was—and still is—a transformative process for me as a leader and a nurse.

The Council of Deans of Health encouraged me, in writing this book, to demonstrate to student nurses the importance of working with other disciplines across organisational and professional boundaries. You will therefore see various case studies beyond nursing. Health is not about health care; today's leaders work in an integrated way and you—our future leaders—have a huge opportunity to look at what is happening beyond your immediate role and think differently about who you can work with to change lives.

My advice is to be yourself, discover your strengths, push yourself, tune into emotions and unconscious thought, enable others, look around you and reflect with a trusted colleague on what's happening. This book is for you, in the hope that my meanderings can help you to get where you want to be in your leadership career a bit more directly than I did.

Heather Henry
Sale, 2022

ABOUT THE AUTHOR

Queen's Nurse Heather is an entrepreneur, writer, social innovator and health policy influencer. Her NHS roles have included cardiothoracic nurse, general practice nurse and director of primary care. She is a trustee for Being There, a Greater Manchester charity that supports people with life-limiting conditions and has an honorary role as a senior lecturer at the University of Salford.

Heather practises a social model of public health, inventing and coproducing solutions with local people. Based on her own severe asthma as a child, her latest innovation is BreathChamps, where children, families and communities learn about breathing in fun ways.

In 2018 Heather won the Sue Pembrey Award for person- and community-centred care, and she has also received the Open University Business School Alumnus Award for her 'Outstanding Contribution to Society'.

Heather lives in Sale and works nationally. She has a stepdaughter Sarah and two grandchildren, Jamie and Sean, a cat called Boo, a dog called Bess and a lovely husband called Keith, who sometimes gets a look in.

ACKNOWLEDGEMENTS

One of the underlying principles of my work is to cocreate solutions to problems, and this is how I tackled the task of writing this book. My hope is that the process of interacting with others made us all stronger and more connected.

The first thing I did when faced with writing a book proposal was to contact @WeStudent-Nurse, a team of student nurses who offer a peer support network, and the founder of the social media 'WeCommunities' network for health professionals, Teresa Chinn, to ask for help. Both agreed to support and advise me in the writing of this book. It has been an absolute pleasure and privilege to work with them.

I would also like to thank the Council of Deans of Health's #150Leaders programme for health students for their guidance and support: Katerina Kolyva, Nadia Butt, Adele Nightingale and Beryl Mansel. Beryl also introduced me to Swansea Leadership Academy, and I have since been invited to do a little work within that programme! I have learnt from Beryl's approach and attempted to share as much of her learning—and her students' success—as I could.

A huge thank you to all the fantastic and inspiring people who have given me advice or agreed to be interviewed and quoted in this book. You give me hope for the future of clinical leadership. They are, in no particular order, Aalijah Buttimer, Joy O'Gorman, Jessica Sainsbury, Brian Webster, Natalie Elliott, Claire Carmichael, Naomi Berry, Sarah Bradder, Alison Booker, Alicia Burnett, Gloria Sikapite, Simon James, Rebecca Lennox, Ian Unitt, Ellie Looker, Rebecca Hollobone, Daniel Branch, Leanne Patrick, Mark Radford, Anne-Marie Dodson, Barbara Stilwell, George Coxon, Lance Gardner, Alicia Clare, Brian Dolan, Zoe Cohen, Victoria McTurk, Gary Mitchell, Ruth Oshikanlu, Joan Pons Laplana, Jennie Aronsson, June Girvin, Nathan Harrison and Jo Odell.

I would not be here writing a book without the support of two longstanding mentors who are always there to help me reflect and learn: Hazel Stuteley and Chris Dabbs. Everyone needs a Hazel and a Chris. I sneaked some tiny examples of our work together into the pages of this book: how to engage communities and improve wellbeing, the Dadly Does It/Salford Dadz-Little Hulton programme and a schools-based initiative called the FACT project, that I adapted as a worked example in the chapter on project planning.

A final thank you to Robert Edwards of Elsevier, who commissioned me to write this book and saw things in me that I didn't see in myself. That was kind and handy when you have a lung condition during a pandemic lockdown and can do little else but think and write.

INTRODUCTION

'You uphold the reputation of your profession at all times. You should display a personal commitment to the standards of practice and behaviour set out in the Code. You should be a model of integrity and leadership for others to aspire to. This should lead to trust and confidence in the professions from patients, people receiving care, other health and care professionals and the public.'

'...Throughout their career, all our registrants will have opportunities to demonstrate leadership qualities, regardless of whether or not they occupy formal leadership positions.'

THE CODE, NURSING AND MIDWIFERY COUNCIL (2018)

As a registered nurse, you will be required to lead others, so maybe you are thinking about how you might start to develop and practice those leadership skills. Maybe you are already in a student leadership role, such as being a course representative at your university, or maybe you are thinking that you would like to lead a project as part of your studies but don't feel equipped to do so. Maybe you want to understand more about leadership in education and research as well as in practice. Maybe you are worried about the idea of being a leader and are looking for ideas.

This book is for you.

It's not only for you, but it's written with the help of fellow nurse, midwife and allied health professional students, newly registered nurses and experienced nurse educators who shared their leadership case studies. They all told me that this book needed to be practical and give real-life examples that you can identify with, of students who are leading in various ways. It covers the questions, concerns and everyday wobbles of undergraduate nurses as well as their successes and, occasionally, failures too. Because if we don't fail we don't learn anything.

The style of this book is intended to be a practical guide rather than a theory-laden textbook, although I have added some theory so you can make sense of the case studies given and you can use relevant theories and models in your clinical and academic work.

But you can't learn about leadership by just sitting in a room reading this book or writing assignments. There are lots of 'time-out' exercises to do. You will get the most out of this book by engaging with them and testing your leadership skills out in the real world and then reflecting upon what you have learnt.

This brings me to mention early on 'imposter syndrome'—feeling that you are not good enough and will be found out. Every student nurse that I have spoken to talked about this—as have many senior nurses too, so there is a big section on this with tips from fellow students to help you to develop your confidence.

When interviewed for this book, Mark Radford, chief nurse at Health Education England, stressed the importance of student nurses developing their leadership skills early on. He sees this as a building block and a way to develop your confidence, especially if you are from a minority ethnic group, so that if you want to step up to different leadership positions you will have good grounding and experiential learning from the start.

Leadership at Every Level

Leadership is a process, not a position. The Nursing and Midwifery Council (NMC) quote above mentions that nurses lead whether they have formal leadership positions or not. Leadership happens at every level, including preregistration. As soon as you walk into a clinical area and engage with a patient you have a leadership role. You will read more about this in Chapter 1.

The Rise of Clinical Leaders

It's useful to reflect on how leadership has evolved in health care so we can see how far we have come, especially as clinical leaders.

Historically, health services operated what is called 'management by consensus': where managers managed, administrators administrated and clinicians led their teams, all within their own hierarchies. They all coexisted within one organisation. But as the cost and complexity of health care increased, in 1983 the government asked Sir Roy Griffiths, a director at Sainsbury's plc, to lead an inquiry into the management of the NHS.

'At no level is the general management role clearly being performed by an identifiable individual. In short, if Florence Nightingale were carrying her lamp through the corridors of the NHS today she would almost certainly be searching for the people in charge.'

GRIFFITHS REPORT (1983)

Management by consensus had led to feudal and fragmented leadership. His report made several recommendations that heralded the introduction of general management into the NHS, based on private sector business principles. General managers became responsible and accountable for their organisations. Boards were established and medical and clinical directors were appointed to them, with the aim of aligning clinical work to the objectives of the organisation.

Throughout the 1990s, the idea that it was important to engage clinicians to ensure effective delivery and avoid doctors in particular from derailing organisational plans was further developed. Today it is recognised that clinically led organisations, where health professionals work in partnership with general managers, perform better.

'Combine your frontline clinical knowledge and experience with leadership skills...to benefit the whole team, benefit the NHS, and benefit the nation.'

MATT HANCOCK, SECRETARY OF STATE FOR HEALTH (2018)

Successive NHS leaders such as the surgeon and reformer Lord Ara Darzi and secretaries of state Andrew Lansley, Jeremy Hunt and Matt Hancock have promoted clinicians as important leaders within the health and care system. The reason for this, according to academics such as Swanwick and McKimm (2017), is that studies have shown that clinical leadership is associated with improved care quality, staff satisfaction, patient outcomes, organisational performance and strategic decision-making.

Clinicians such as nurses know how things work. They are in touch with staff, patients, families and communities, and they can therefore influence service delivery and research priorities in ways that make sense. Clinical leadership works best when it is multidisciplinary and helps engage fellow clinicians to set the direction that an organisation should take.

In 2011 the NHS Leadership Academy was established with the aim of delivering excellence in leadership to improve patient care. It developed a clinical leadership competency framework and a healthcare leadership model, setting out the evidence-based leadership behaviours for everyone working in the NHS.

Leadership development in the NHS is now seen as a career-long process. Programmes of leadership development now operate from undergraduate level through to early career, middle/senior management and at executive level.

In the past, many universities didn't include leadership development on their nursing course curricula, and, for those that did, it was often an academic approach focusing on teaching leadership theory. This meant that at the point of registration, newly registered nurses were often poorly prepared for activities such as leading a ward team.

There are a lot of factors that have recently driven the development of student nurse leadership skills. In 2018, the NMC consulted on and then published the proficiencies expected within an undergraduate nursing curriculum. Platform 5 of this document is wholly concerned with leading and managing nursing care and working in teams:

> 'Registered nurses provide leadership by acting as a role model for best practice in the delivery of nursing care. They are responsible for managing nursing care and are accountable for the appropriate delegation and supervision of care provided by others in the team including lay carers. They play an active and equal role in the interdisciplinary team, collaborating and communicating effectively with a range of colleagues.'
> FUTURE NURSE: STANDARDS OF PROFICIENCY FOR REGISTERED NURSES, NMC (2018)

Around the same time, Health Education England (HEE) published *Maximising Leadership Learning Within the Pre-Registration Healthcare Curricula* (2018). The aim was to prepare students with the skills to lead from the very start of their careers. It sets out guidelines to help education providers to maximise leadership learning in the preregistration health care curricula.

In 2020, at the height of a global COVID-19 pandemic when the quality of NHS leadership was being scrutinised, the NHS People Plan was published. At its heart were three things: more people, working differently, in a compassionate and inclusive culture. This plan signalled the importance of leaders understanding and supporting people: being 'more human'—looking after its people, embracing diversity and giving everyone a sense that they belong, a far cry from the general management concepts of a man from Sainsbury's. There has been a move to more inclusive leadership with 'permission to act', meaning local organisations having more autonomy and leaders at all levels given licence to act in creative and innovative ways. The People Plan also introduced coaching and mentoring and 'leadership support circles', online sessions offering time and a reflective safe space for those with responsibility for managing others. It also set goals to ensure diversity in leadership across all the protected characteristics.

Shaping Student Leadership: The #150Leaders Programme

This book has been hugely influenced by the approach and learning from the #150Leaders programme, which was established in 2018 by the Council of Deans of Health and the Burdett Trust for Nursing, who funded the programme. This was a 2-year UK-wide student leadership programme targeted at health care students from a variety of disciplines. It offered 150 students of nursing, midwifery and a variety of allied health professional courses across the UK the opportunity to be exposed to leadership development through role modelling, reflection, networking and mentoring. Most of the students and newly registered nurses interviewed for this book have attended this programme and were able to reflect on how it had helped them.

The aim was to 'promote student leadership as a key capability within education and research and promote innovation in healthcare higher education' (Kolyva et al, 2018). Not only were the approaches to developing leadership capabilities evidence based, but they were also codesigned and cocreated by students themselves. This enabled the students to become advocates for undergraduate leadership development opportunities. They were encouraged to attend high-level policy meetings and events to help change the status quo. Although a challenging experience, students experienced first hand the power of leaders listening to them. They also gained exposure to the sort of environments that they will operate in as future health care professionals.

The #150Leader participants wanted interactive leadership programmes (rather than theory), networking opportunities, and mentorships. They wanted to be supported to reflect on what makes a good leader and what shaped the leadership journey of others. They wanted to understand and develop their personal leadership style and how it might differ from, and be complementary to, others.

The Council of Deans of Health consider that part of the programme's success lies in it being UK-wide and interdisciplinary. Therefore, a key consideration, as you ponder your leadership journey, is diversity and inclusion. Think about engaging with fellow student leaders across the four nations of the UK. This can be done via social media, listening to podcasts, reading blogs as well as attending events. Be curious and engage with other disciplines. For example, I recently attended an online discussion with physiotherapists discussing pulmonary rehabilitation. As a public health nurse, I am curious about the contribution of the housing sector to health and wellbeing, and spend as much time as I can collaborating with them.

How to Use this Book

The HEE document *Maximising Leadership Learning Within the Pre-Registration Healthcare Curricula* describes three stages of developing as a leader. This book is structured in the same three ways, and you will get the most out of it by working through it from beginning to end, rather than dipping into it.

Our leadership journey starts by understanding ourselves and appreciating who we are and what we can offer. We need to reflect on what good leadership looks like and connect to mentors, coaches and networks who will help us to understand ourselves and offer support. We need to reflect on progress and learn to manage our emotions, notice the emotions of others and manage the pressures we face. This will be covered in Section I.

The second stage is then how we start to work with others, begin to appreciate our differences, start to codesign solutions, be courageous and decisive, communicate with our team and know how to influence them. We cover this in Section II.

And the third stage is to start to understand how organisations and the wider health and care system work, so that we can start to think about how to improve health and care, how we can be creative and innovative and how we can handle challenging and risky situations.

These three stages are sometimes termed 'comprehensive leadership'.

Tips to Reflect on Your Learning

Katerina Kolyva, chief executive of the Council of Deans of Health has this advice to students reading this book about how to maximise your learning:

- Write a letter to yourself to open at the end of the book. This might include:
  - asking yourself questions such as 'Why do you want to be a leader? What do you hope to achieve?'
  - talking about who you are now, your thoughts and fears, your skills and abilities and your goals and hopes;
  - adding things that you want to stop, start or continue doing such as 'Stop speaking negatively to yourself, you're too much of a perfectionist';
  - giving yourself advice: 'Take a risk; you're good enough to cope';
  - sealing the letter, storing it safely and setting a date on your phone for when you want to open it. Give yourself enough time—somewhere between 1 and 5 years.
- Keep a reflective diary of your thoughts and feelings as you study this book and complete the exercises.
- Use your diary to write a blog or article for a nursing journal on your undergraduate leadership journey: how did you feel, what did you learn, what did you change, what did you take away. It may be helpful to use a model of reflection to structure this.

If you'd like to let me know how you are doing, please send me a tweet at
@heatherhenry4. You can also Tweet #150Leaders at @150Leaders and
@WeStudentNurse—it's a very active leadership community and you will expand your
leadership network!

References

Griffiths Report, 1983. NHS Management Inquiry. Department of Health and Social Security, London.
Hancock, M., 2018. Speech: Leadership within the NHS. Department of Health and Social Care.
Kolyva, K., Butt, N., Eames, J., 2018. #150Leaders: Fostering Student Leadership. Council of Deans of Health
NHS England, 2020. We are the NHS: People Plan for 2020/2021 – Action for us all.
NHS Leadership Academy, 2011. Clinical Leadership Competency Framework.
NHS Leadership Academy, 2013. Healthcare Leadership Model.
Nursing and Midwifery Council, 2018. Future Nurse: Standards of proficiency for registered nurses.
Nursing and Midwifery Council, 2018. The Code.
Swanwick, T., McKimm, J., (ed), 2017. ABC of Clinical Leadership. Wiley and Sons.

Know Yourself as Leader

What Is a Leader?

OBJECTIVES

After reading this chapter and completing the activities, you should be able to:

- Describe the main differences between leadership and management
- Explain why both leadership and management are needed to deliver high-quality care
- Appreciate transferrable knowledge, skills and experience that you already have
- Identify leadership activities that you already carry out
- Support fellow students to recognise their own leadership abilities.

Relevance to the Nursing and Midwifery Council (NMC) Code

Promote Professionalism and Trust
Paragraph 25:
Provide leadership to make sure people's wellbeing is protected and to improve their experiences of the health and care system.
Throughout their career, all our registrants will have opportunities to demonstrate leadership qualities, regardless of whether or not they occupy formal leadership positions.

The Culture of Nurse Leadership Preregistration

The genesis to becoming a leader for many student leaders interviewed for this book came from a desire to help others—whether this be patients, peers or the wider system. The realisation that, in stepping up and making a change, they were in fact leaders was resisted by many because of their understanding of what leadership meant: hierarchy, being in charge, knowing more than others, maybe even thinking of themselves as better than someone else. There is a lot of confusion between management and leadership, which this chapter will start to tease out.

■ Time Out

What motivates you to read this book?
How do you feel about the idea of being a leader?

There is still a pervading culture that exists in clinical placements that you are 'the student'—not even a name, here to learn—and the thought that you may somehow be a leader goes against the grain of students' thinking.

'You have that idea in your head [about leadership] *that you're at the top and everyone else is behind you, following you. Personally, I would never even as a nurse put myself in that position because there's always someone who can lead a situation.'*

ELLIE LOOKER, UNIVERSITY OF PLYMOUTH

Student life is generally a very democratic one, and the student leaders interviewed were quite often at pains to emphasise the role of others in the team. Some were able to articulate that leaders are often not the ones at the front but can be the enablers of change in the background. There are many different styles of leadership, and it is for you to find the right style that suits your personality. Students often reported that they identified, followed or befriended more senior leaders whose style they identified with.

And yet, despite this 'in charge' view of leadership, many stepped forward because of that passion and a desire to 'give it a go', get out of their comfort zones and learn something new. At this point students talked about imposter syndrome and not being good enough to be a leader. Again, this will be an important theme for the book, with students and senior nurses sharing tips on how they manage it: because it does not go away for most of us, it requires continuous work.

'I find it quite challenging speaking up and being visible. I often feel that I'm taking up too much space and I don't have the right to be there, so some of that for me was about learning how to navigate that.'

AALIJAH BUTTIMER,
DUAL MENTAL HEALTH/
ADULT NURSING PROGRAMME,
SPEAKING ABOUT PARTICIPATING
IN THE *#150LEADERS PROGRAMME*

The students interviewed were reluctant to declare themselves a 'leader' at first. This was overcome by the desire, primarily, to make a difference. The stretching that came with giving it a go was rewarded by their learning through trial and error and the confidence that they gained through experience. They talked about how they grew to accept the idea of being called leaders and describing themselves in this way.

So nursing, even at undergraduate level, gives you a great platform to practise your leadership skills. This is because:

■ You are the first point of contact for your patients and their families when they are most vulnerable.
■ You are your patient's advocate in the interprofessional team.

Leadership therefore is not about your position in the hierarchy. We are all leaders in one way or another. By choosing to be a health professional you have confirmed that to yourself.

The elephant in the room is the desire for power, money or attention. These are poor reasons to take on leadership skills and are usually obvious to observers. Many people equate power with position, but there are in fact many ways to exert power and influence as a student nurse. We shall look at this in Section 2 of this book.

What Is a Leader?

'Management is doing things right; leadership is doing the right things. Management is efficiency in climbing the ladder of success; leadership is about determining whether the ladder is leaning against the right wall.'

PETER DRUCKER, MANAGEMENT THEORIST

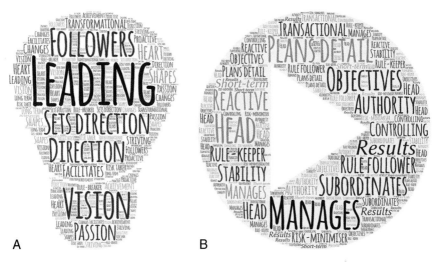

Fig. 1.1   Word cloud showing the differences between leaders and managers.

WHAT'S THE DIFFERENCE BETWEEN LEADERSHIP AND MANAGEMENT?

Refer to Fig. 1.1, which shows word clouds incorporating words commonly associated with leadership and management.

■ Time Out

Organise this list of activities under two headings: *(i)* those that you think are management activities, *(ii)* those that you think are leadership activities:

1. Compiling the staff rosters
2. Dealing with complaints
3. Enforcing uniform policy
4. Mentoring a more junior staff member
5. Wearing your uniform correctly every day
6. Managing a ward budget
7. Helping a patient to understand their medications
8. Handing over from one shift to the next
9. Sharing a new idea about preventing falls
10. Acting as a course representative at your university
11. Delegating staff to work in certain clinical areas
12. Reflecting on what has been learnt from a failed task
13. Writing up reports for your manager
14. Reporting an adverse drug reaction
15. Standing up for a colleague
16. Writing a blog to help fellow students
17. Checking the controlled drugs record
18. Accompanying the consultant on their ward round
19. Giving a presentation at university on a topic you know
20. Attending a meeting of your professional body and reporting on issues you've seen

It Is Not Easy – Is It?

Consider which are about *doing the right thing* and which are about *doing things right*. Think also about when nurses act as role models and when they are changing things for the better—classic leadership skills. Leadership is also about having a *vision* for where we should be going; setting the *direction* of a group, team and organisation; and creating the *values* of the team or organisation (West et al., 2015). Conversely, management is about directing people and resources to deliver on agreed aims, strategies and targets.

The two roles are complementary—you cannot have management without leadership and you cannot have leadership without management. Complex organisations need both wise leadership and consistent management to flourish, to deliver quality care, to innovate and make improvements. Roles often have leadership and management responsibilities depending upon the task in hand, including the roles of student nurses.

Refer to Table 1.1 for how the earlier list might look.

There are some activities on this list, however, that might include both leadership and management. What if, during or after the routine ward round, you drew the consultant's attention to a piece of research that might improve the way that patients are treated? What if you are using delegation to strategically develop the skills of particular members of staff in managing arterial ulcers as part of a new project to improve wound care? What if the presentation was not about sharing new information but on something that all your peers understood and you were just being assessed on how well you communicated? Would that be leadership? Probably not.

Most nurses carry out activities from both lists, making arbitrarily designating roles into leadership and management unhelpful. It is also not helpful to see leadership as a superior role to management: they both work together. Here is how one clinical leader describes it:

> '*Think of a ship setting out on a journey; while it is vital to set direction and motivate the sailors to cope with challenging situations (the leadership aspects), the ship will not reach its destination if it is not watertight and doesn't have enough fuel, provisions or people to sail it (the management activities).*'
> ANDREW LONG, CONSULTANT IN PAEDIATRICS,
> GREAT ORMOND STREET HOSPITAL, 2018

TABLE 1.1 ■ **Leadership and Management Activities in Nursing**

Leadership—Doing the Right Things: Direction, Vision, Values, Role Modelling	Management—Doing Things Right: Directing People and Resources
Change and Movement	***Order and Consistency***
Mentoring a more junior member of staff	Compiling staff rosters
Helping a patient to understand their medications	Dealing with complaints
Wearing your uniform correctly every day	Enforcing uniform policy
Sharing a new idea about preventing falls	Managing a ward budget
Acting as a course representative at your university	Handing over from one shift to the next
Reflecting on what has been learnt from a failed task	Writing reports for your manager
Standing up for a colleague	Reporting an adverse drug reaction
Writing a blog to help fellow students	Checking the controlled drugs record
Attending a meeting of your professional body and reporting on issues you have seen	Accompanying the consultant on their ward round
Giving a presentation at university on a topic you know about	Delegating staff to work in certain areas

Followership

Another important and often underappreciated role in relation to leadership is followership. More recent views on leadership have appreciated the interrelationship between leaders and followers, and that in some cases leadership can be seen as a collaboration. We shall cover collaborative styles of leadership later on in this chapter and talk more about the importance of followership in Section 2.

Responsibility and Accountability

The other terms that often confuse people are the difference between being responsible and being accountable. Responsibility is something that can be shared, for example, if you all jointly prepare a presentation at university. Being accountable means that the buck stops with you, you are literally 'called to account' and you are the only one that has this role, such as the chief executive of an NHS Trust. Accountability also occurs at the end of a task, whereas responsibility is continuous.

The Importance of Diverse and Distributive Leadership

Over the last few years and certainly during the COVID-19 pandemic, we have seen a move away from the idea of the leader being at the front, being the one 'in charge,' who tells people what to do. Increasingly the pandemic has taught us that it is people on the ground who know what needs doing. The centralised command-and-control style of leadership has given way to distributive leadership, with permission from the organisation to make local decisions quickly.

Remote boards of directors, who may be predominantly White middle-class males, are now a thing of the past. Good leadership requires diversity of thinking, interdisciplinary working and the involvement of everyone from the most junior to most senior. Diversity of backgrounds and cultures is also especially important so that the workforce reflects the culture and behaviours of the communities that are served.

Leadership at Every Level

Leadership development in the NHS has now come to be seen as an essential feature of staff development from the very start of people's careers.

Students interviewed for this book stressed the importance of leading from whatever level they are, as a student or health care associate for example.

'It's about looking at how we can influence change from our level, which is different to how we can get as high up as we can.'

AALIJAH BUTTIMER,
DUAL MENTAL HEALTH/
ADULT NURSING PROGRAMME

The most fundamental leadership role is to be a role model for our patients. This is the subject of a vlog by Claire Carmichael, a newly registered nurse working in general practice, who explains that student nurses should be their best selves and who role models things such as healthy eating and encouraging patients to work with caregivers on care plans.

'And if we're not that person that they [the patients] *can trust, can follow, can listen to they're not going to follow our advice.'*

CLAIRE CARMICHAEL,
LEADERSHIP IN NURSING VLOG

Claire looks forward to when students become registered nurses and become mentors, practice supervisors and practice assessors, and encourages students to start developing their leadership skills in preparation.

'Leadership could be about something as simple as teaching a more junior student about how to wash their hands properly.'
ALICIA BURNETT, CHILDREN'S NURSE AND STUDENT MIDWIFE

Ann-Marie Dodson, a senior lecturer at Birmingham City University and an intensive care nurse, gives the leadership example of teaching her patients breathing exercises and 'bed aerobics' in the early stages of recovery.

'We need to show how we are being a leader at every level and why that's important. Because at every stage in your life or in your career you're being a role model for someone.'
SARAH BRADDER, NEWLY REGISTERED THERAPEUTIC RADIOGRAPHER

Being part of a small group of allied health professionals has led Sarah to be invited to speak about her role as a therapeutic radiographer as part of school careers guidance. She became a school ambassador for STEM (science, technology, engineering and mathematics) careers and has appeared on The WOW Show, a YouTube channel that promotes different careers, to explain her role.

Practising leadership early on can help set you up for more senior roles later in your career. Ann-Marie Dodson talks about the importance of 'serving time on the shop floor' and 'working your way up' and the credibility this gives.

■ Time Out

Looking back at Table 1.1, make a list of activities that you undertook in the last week that exhibit leadership.

There are also clear examples in this book of students who 'hand on the baton' of leadership to less experienced students. An example of this is how students manage and run a Twitter account to offer peer support and how they recruit 'interns' and show them the ropes of managing the account before handing over to them.

Transferrable Leadership Skills

What shapes you as a leader is also important. Each student interviewed for this book was asked about their life before they entered university. Many had fought to get their place and adversity seemed to drive them onwards, as did personal experience of poor health in themselves or their families. When asked about past careers involving leadership and whether they had transferrable skills however, many of them were reluctant to recognise this. When asked, they admitted that they were so overwhelmed with the unfamiliarity and the responsibility of clinical work (and perhaps because they were referred to as 'the student') that it felt as if they had no right to bring in the skills that they had.

Prior experience in a health care role before starting their course was also highly prized, and those who had come into nursing without any experience felt disadvantaged. Those who returned to studying later in their careers felt less confident, they said, when they compared themselves to those who had studied more recently.

What is important is to focus on the positive leadership characteristics that you have rather than what you have not. This book emphasises a glass half full or asset-based approach, highlighting the strengths, skills and talents that you have, rather than just teaching you what you need to know.

Listening to each other and gaining strength from what each of you have achieved are vitally important. It is no mistake that I chose to collaborate with students to write this book. It would have been impertinent to have done otherwise, having not been a student for 37 years! A key message is that each of you will have talents and skills that are different to the next person.

Fresh Eyes in Leadership

Someone with no prior experience in health and care has no expectations and will view their experience through fresh eyes, something that is incredibly valuable. Someone who has been an inspector on the railway before entering nursing will know how to read people and situations. Someone who has been an accountant will have an eye for detail. Someone who has been a lawyer will be able to see things from many angles. Someone who has been a patient will know what might need changing in the system. Someone who is a parent or a carer will know how to prioritise. These are all transferrable leadership skills, and looking through the lens of prior experience at this new experience of health care is a definite advantage.

■ Time Out

Reflect on your experiences prior to entering your nurse training. Make a Post-it note list of the skills and strengths that you have that will be valuable to you as a student nurse leader. Put it on your bathroom mirror to remind yourself.

Summary

Leadership is no longer connected to your position in the hierarchy. Everyone can be leader, and the NHS now recognises that leadership development should take place from the very start of your career.

A lack of confidence in leadership ability is extremely common among student nurses, but many have found many ways to combat this and have shared their top tips.

Leadership and management often get confused. Leadership is about setting direction, having a vision, articulating values, role modelling and managing change. Management is about directing people and resources to achieve that vision and direction; it is more about doing things in an orderly and consistent way.

Both leadership and management are essential for the smooth functioning of high-quality health and care services. Staff roles include both.

Everyday nursing duties, such as role modelling how to wear your uniform correctly or teaching someone else how to wash their hands, is an example of leadership.

Everyone has transferrable strengths and skills that can be used to lead.

References

The WOW Show, 2020. YouTube. Career Guide: want to be a therapeutic radiographer? <https://www.youtube.com/watch?v=ZZO05ceGZpY> (Accessed: 09 June 2021).

West, M., Eckert, R., Armit, LL., Lee, A., 2015. Leadership in Health Care: A Summary of the Evidence Base. Faculty of Medical Leadership and Management, The King's Fund and the Center for Creative Leadership.

CHAPTER 2

Recognising Effective Leadership Models and Theories

OBJECTIVES

After reading this chapter and completing the activities, you should be able to:
- Name the main leadership models and theories promoted/used in the NHS today
- Identify key documents that promote and explain these models
- Give examples of where they are being/have been used by student nurses and current nurse leaders.

Relevance to the Nursing and Midwifery Council (NMC) Code

Practise Effectively
Paragraph 6:
Always practise in line with the best available evidence
To achieve this, you must:
6.1 make sure that any information or advice given is evidence based, including information relating to using any health and care products or services
6.2 maintain the knowledge and skills you need for safe and effective practice

Promote Professionalism and Trust:
Paragraph 25:
Provide leadership to make sure people's wellbeing is protected and to improve their experiences of the health and care system

The Evidence for Leadership Development

The leadership style of an organisation is the major determinant of the culture of that organisation—something that will be explored further in Section 3. As current or future nurses, we all practise evidence-based clinical approaches. However, the same is not true when it comes to leadership development and practise.

Commentators on the health system such as academics West and colleagues (2015) and Swanwick and McKimm (2018) describe how leadership development, critical for the delivery of high-quality care, has been developed based on fads and fashions. They call for evidence-based approaches to leadership development using models, styles of leadership and the accompanying attributes and behaviours that are most likely to be effective.

An evaluation conducted by West and his colleagues in 2015 found that good leadership is required to ensure the commitment, alignment and direction needed to deliver high-quality compassionate care. Good leadership supports staff and promotes kindness, altruism, fairness, accountability and optimism. However, there are gaps in the evidence for what makes an effective leader.

The aim of this chapter therefore is to help you 'learn the jargon' and be able to differentiate between outdated models or styles of leadership and models that we know (so far) are more effective in leadership. These include:

- Collective leadership
- Collaborative leadership
- Compassionate leadership
- Authentic leadership
- Transformational leadership

There are also behaviours (rather than models) that have been cited positively in leadership literature:

- Emotional intelligence—to be aware of and handle one's own emotions and to handle relationships judiciously
- Empathetic and authentic leadership—being self-aware and genuine

These shall be covered in the next chapter when we discuss leadership behaviours and how you as a student nurse can start to develop those skills and behaviours.

Leaders should also be able to adapt their leadership style depending on the situation. For example, a more autocratic style may be used during a crisis and a more collective approach at other times. This is called 'situational leadership' (Goleman 2020). If you want to know more about different models and styles—maybe for an assignment—I have added references for you to read in more depth.

In the next chapter you will have the opportunity to reflect on these styles of leadership and start to understand yourself as leader. Everyone is different and it is for you, over time, to consider which style of leadership suits you personally, rather than try to emulate someone else (Kirkham 2020).

Practising Leadership Is the Best Way to Hone Your Skills

Leadership skills are best honed via experience and so practising leadership, with appropriate support, is the best way to develop your skills. Throughout this book therefore I will be encouraging you to be active in your leadership by completing the 'Time Out' exercises, identifying and using role models, finding mentors and coaches, as well as working with your peers to offer each other support.

The Fads and Fashions of Leadership Over Time

There is no such thing as a unifying framework for leadership. The types of leadership models or theories we have are generally a product of the socio-political system and the culture of their time. Take for example Winston Churchill, who had exactly the right qualities needed to lead a nation through the second World War but failed as a leader during peacetime when different leadership skills were required.

▪ Time Out

Think about the historical nursing leaders that we know. What leadership qualities or models did they exemplify? How much were they products of their time?

Perhaps the first person you thought of was Florence Nightingale and her work during the Crimean War. Her style has often been described as transformational because of the inspirational changes that she introduced. This may have been because a war situation or indeed any crisis often provides a unique opportunity to be visionary and introduce innovative practices. On the flip side she could also be autocratic, especially when people disagreed with her!

Mary Seacole by contrast was perhaps more of a rebel leader. With no formal nurse training and rejected from the official Crimean nursing service, she still funded herself to set up camp close to the front line. We shall talk more about rebel leadership and how to survive in Section 2.

Trait Theory

In the late 19th and early 20th centuries came the idea of trait theory or 'great man' (for it was often about men): the idea that leaders were born that way and had special characteristics that made them leaders. But as the century wore on, doubt was cast over whether leaders had inherent personal characteristics. Trait theory was often accompanied by the idea of charismatic leadership—people who may have exceptional power and influence over others.

Trait theory gave rise to the development of psychometric tests that measured whether you had the desired qualities to be a leader.

Behavioural Theories

In the 1950s behavioural theories suggesting that leadership skills can be learned became popular. This followed a huge study by Stogdill and Coons (1957), which administered the 'Leaders Behaviour Description Questionnaire' measuring nine dimensions of leadership. This identified two groups of behaviours that were strongly correlated: consideration (people-oriented behavioural leaders) and initiating structure (task-oriented leaders). People-oriented leaders focus on the needs of staff and listen, coach and encourage, whereas task-oriented leaders, whilst aware of staff motivation, are primarily concerned with keeping control and following standard operating procedures. These theories suggested that a leader needed to adapt their style to the situation. For example, forming a new nursing team would suggest a people-oriented style, whilst managing a cardiac arrest would require a task-oriented style (situational leadership).

Autocratic, Democratic and Laissez-Faire

These three leadership styles were put forward and used in psychological experiments by Kurt Lewin in the 1930s, and their titles are self-explanatory.

In an autocracy (also referred to as monothetic or authoritarian leadership), the leader is strong, trusted and confident. Decisions are made without consultation and followers are motivated by fear, threats of punishment and awards.

Laissez-faire comes from the French 'leave alone' and means hands off or delegated leadership that may be perceived as the absence of leadership. Team members have complete freedom to act and make decisions.

In democratic or participative leadership, the opinions and suggestions of subordinates are given credence. Staff are kept informed of issues affecting them and there are open lines of communication within the organisational structure. The democracy ensures freedom of expression, independent thought and participative decision-making.

■ **Time Out**

When might an autocratic style of leadership be appropriate?
What might be the advantages of laissez-faire leadership?
Think of any examples that you may have seen of these styles being used.

An autocratic style offers clarity of purpose and fast decision-making, which make it a suitable style for leading in a crisis. You may see this in critical situations such as during the management of a cardiac arrest or by a commander in the fire and rescue services attending a fire or car crash. In these situations, you really would not want to debate much or leave it to staff to decide what to do—the most senior person takes charge. The disadvantages of autocracy are that staff are not empowered and a dependency on a single leader is risky if anything happens to that leader.

There are some advantages to laissez-faire leadership in that team members are able to exercise significant speed and freedom over how work is done, and this may lead to more creativity. You may be more likely to see this style in community and voluntary settings. Take, for example, neighbours coming together to help each other during the COVID-19 pandemic.

Over a longer term laissez-faire leadership can lead to problems in productivity, a perception that the leader does not care, or confusion about roles, purpose and direction. For example, during the COVID-19 pandemic we witnessed the freedom of laissez-faire leadership allowing informal neighbour support, which then developed into a formalised NHS Volunteer Responders Scheme.

Theory X and Theory Y

The ideas behind autocratic and democratic leadership are driven by McGregor's (1960) 'theory X and theory Y,' which describes how leaders are motivated.

Theory X represents the authoritarian style of manager. The assumptions underpinning their motivation are:
1. The average person dislikes work and will avoid it if possible.
2. Therefore, most people must be forced with the threat of punishment to work towards organisational objectives.
3. The average person prefers to be directed and to avoid responsibility; they are relatively unambitious and want security above all else (Tips Box 2.1).

Theory Y by contrast aligns with more democratic styles of leadership, where the assumptions are:
1. Effort in work is as natural as work and play.
2. People will apply self-control and self-direction in the pursuit of organisational objectives, without external control or the threat of punishment.
3. Commitment to objectives is a function of rewards associated with their achievement.
4. People usually accept and often seek responsibility.
5. The capacity to use a high degree of imagination, ingenuity and creativity in solving organisational problems is widely (not narrowly) distributed among the population.
6. In industry, the intellectual potential of the average person is only partly utilised.

TIPS BOX 2.1

Coping With an Autocratic 'Theory X' Leader

If you end up working with an autocratic, logic-driven mentor, tutor or ward manager, the following tips may help:

- Theory X are results oriented, so focus your discussions on, for example, what you can deliver and when; e.g., 'Give me a week and I can get you a detailed list of feedback for our course representatives meeting,' not 'I've been off sick and need another week to do this.'
- They are interested in facts and figures, not incidentals, so be able to measure and substantiate what you say; e.g., 'Twelve students got their rotas 4 weeks in advance. The remaining 50 got theirs only a week or less in advance,' not 'It's really unfair that most students aren't getting their rotas in good time.'
- They may not be interested in human factors. This means managing yourself well and what you can achieve, and setting your objectives to meet organisational aims; e.g., you establish monthly dates for peer assistance learning sessions because you have family commitments, rather than fortnightly and then having to cry off because your partner has started to complain that you are not pulling your weight at home.
- Always deliver on your commitments and promises. If what is expected is unrealistic, state solid reasons why. Stand up for yourself but avoid confrontation. Be constructive and never negative; e.g., 'The bays assigned to me include Mrs Stoddard and Mrs Ahmed, who each need on average an extra 10 minutes to help them dress and have breakfast because of their multiple sclerosis. This means I won't be free to accompany Miss Arif to X ray at 10.00 am, but I've spoken to Student Nurse Roberts and she is happy to do this.'
- Never threaten to go over their heads; this will escalate problems in your relationship.
- If asked to do tasks in a way that you are uncomfortable with, confirm the end result and check if it is okay to 'get things done more efficiently/safely' so you have control over what, but not how. I was once told off for taking too long to admit patients for a day procedure, but once I explained that I was making sure that the patients were completely safe to undergo a general anaesthetic and enquired if the surgeon wanted me to compromise his work, I was left to get on with it.

Adapted from Chapman 2020.

The Psychological Contract

McGregor's ideas relate to a concept known as the 'psychological contract,' which in its simplest terms is a tacit agreement between employer and employee about what each gets from the other. This term is still used by managers and human resources teams. On the employer side the contract is about treating the employee fairly, and in return the employee performs the role expected of them. This is an unwritten understanding based on trust and relationships.

Transactional and Transformational Leadership

Later in the 20th century, behavioural theories such as transactional leadership and motivational theories such as transformational leadership came more to prominence (Tannenbaum et al. 2013). Transactional leadership resembles management and is described as organisation-driven and top down, focusing on reward and punishment. Transformational leaders are described as those who inspire positive changes in their followers. They are visionary and work with teams to identify and execute the needed change, producing remarkable results. Rather like task- and people-oriented leaders, later theorists suggested that good leaders could adapt their style between transactional and transformational.

■ Time Out

Can you think of examples of nurses who may be described as transformational leaders who inspire others to make remarkable changes?

You may be able to think of nurses or fellow students who you have seen on your placements, read about in books and journals or met via social media. Transformational leadership can emerge when you least expect it, including, for Brian Dolan (2017), during a chat on Twitter:

'Nursing was born in the church and raised in the army, so leaving patients in pyjamas is their "uniform"'
#Letsfixthat

BRIAN DOLAN

When entrepreneur and former accident and emergency nurse Brian Dolan first tweeted this phrase on social media, he had no idea of the life it would take on in hospitals, care homes and conversations amongst nurses and allied health professionals.

Within a few days #Letsfixthat became #endPJparalysis and a movement was born (we will talk more about social movements and power in Section 2). #EndPJparalysis has now become a global movement embraced by nurses, therapists and medical colleagues aiming to get patients out of bed and dressed to avoid immobility, muscle deconditioning and dependency, and at the same time protect cognitive function, social interaction and dignity. In doing so, he originated a genuine social movement in health care.

Nottingham University Hospitals were one of the first trusts to pick up on the campaign via Deputy Director of Nursing (and now Chief Nurse at University Hospitals North Midlands) Ann-Marie Riley and colleagues, and others got involved very quickly.

'While I may have initiated the term #EndPJParalysis I'm keen to stress to people that I don't "own" it; my rationale being that if no one owns it we can all "own" it and no one needs "permission" to do what they will with it.'

BRIAN DOLAN

What became clear from this movement was that the power and control about how health and care staff interpreted this idea of ending PJ paralysis lay with the followers. Neither Brian nor Ann-Marie set up standard operating procedures or performance targets, but rather they trusted that people would interpret ideas in their own ways.

Brian went on to take up honorary and visiting professorships and was awarded an OBE in 2019. You can view and join the movement at https://endpjparalysis.org/.

Action-Centred Leadership

Adair (1984) describes the leadership role as being comprised of three interdependent elements: the team, the task and the individual. The leader delivers the task by building and developing the team and developing individuals within that team. The key is to focus not only on the task but also on the human elements of the team and the individual, and to balance all three activities.

We shall move on now to contemporary leadership models that are frequently referenced as effective.

Collective and Inclusive Leadership

The culture of leadership in the NHS in the 21st century has significantly moved away from the idea of a single leader and the development of individuals as leaders. Organisations are now extremely complex, and the system now comprises of many organisations working across many boundaries. 'Heroic' leaders can end up being derailed by failing to recognise that answers may lie within their teams, patients and communities. Today the emphasis is on the idea that leadership is a collective effort and that everyone, at any level, has a part to play and so we must develop the capabilities of everyone (West et al. 2014).

Power is distributed to wherever the expertise, capability and motivation lies, and so leadership and followership shift according to the situation. West (2015) gives an example of this when he talks of a ward clerk passing a patient in a corridor where the bedclothes have slipped off the patient. The ward clerk stops, covers and settles the patient before letting the responsible person know of what happened so the situation can be avoided in future.

This in effect is an 'ethos' rather than a model or style of leadership. Collective and inclusive leadership strategies in organisations will in turn develop healthy organisational cultures that will enable compassionate, high-quality care for all. In terms of inclusivity, it is crucial that organisations mirror the values and diversity of the community they serve. Board-level commitment is needed to empower staff and ensure that this diversity is adequately represented and developed.

Patient-Centred Leadership

Linked to the idea of collective leadership is the idea that patient leaders are an asset that can work collectively alongside NHS leaders (Centre for Patient Leadership and FPM 2013). This idea came to prominence in the wake of the Francis Report of 2013 into the care failures at Mid Staffordshire NHS Trust. We shall discuss ideas of patients and communities co-creating solutions further in Section 2.

Collaborative Leadership

Whilst we have just discussed leadership as a collective effort (all in it together), another important trend is that effective leaders also collaborate (all working together).

Collaboration means including everyone in problem solving and decision-making. It is more appropriately defined leadership of a process, rather than what leaders do. It often starts off as an open process, with the end point being worked out by the members who collaborate with no defined goal in mind.

There are essentially two definitions of a collaborative leadership: leadership of a collaborative effort and leadership in a collaborative effort. Modern NHS leadership emphasises 'integrated care', meaning that parts of the system work seamlessly together across discipline, team and organisational boundaries. A classic example here is where people move between health care and social care. The NHS, social services and independent care homes need to work together to provide personalised care. This leads us the idea of collaborating in our leadership endeavours. In 2019 for example, NHS England published the Long-Term Plan (www.longtermplan.nhs.uk), a strategy to enable the NHS to be fit for the future, with this idea of collaboration and integration at its heart. This is leadership of a collaborative process, where the leadership lies in coordinating the process by which the collaboration partners decide upon and carry out actions to achieve its goals.

Leadership in a collaborative effort means that the leader is not in control but acts as a guide and support for equal partners who together make decisions and take actions. An example of this is the development of a social media support group called @WeStudentNurse.

CASE STUDY 2.1 @weStudentNurse

@weStudentNurse is an example of collaborative leadership involving a group of student nurses curating a Twitter account to offer peer support and self-care tips to student nurses.

It started when Leanne Patrick, then a student mental health nurse, approached Teresa Chinn, the founder of a Twitter chat-hosting community called WeCommunities, about the idea of hosting regular tweet chats for student nurses.

Teresa is a professional social media community development specialist, blogger, speaker, presenter, social media consultant and nurse. Whilst working as an agency nurse she saw an opportunity in the form of social media, particularly Twitter, to help nurses to connect and learn together. Through developing nurse Twitter chats with a previous employer, Teresa knew that the emerging community needed more than chats—they needed support to change the way they use social media and help to ensure their colleagues and employers could see the value too.

Now she enjoys offering support to nurses connecting via Twitter, and working with NHS Trusts, the Department of Health, Public Health England, Plymouth University and the Nursing and Midwifery Council (to name a few) to support the ongoing creation of the value that social media brings to nurses and health care.

Leanne was treading a familiar path. Many other health professionals and managers from a wide variety of disciplines had approached Teresa over the years to set up their own professional Twitter networks: health visiting, finance, midwifery and allied health professionals to name but a few, each run by a team of enthusiastic volunteers and hosted by Teresa's online platform. You can see the whole range of Twitter groups and find out more by visiting www.wecommunities.org.

But there was resistance from nurse leaders to students having their own social media platform: would they remember to refer to the Nursing and Midwifery Council's social media guidelines? Would anything they said reflect badly on universities or trusts? Teresa helped Leanne to set up @weStudentNurse and mentored her and three other students to manage the account and run their first tweet chats until they found their feet.

In terms of a leadership model, initially there was no main leader. Decisions were reached by consensus, but slowly the group realised that they needed someone to bring the group together and help them to take decisions, so it did not become, as Leanne said, them 'jumbling together, fumbling for ideas'. The group looked to Leanne to do this role, as the 'most naturally enthusiastic'.

Leanne started @weStudentNurse with just three others, but by the time that she was reaching the end of her course there were 20 students from different fields supporting @weStudentNurse. Leanne wanted to hand over the reins and was keen that the leadership style of 'just having someone to guide the group, and pull things together', such as arranging meetings, would continue. It was put to the group and Joy O'Gorman, an adult nursing student, agreed to take over. Since then, Natalie Elliot has taken over from Joy, and the same style of consensus leadership has prevailed.

Leanne describes the handover to Joy via Skype as a discussion about what to expect, particularly the unseen parts of the role and the challenges and successes that had been experienced along the way. However, because @weStudentNurse had always been a group effort and was very transparent, handover was not onerous. Joy was already part of the leadership, making decisions with the other members. The main thing, as Joy herself describes in the handover to Natalie, was to develop confidence and feel like she had peer support to help her to do a good job.

Each generation of @weStudentNurse account curators have built on the shoulders of their predecessors, and various initiatives have bloomed. Examples include introducing a Student Nurse Mental Health Day (more on this in Section 3 on innovation), a student nurse podcast (available on Spotify as WePods), revision polls and an environmental awareness initiative called #WeGoGreener.

The @weStudentNurse initiative reflects the whole 'We' ethos that Teresa developed, emphasising a collaborative leadership approach and the sustained development of the student account. It is literally about 'we students' and not individuals. The groundwork undertaken by Leanne and her first team and the successive guidance of peers by Joy and Natalie has resulted in the account now having over 15,000 followers and a strong social media presence, offering peer-to-peer support to student nurses within the United Kingdom.

■ **Time Out**

Write down what you think might be the advantages of collaborative leadership, based on this case study.

Advantages include:

- Buy in—everyone is involved in making decisions and so feels ownership of the process.
- Investment in success—because team members have taken decisions, this makes them more likely to want to implement decisions successfully.
- Empowerment and development—everyone involved in curating the Twitter account and leading various initiatives feels empowered. By sharing leadership, the curators of @WeStudentNurse develop their leadership skills.
- Trust—collaborative leadership requires open dialogue that builds relationships and trust.
- Harmony—because everyone's concerns are heard and decisions are taken together.

Servant Leadership

Servant leadership moves away again from the idea of the leader being the one in charge and identifies leaders who are in a more interdependent relationship with their team. Here the desire of the leader is first to serve and to put the needs of the team first (Ellis 2019).

CASE STUDY 2.2	Rebecca Lennox, Robyn Mills and Colleagues

'I want to be the leader that inspires others to chase their dreams, to do their best.'
                                                                                                               REBECCA LENNOX

Communicating clearly with patients is integral to the delivery of safe and effective nursing care. The Nursing and Midwifery Council Code states that reasonable steps must be taken to meet people's language and communication needs.

Deaf with a capital 'D' refers to people who have been deaf all their lives or since before they started to learn to talk—they are prelingually deaf. The word 'deaf' is used to describe or identify anyone who has a severe hearing problem, or is severely hard of hearing.

Rebecca Lennox is a student nurse at Liverpool John Moores University (LJMU) who has been extremely hard of hearing in her left ear for many years and wears a hearing aid. When she was on maternity leave, she met a mother called Jen who had a little son, Alex, who was then aged 4 months and another mother called Lyndsey whose little girl, Lucy, was then aged 9 years. Both children were and are profoundly Deaf. The little girl, Lucy, only uses sign language to communicate. Rebecca started to appreciate the struggles of D/deaf people, especially those who, in Rebecca's words, did not have that 'Deaf voice' (speech that indicated that deaf people could not hear what they sounded like), so others assumed that they could hear. When Lucy was ready to start secondary school, Lyndsey had to search across both England and Wales to find a suitable school that could meet Lucy's needs. Lyndsey felt her daughter would be isolated in a mainstream school as the only signing child, so she wanted a school with peers who also signed to ensure that this did not happen.

Robyn, a fellow student nurse, had a boyfriend who is also Deaf. Robyn found that she had to help him on occasions, such as making telephone calls on his behalf to check hospital appointments. Robyn felt that he should be able to manage his own life, and both student nurses had a desire to raise awareness of the needs of D/deaf people in health services.

Rebecca started to attend a basic British Sign Language (BSL) course with Jen, who wanted to use BSL to communicate with Alex. She then progressed to start a level 1 course. Rebecca's aim was to complete a qualification in BSL.

Rebecca and Robyn gained approval from the Student Union to start a university student society open to any student on campus. Their eventual aim was to include D/deaf awareness as part of the undergraduate student nurse curriculum, but they decided to start small by offering two 1-day D/deaf awareness masterclasses for both staff and students. They contacted Merseyside-based charity Deaf Active to deliver the masterclasses because it is important that BSL and D/deaf awareness are taught by an expert. The chief executive Thomas Maher himself came to run the courses and about 30 people attended, including the disability staff lead at the university (Fig. 2.1). They followed up with two more events—one at an introductory level and the second slightly more advanced to allow progression. Their aim was to continue to offer two masterclasses every semester, but the disruption caused by the COVID-19 pandemic meant that it had to be put off.

The Society set up a Facebook page called LJMU Deaf Awareness Society to help cultivate D/deaf awareness and to practice some of the signs.

CASE STUDY 2.2   Rebecca Lennox, Robyn Mills and Colleagues—cont'd

Many people said they did not expect to learn so much in such a short time and have felt confident enough to communicate with D/deaf people and sign basic phrases like 'hello my name is...' and 'do you want a drink?'.

Rebecca and Robyn developed a team of people, each with different skills, who now run the Society. For example, Rebecca is less confident about using technology, and Robyn's skills are around technology and wording communications effectively. They were joined by Sanjeev Singh who is on an education course, is deaf, uses hearing aids and communicates by BSL. The three of them meet up regularly to discuss what they wanted to do with the Society and to plan the masterclasses. They were later joined by a member of the Society, mental health student nurse Laura Knowles, who has an interest in sign language.

Rebecca also set up a YouTube channel called *Becca Lennox* to encourage others to use BSL. She demonstrates signs and explains them in a bit more detail, such as the direction that the hands take in a handshake.

The Society won John Moores Student Union society of the year and event of the year awards in the 2019/2020 society awards.

(Consent has been given to use real names in this case study.)

▨ Time Out

What type of leadership style or styles are featured in this case study?

Rebecca and Robyn are displaying servant leadership. The servant leader is often described as the 'first among equals', someone who does not consider themself above those they lead. That is, they see those they lead as peers to teach and to learn from. They are willing to lead others to reach an agreed-upon goal but do not believe that they are any better than anyone else.

Servant leaders are team builders. Rebecca and Robyn drew on the strengths of followers and became followers themselves when appropriate. A servant leader gauges each situation and responds to each individually. We can see in this case study that Rebecca and Robyn engage others to lead where necessary and work with people's strengths.

Rebecca also leads by example and seeks to inspire others through her YouTube channel (which she also shares effectively on Twitter at @stnbecca2). She has a clear vision for what she wants: for BSL to be part of the undergraduate nursing curriculum. It might be argued that she is therefore showing signs, by inspiring others with her values, of becoming a transformational leader as well as a servant leader, using different leadership styles in different contexts.

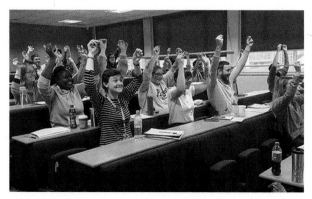

Fig. 2.1   Photo: One of the British Sign Language masterclasses at Liverpool John Moores University. (Rebecca Lennox, with permission.)

Compassionate Leadership

The King's Fund think tank has strongly influenced NHS system leaders over the last few years to see compassion and compassionate leadership as a core value in health and care. They argue that compassion creates a work environment where staff can feel listened to, valued and supported. Where staff are able to identify new ways of working and innovation, this can encourage service improvement (West et al. 2017).

There are four central behaviours exhibited by the compassionate leader: attending, understanding, empathising and helping (Atkins and Parker 2012):

- Paying attention to the other and noticing their suffering—attending
- Understanding what is causing the other's distress, by making an appraisal of the cause—understanding
- Having an empathic response, a felt relation with the other person's distress—empathising
- Taking intelligent (thoughtful and appropriate) action to help relieve the other person's suffering—helping

This idea of compassion is linked to the importance of 'looking after our people' in the NHS People Plan (2020). In the next chapter we shall explore in more detail what it means to be a compassionate leader in nursing.

Summary

Good leadership is needed to ensure the commitment, alignment and direction needed to deliver high-quality compassionate care. Good leadership supports staff and promotes kindness, altruism, fairness, accountability and optimism. It is the major influence on the culture of teams and organisations.

There have been many fads and fashions in leadership development, and these often reflect what is happening in society. The emerging evidence base for which models, skills and behaviours are effective is not always referred to when developing leadership programmes. This chapter gives you a start in terms of understanding where to look for your leadership inspiration and be able to think through which style or styles you might adopt.

As health care increases in complexity, the idea of a heroic leader at the top of a hierarchy becomes less and less tenable. Today's leaders are found at every level in the organisation and are encouraged to be authentic and compassionate. The vision today is that power and responsibility are dispersed throughout organisations—that idea of collective leadership. Staff and teams are also urged to deliver person-centred care and, to achieve this, they collaborate to integrate care across disciplines and boundaries.

More recently, national events such as the COVID-19 pandemic have highlighted the need to look after the people who work in and around the NHS and be compassionate towards each other.

Resource

Let's talk leadership podcasts www.letstalkleadership.org

References

Adair, J., 1984. Action Centred Leadership. McGraw Hill, London.
Atkins, P.W.B., Parker, S.K., 2012. Understanding individual compassion in organisations: the role of appraisals and psychological flexibility. Academy of Management Review 37 (4), 524–546.
Centre for Patient Leadership and FPM, 2013. Bring it on: 40 steps to support patient leadership. <http://engagementcycle.org/wp-content/uploads/2013/03/Bring-it-on-40-ways-to-support-Patient-Leadership-FINAL-V-APRIL-2013.pdf>.

Chapman, A., 2020. What is X-Y theory of management. <https://www.businessballs.com/improving-workplace-performance/mcgregors-xy-theory-of-management/>.

Dolan, B., 2017. #EndPJparalysis is about trusting nurses and valuing patients' time. Nursing Standard. <https://rcni.com/nursing-standard/opinion/comment/endpjparalysis-about-trusting-nurses-and-valuing-patients-time-119766>.

Ellis, P., 2019. Leadership, Management and Team Working in Nursing. Sage, London.

Francis, R., 2013. Report of the Mid Staffordshire NHS Foundation Trust Public Inquiry. Stationary Office.

Goleman, D., 2020. Leadership that gets results. Harvard Business Review 78 (2), 78–90.

Kirkham, L., 2020. Understanding leadership for newly qualified nurses. Nursing Standard 35 (12), 41–45.

Lennox, R., Mills, R., 2020. Why all nursing students should learn basic British Sign Language. Nursing Standard. Posted 11 December 2020. <RCNi.com>.

Lewin, K., Lippitt, R., White, R.K., 1938. Patterns of aggressive behavior in experimentally created social climates. Journal of Social Psychology 10 (2), 271–301.

McGregor, D., 1960. The Human Side of Enterprise. McGraw Hill Book Company, Inc., New York.

NHS England, 2020. We are the NHS: People Plan for 2020/21 – action for us all.

Stogdill, R.M., Coons, A.E. (Eds.), 1957. Leader Behavior: Its Description and Measurement. Ohio State University, Bureau of Business, Columbus.

Swanwick, T., McKimm, J., 2018. ABC of Clinical Leadership. Wiley, Chichester.

Tannenbaum, R., Weschler, I.R., Massariki, F., 2013. Leadership and Organisation: A Behavioural Science Approach. Routledge, London.

West, M., 2015. Why teams? Creating collective leadership. YouTube.

West, M., Collins, C., Eckert, R., Chowla, R., 2017. Caring to change: how compassionate leadership can stimulate innovation in health care. The King's Fund.

West, M., Eckert, R., Armit, L.L., Lee, A., 2015. Leadership in Health Care: A Summary of the Evidence Base. Faculty of Medical Leadership and Management, The King's Fund and the Center for Creative Leadership.

West, M., Eckert, R., Steward, K., Pasmore, B., 2014. Developing Collective Leadership for Health Care. The King's Fund and the Center for Creative Leadership.

CHAPTER 3

Understanding and Developing Your Leadership Behaviours

OBJECTIVES

After reading this chapter and completing the activities, you should be able to:
- Identify the leadership behaviours that are most effective
- Identify national leadership frameworks that promote these behaviours
- Undertake a range of inventories that will help you to understand yourself as a leader.

Relevance to the Nursing and Midwifery Council (NMC) Code

Prioritise People
Paragraph 1:
Treat people as individuals and uphold their dignity
To achieve this, you must:
1.1 treat people with kindness, respect and compassion
Paragraph 2:
Listen to people and respond to their preferences and concerns
To achieve this, you must:
2.1 work in partnership with people to make sure you deliver care effectively
2.6 recognise when people are anxious or in distress and respond compassionately and politely

Practise Effectively
Paragraph 8:
Work cooperatively
To achieve this, you must:
8.1 respect the skills, expertise and contributions of your colleagues, referring matters to them when appropriate
8.4 work with colleagues to evaluate the quality of your work and that of the team

Relevance to the Nursing and Midwifery Council (NMC) Code—cont'd

8.7 be supportive of colleagues who are encountering health or performance problems. However, this support must never compromise or be at the expense of patient or public safety

Paragraph 9:

Share your skills, knowledge and experience for the benefit of people receiving care and your colleagues

To achieve this, you must:

9.1 provide honest, accurate and constructive feedback to colleagues

9.2 gather and reflect on feedback from a variety of sources, using it to improve your practice and performance

9.3 deal with differences of professional opinion with colleagues by discussion and informed debate, respecting their views and opinions and behaving in a professional way at all times

9.4 support students' and colleagues' learning to help them develop their professional competence and confidence

Promote Professionalism and Trust

Paragraph 20:

Uphold the reputation of your profession at all times

To achieve this, you must:

20.1 keep to and uphold the standards and values set out in the Code

20.2 act with honesty and integrity at all times, treating people fairly and without discrimination, bullying or harassment

20.3 be aware at all times of how your behaviour can affect and influence the behaviour of other people

Good Leaders Understand Themselves

So far in this book we have learnt that leadership is probably the most important determinant of culture and that the culture of an organisation is important when it comes to quality and safety in health care.

We also know that leadership today is less about hierarchy and more about collective responsibility. We are all leaders, both in universities and in our clinical placements. We can lead from the front, inspire and take charge, especially in a crisis, but we can also lead in an enabling and facilitative way, for example by being a 'servant leader'—so the word 'lead' can sometimes be a red herring.

Just as we know from research which leadership models are most effective, we also know which leadership behaviours are most helpful, so we shall start to explore these in this chapter and you can read up more if you wish. However, the other factor that is important as you start to lead is to know yourself. Here is how one experienced nurse educator describes it:

> '...take steps to learn about yourself. What excites and motivates you? What presses your anxiety buttons? What have been the situations where you feel you have made an impact? What were the disappointments? Explore these things—with help if necessary—and work out how you react in different situations and how you can learn to react in a steady and positive way, whatever the stimulus might be. Knowing yourself really well is never time wasted—and it's essential as you become more senior.'
>
> JUNE GIRVIN, PROFESSOR EMERITUS,
> INTERVIEWED BY BRIAN WEBSTER,
> ADULT STUDENT NURSE FOR THE WEBSITE THINK THEORY19
> (HTTPS://THINKTHEORY19.WIXSITE.COM/WEBSITE)

As leaders we need to learn more about ourselves—how we appear to others and how we engage with others to achieve common goals. As a student nurse you are entering a rapidly changing environment. What will help is to understand and draw upon your core values, what you are trying to achieve and why, and then consider what personal skills and qualities you have, to achieve lasting and meaningful change.

In the previous chapter for example, we saw two student nurses Rebecca and Robyn highlight the importance of D/deaf awareness based on their own experience and values. They understood and brought out the strengths in each other and their wider team. They were clear about their aim of having D/deaf awareness included in the undergraduate curriculum.

The Development of the NHS HealthCare Leadership Framework

The modern NHS focus on developing the most effective leadership competencies came about because of the Francis enquiry in 2013 into the care scandals at Mid Staffordshire NHS Foundation Trust. Robert Francis reported on the toxic culture at the trust and that this came from leaders who were more concerned with hitting targets rather than supporting staff to enable them to care effectively for their patients.

Francis made several recommendations about the importance of good leadership, which led to the development of a healthcare leadership model, or HLM. This is a nine-dimension tool developed by the NHS Leadership Academy that reflects the values of the NHS and sets out what good leaders do. The HLM is intended for anybody at any level and is a good resource for students to use.

■ Time Out

It is a good idea at the start of your leadership career to get familiar with this HLM, and as you get closer to registration to carry out a self-assessment against the nine leadership dimensions.

Search for 'healthcare leadership model' on the internet and download the document from the NHS Leadership Academy website.

Each dimension is briefly described, alongside why it is important. There are also behavioural indicators which are presented as a series of questions written in the 'first person' (Do I/Am I...?). The statements build from essential performance to exemplary, so you can gauge the level that you are working at now and could aspire to, for example,

- Essential—Am I visible and available to my team?
- Proficient—Do I help people to see the vision as achievable by describing the 'journey' we need to take?
- Strong—Do I encourage others to become 'ambassadors' for the vision and generate excitement about long-term aims?
- Exemplary—Do I describe future changes in a way that inspires hope and reassures staff, patients and the public?

Open your reflective diary and reflect on these questions. They are not meant to be answered 'yes' or 'no', but instead should help you explore your intentions and motivations and see where your strengths and areas for development may lie.

You may feel that some of the dimensions are not applicable to your current practice as a student, but they may be something you return to as a newly registered nurse.

You also have the option of registering with NHSx (a national team driving digital care delivery) and using an electronic self-assessment tool with the HLM. Later in your career you have the opportunity of doing something called a 360-degree assessment, which is where you receive feedback from the people around you about your leadership skills, such as a manager, a peer and a team member. The feedback is collated and fed back to you by someone (usually a human resources manager) who is trained to offer you the feedback and help you to think through how to use it.

Personality and Leadership

In the age-old debate about whether leaders are born or made, the conclusion seems to be that both are important. Our personality traits may give us a natural propensity to inspire or be visionary, but the fact is that anyone can develop their skills as a leader. Our predispositions may lead us to behave in certain ways, so it is important that we start to understand our own strengths and limitations.

THE BIG FIVE

Personality research over the decades has helped identify what is called the 'Big Five' dimensions of personality (Barrick and Mount 1991), known by the mnemonic OCEAN:
- Openness: originality, openness to new experience
- Conscientiousness: will to achieve, focus, organise
- Extroversion: sociability, enthusiasm and activity
- Agreeableness: adaptability and cooperation
- Neuroticism: need for stability, emotional reactivity

■ Time Out

Search the web to find and complete a free version of an OCEAN 'Big Five Personality Test'. Open your diary again and jot down your results and reflect on what you learnt about yourself.

Judge et al. (2002) found a correlation between certain OCEAN scores and leadership success. Good leaders exhibit:
- Conscientiousness (focused, dutiful and organised),
- Emotional stability (resilience to stress and setbacks),
- Extroversion (sociable, assertive and energetic), and
- Openness to experience (intellectually curious, adaptable to change and empathic).

One difficulty that clinical leaders may experience, according to Lake and King (2018), is that they are often altruistic and agreeable, and they may have difficulty challenging others, managing conflict and driving through needed changes. An example here may be that you need to manage a prescribing budget and formulary, but fellow nurses may complain that the budget is insufficient or that a particular patient requires an expensive, off-formulary wound dressing. Having an awareness of this potential trait conflict is important so that you can recognise if it applies to you so that you find ways to manage it.

MYERS BRIGGS TYPES

'If you don't know what an extrovert thinks, you haven't been listening. If you don't know what an introvert thinks, you haven't asked them!'

ISABEL BRIGGS MYERS

The Myers Briggs Types Indicator (MBTI) is another well-known personality inventory (Fig. 3.1). It enables the psychological types described by Karl Jung to become more understandable and useful in everyday life. It was developed by mother and daughter Katharine Briggs and Isabel Briggs Myers.

They explain that seemingly random behaviour is consistent and ordered, based on the preference of individuals to behave in certain ways. They identify four dimensions:
- Energy source—do you prefer the outer world (extroversion, denoted as E) or inner world (introversion, denoted as I)?
- Information—do you prefer to focus on the basic information you take in (sensing, denotes as S) or do you prefer to interpret and add meaning (intuition, denoted as N)?
- Approach to life—in dealing with the outside world, do you prefer to get things decided (Judging, denoted as J) or do you prefer to stay open to new information and options (perceiving or P)?

What's Your Personality Type?

Use the questions on the outside of the chart to determine the four letters of your Myers-Briggs type.
For each pair of letters, choose the side that seems most natural to you, even if you don't agree with every description.

1. Are you outwardly or inwardly focused? If you:

- Could be described as talkative, outgoing
- Like to be in a fast-paced environment
- Tend to work out ideas with others, think out loud
- Enjoy being the center of attention

then you prefer

E
Extraversion

- Could be described as reserved, private
- Prefer a slower pace with time for contemplation
- Tend to think things through inside your head
- Would rather observe than be the center of attention

then you prefer

I
Introversion

2. How do you prefer to take in information? If you:

- Focus on the reality of how things are
- Pay attention to concrete facts and details
- Prefer ideas that have practical applications
- Like to describe things in a specific, literal way

then you prefer

S
Sensing

- Imagine the possibilities of how things could be
- Notice the big picture, see how everything connects
- Enjoy ideas and concepts for their own sake
- Like to describe things in a figurative, poetic way

then you prefer

N
Intuition

3. How do you prefer to make decisions? If you:

- Make decisions in an impersonal way, using logical reasoning
- Value justice, fairness
- Enjoy finding the flaws in an argument
- Could be described as reasonable, level-headed

then you prefer

T
Thinking

- Base your decisions on personal values and how your actions affect others
- Value harmony, forgiveness
- Like to please others and point out the best in people
- Could be described as warm, empathetic

then you prefer

F
Feeling

4. How do you prefer to live your outer life? If you:

- Prefer to have matters settled
- Think rules and deadlines should be respected
- Prefer to have detailed, step-by-step instructions
- Make plans, want to know what you're getting into

then you prefer

J
Judging

- Prefer to leave your options open
- See rules and deadlines as flexible
- Like to improvise and make things up as you go
- Are spontaneous, enjoy surprises and new situations

then you prefer

P
Perceiving

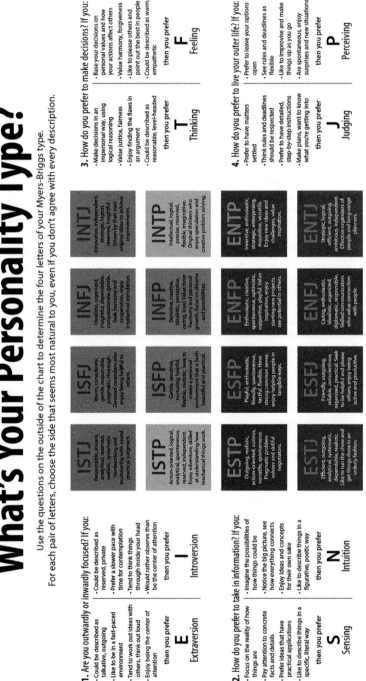

ISTJ — Responsible, sincere, analytical, reserved, realistic, systematic. Hardworking and trustworthy with sound practical judgment.

ISFJ — Warm, considerate, gentle, responsible, pragmatic, thorough. Devoted caretakers who enjoy being helpful to others.

INFJ — Idealistic, organized, insightful, dependable, compassionate, gentle. Seek harmony and cooperation, enjoy intellectual stimulation.

INTJ — Innovative, independent, strategic, logical, reserved, insightful. Driven by their own original ideas to achieve improvements.

ISTP — Action-oriented, logical, analytical, spontaneous, reserved, independent. Enjoy adventure, skilled at understanding how mechanical things work.

ISFP — Gentle, sensitive, nurturing, helpful, flexible, realistic. Seek to create a personal environment that is both beautiful and practical.

INFP — Sensitive, creative, idealistic, perceptive, caring, loyal. Value inner harmony and personal growth, focus on dreams and possibilities.

INTP — Intellectual, logical, precise, reserved, flexible, imaginative. Original thinkers who enjoy speculation and creative problem solving.

ESTP — Outgoing, realistic, action-oriented, curious, versatile, spontaneous. Pragmatic problem solvers and skillful negotiators.

ESFP — Playful, enthusiastic, friendly, spontaneous, tactful, flexible. Have strong common sense, enjoy helping people in tangible ways.

ENFP — Enthusiastic, creative, spontaneous, optimistic, supportive, playful. Value inspiration, enjoy starting new projects, see potential in others.

ENTP — Inventive, enthusiastic, strategic, enterprising, inquisitive, versatile. Enjoy new ideas and challenges, value inspiration.

ESTJ — Efficient, outgoing, analytic, systematic, dependable, realistic. Like to run the show and get things done in an orderly fashion.

ESFJ — Friendly, outgoing, reliable, conscientious, organized, practical. Seek to be helpful and please others, enjoy being active and productive.

ENFJ — Caring, enthusiastic, idealistic, organized, diplomatic, responsible. Skilled communicators who value connection with people.

ENTJ — Strategic, logical, efficient, outgoing, ambitious, independent. Effective organizers of people and long-range planners.

Fig. 3.1 Chart detailing all Myers Briggs personality types. (Source: Jake Beech, 2014. <https://en.wikipedia.org/wiki/Myers%E2%80%93Briggs_Type_Indicator#/media/File:MyersBriggsTypes.png>)

- Decisions—when making decisions, do you prefer to look first at logic and consistency (thinking or T) or first look at the people and special circumstances (feeling or F)?

Once someone has completed the inventory in relation to each dimension, they will discover which of the 16 personality types is their particular preference.

Undertaking the MBTI assessment of your preferences will help you to understand your behaviour and give insight into your communication habits. It will also help you to understand other people, especially if they have also done an MBTI assessment. In health care teams, often all members take the assessment and share their preferences. By understanding each other's preferences, this can help team members to know each other, use each other's strengths and reduce team conflict.

Note that these are preferences, or preferred ways of working. More sophisticated assessments can tell you how strong your preferences are. For example, I know that I am ENTJ but that my judging score is not very dominant, so I am somewhere in the middle between getting things decided (J) and being open to new options (P).

Sometimes I have had to work against my 'judge' to get certain jobs done well. For example, I was asked to investigate staff complaints about a rather domineering ward sister (my first reaction—J) and had to keep an open mind (P) about what was happening. By interviewing and listening to every staff member, including the sister, I discovered much more about how staff interpreted this sister's behaviour. For example, a newly registered male nurse considered her actions to be bullying and biased against men, when in fact she behaved the same way towards everyone, justifying that her standards were high and that she expected people to respect that. Seasoned staff tolerated her behaviour and normalised it. She had no malicious intent and indeed had not recognised how her approach upset her team. When I fed back to her what I had found, this sister was devastated and got help to change her behaviour. Had this sister understood her MBTI type and engaged with her team to understand and work with each other's behaviour preferences, maybe what happened would not have occurred.

■ Time Out

Complete your own MBTI assessment and make some notes in your diary about what the results tell you.

Search the web for a 'free MBTI personalities test'. There are plenty on offer. These are free but unofficial versions of the test.

For an official version search for https://www.mbtionline.com/, for which there is a small charge, but you get free guides and lifetime access. The site itself gives a great deal of background information on MBTI.

If you wish to have help in interpreting your MBTI result, the Myers and Briggs Foundation recommends that you contact a qualified practitioner to help you. Many NHS organisations do exactly that when undertaking team Myers Briggs exercises.

There are many other personality tests that can be taken; however, be careful that they have strong evidence base behind them. We shall consider a couple more in relevant chapters, such as the Kirton Adaptation-Innovation Inventory in the chapter on innovation and entrepreneurship.

Emotional Intelligence

The new Nursing and Midwifery Council (2018) standards of proficiency for registered nurses acknowledge the importance of developing emotional intelligence (EI) in nurses. Most NHS leadership programmes now include EI as a central leadership competency. It is about being able to recognise your own emotions and those of others around you, discern different feelings and emotionally regulate yourself.

As soon as I think about EI I think back to the days when my reaction to any constructive feedback was always to be defensive. I can see my boss, the chief executive, remarking on it (which made me defensive about my defensiveness) and I remember thinking 'well isn't that what everyone does when they are criticised?' Apparently not.

The chief executive encouraged me to complete a leadership programme that had EI at its core. Nowadays in any situation I am tuned in to how I am feeling and how I think other people are feeling too. I try to stay curious about why somebody reacts in a way that I do not expect and I think through all the different ways that I can respond. It is not always easy and I am still learning.

First recognised in 1964, EI was brought to prominence by Daniel Goleman in a 1995 best-selling book called *Emotional Intelligence.*

In his follow-up book *Working with Emotional Intelligence* (1998), Goleman describes EI as 'a different way of being smart'. He cites evidence from his predecessor David McLelland, whose 1973 studies demonstrated that good school grades and traditional academic aptitude did not guarantee success in your career or in life. Instead, he noted specific competencies that distinguished the most successful from those who are just good enough at their jobs.

Goleman gives an example of an air steward's EI, using an incident which took place on 'Super Bowl Sunday', the US equivalent of our FA Cup final, when most right-thinking American football fans want to be at home to watch the game. The plane she was working on had been delayed and the travellers were becoming increasingly restless to get home. As the plane taxied to the gate, the passengers began to get up and gather their belongings.

Instead of reminding them of federal regulations against moving before the doors opened, she took to the intercom and said 'You're staaaaanding!' in a sing-song voice, to which the passengers laughed and sat down again. She had successfully defused the situation.

Goleman (1998) describes an emotional competency framework (Box 3.1) consisting of five competencies, three of which are personal competencies (how we manage ourselves) and two that are social competencies (how we handle relationships).

BOX 3.1 ■ The Emotional Competency Framework

Personal Competencies

Self-Awareness

- Emotional awareness: recognising your emotions and their effects
- Accurate self-assessment: knowing your strengths and limits
- Self-confidence: a strong sense of your worth and capabilities

Self-Regulation

- Self-control: keeping disruptive impulses and emotions in check
- Trustworthiness: maintaining high standards of integrity and honesty
- Conscientiousness: taking responsibility for personal performance
- Adaptability: flexibility in handling change
- Innovation: being comfortable with novel ideas, approaches and new information

Motivation

- Achievement drive: striving to improve or meet a standard of excellence
- Commitment: aligning with the goals of the group or organisation
- Initiative: readiness to act on opportunities
- Optimism: persistence in pursuing goals despite obstacles and setbacks

---

BOX 3.1 ■ The Emotional Competency Framework—cont'd

Social Competencies

Empathy

- Understanding others: sensing others' feelings and perspectives
- Developing others: sensing others' development needs and bolstering their abilities
- Service orientation: anticipating, recognising and meeting customers' needs
- Leveraging diversity: cultivating opportunities through different kinds of people
- Political awareness: reading a group's emotional currents and power relationships

Social Skills

- Influence: wielding effective tactics for persuasion
- Communication: listening openly and sending convincing messages
- Conflict management: negotiating and resolving disagreements
- Leadership: inspiring and guiding individuals and groups
- Change catalyst: initiating or managing change
- Building bonds: nurturing instrumental relationships
- Collaboration and cooperation: working with others towards shared goals
- Team capabilities: creating group synergy in pursuing collective goals

From Goleman, D., 1998. Working with Emotional Intelligence. Bloomsbury Publishing Inc., London.

Goleman (1998) explains that certain occupations may emphasise certain EI capabilities. He states that for nurses it is a sense of humour! As you rise up through the ranks then EI will become increasingly important, especially the competencies relating to understanding and managing the politics of your organisation.

■ Time Out

Spend some time getting to know yourself, what your emotional triggers are and how you are likely to respond in particular situations. So, for example, when I was a junior manager I was very defensive and this stopped me from admitting that others had suggestions that could help me. I learned to admit that I could be wrong and this helped me to listen and to build relationships that would help me.

The first step is to notice your emotions and recognise what they are—are you threatened, jealous, worried or over-tired, for example?

How do these emotions drive you to respond?

How do people react to you?

What have you learnt about what triggers you, and what can you do differently next time?

Until recently, there was little evidence about the application of EI in nursing leadership. In 2019 Mansel and Einion of Swansea University discovered that nurse leaders reflected some of the core capabilities of EI. Their ability to do this however was hampered by low staffing levels, the pressures of the job and competing priorities.

During interviews with nurse leaders, Mansel and Einion found that nurse leaders can actively develop the EI of nurses around them:

'An awareness. You can nurture it in somebody, if you can pick up that somebody is showing these tendencies, that they can come tell you, look something is not right with so and so this morning, keep an eye, see if you can have a word with them later.'

NURSE LEADER INTERVIEWEE 2. MANSEL AND EINION (2019)

CASE STUDY 3.1 **Rebecca Lennox, Student Nurse, Liverpool John Moores University**

Rebecca originally planned to join the RAF (Royal Air Force) as a medic but had to put it off due the death of her grandfather. She subsequently acted as a carer for her grandmother and ended up in various jobs.

Just as she started her midwifery training, she suffered a miscarriage and withdrew from her course, but eventually she started her nurse training. It was fair to say that at a young age, Rebecca had plenty of life experience.

In her first year she was nursing a pregnant woman who had extensive cancer and was admitted for a medical termination of her pregnancy and palliative care. Reflecting on her own experience, Rebecca noticed that the ward staff were focusing on the palliative care and that nobody had spoken to the mother or her husband about the loss of a child. She observed that the ward staff were extremely busy and perhaps had not had time to think through the needs of grieving parents.

Rebecca approached the bereavement service at the hospital, who had expertise in giving advice and counselling in such situations, to see how they could help. She took the information to her mentor to ask for advice about approaching the mother to see if she wanted to talk about what happened, and she got permission to approach the mother.

Rebecca gently asked if the mother wanted to talk about what had happened and left some information. Both parents were thankful for this and took up Rebecca's offer. This helped the parents to talk together about their loss. The father told Rebecca that he felt that he now had permission to grieve for his child after his wife had died.

■ **Time Out**

Look back at Goleman's emotional competency framework.
In what ways did Rebecca exhibit emotional intelligence?

Rebecca showed self-confidence. As a student, she still felt able to initiate support for this family. She showed self-awareness and empathy; she remembered how a miscarriage had affected her and considered how the loss of a child would affect the parents.

Rebecca showed initiative: knowing that staff were busy, she made some investigations and brought it back to her mentor. She approached the parents with real sensitivity, recognising that they might not want to talk, but with her instinct telling her that they would.

Empathy

Goleman identifies empathy as a component of EI. Empathy is about being able to identify with the feelings and thoughts of others. As a nurse, you understand that patients are often afraid, sick and in pain. As such, they may appear difficult, angry or rude. Just as we understand empathy when nursing, we also need to use it when leading.

In practicing empathy, you are trying to understand why people are acting that way. Empathy is not agreement; it is about understanding the feelings of those you lead. Get to know the people you work with; their home circumstances, what makes them tick, what worries them, what they might be striving for. That emotional connectedness is a crucial factor for all nurse leaders to practise.

When nurse leaders 'manage at a distance' this may be perceived as a lack of empathy, according to participants in Mansel and Einion's research. This can lead to staff not feeling valued and understood as individuals.

In his 2017 TED talk, *Empathy—Best Speech of All Time*, Simon Sinek says that the job of a leader is not being in charge but taking care of people in our charge. When faced with someone who is underperforming in their role, Simon suggests that leaders use empathy. Instead of berating the staff member, leaders should enquire whether all is well and offer them help to do their job well. This relating to what others are going through will encourage a culture of openness he says, where people are more willing to ask for help, admit mistakes and share their worries.

Sinek describes how many managers used to do the jobs that their staff now do and end up micromanaging them. He explains that leaders need to go through a transition period, where they start to realise that they are not responsible for the job but rather they are responsible for the people who are responsible for the job. In the same way, he considers that chief executives are not responsible for the customer (in our case, the patient) but instead are responsible for the people who are responsible for the customer. In the business world, especially during the 1980s and the 1990s, maximising shareholder value was the name of the game. Sinek explains that this is like prioritising the needs of the fans over the needs of the players. In the same way in the health system, in the past we have seen chief executives and boards prioritising the delivery of NHS targets and universities focus on maximising student numbers, without necessarily considering what would help their staff to do their jobs.

Authentic Leadership

'You kind of hold these people on a pedestal and think they've gone from success to success, whereas every single one of them had had some kind of failure like not getting a job or publications that haven't been accepted. And it's always kind of stuck out in my head that the only way to be a good leader and to be someone that you want people to look up to is to be honest, because it makes you more real. It makes people more likely to trust you if you're being authentic. I think it inspires people more ... because they don't just see all this shiny amazing stuff that looks so unattainable on its own.'

SARAH BRADDER,
NEWLY REGISTERED THERAPEUTIC RADIOGRAPHER,
TALKING ABOUT SENIOR LEADERS WHO HAD TOLD THEIR LEADERSHIP
STORIES ON THE #150LEADERS PROGRAMME

Authentic leadership is a relatively new concept in nursing. It is about developing a strong sense of self, and knowing and communicating your ethics, values and beliefs. To be authentic is to be real and genuine about who you are—to show your individual character openly and transparently (Long 2020) (Tips Box 3.1).

TIPS BOX 3.1

How to Develop the Four Components of Authentic Leadership

1. Self-awareness
   It is important for authentic leaders to have a strong sense of self, including weaknesses as well as strengths. You must know who you are. This also helps your colleagues to feel that you are not hiding anything and so build trust.
   * Seek feedback from trusted colleagues.
   * Use self-reflection to understand your behaviour better.
   * Practise self-observation of your feelings 'I am really nervous about this meeting. Why? What can I do to feel better?'
2. Relational transparency
   * Practise being genuine, straightforward and honest with colleagues.
   * Aim for constructive feedback rather than passive aggression or subtle messaging.
3. Seek opinions
   * Seek out people's views before making decisions.
   * Make sure to include opposing views to help reveal pitfalls in your arguments.
4. Do the right thing
   * Take actions that benefit the wider organisation rather than you. For example, tweet your support for other students' ideas rather than always try to shine.
   * Practise what you preach: For example, turn up on time if you want others to do so.

Adapted from Caroline Forsey's blog on Hubspot.com (undated).

Authentic leaders lead by example and in doing so present as genuine, trustworthy, reliable and believable. In her 2020 TEDx Talk, Nashater deu Solheim, a clinical psychologist, talks about how she approached the assessment of a psychopathic killer. She needed to create a safe space for the offender to be able to share his feelings—a concept called psychological safety.

She explains how she undertook her clinical assessment in an empathic way by understanding what led up to the killings and understanding the killer's current situation and feelings. To do this she needed to build trust. Crucially, she explains her concept of authenticity and how she subtly interpreted this as being about sharing the professional part of herself as a psychologist rather than showing all of her true self, her feelings and judgements about his crimes. She calls this 'authenticity with empathy'. This enabled her to undertake her assessment as to whether he remained a danger to people.

Solheim warns that sometimes 'authentic leadership' is interpreted as being brutally honest about oneself 'this is me—take me as I am'. This can lead to behaviours such as conducting meetings from behind computers or giving feedback in red pen. She warns that this level of authenticity kills motivation, trust and cooperation (Tips Box 3.2).

TIPS BOX 3.2

Showing Authentic Leadership With Empathy

- Stay within your role—you are there as a leader, not a friend.
- Understand and get to know your team members, their desires and motivation, and hook into these desires.
- Remain curious rather than be judgemental or critical, especially of team members who you do not like.

Adapted from Solheim (2020).

■ Time Out

Invite a senior leader who you consider to be a role model to come to your nursing society or talk to your year group and tell you their leadership story. Ask them to be open and honest about their journey. Reflect in your diary about what you heard, particularly what you learnt about authenticity and emotional intelligence.

What might you do differently as a result?

Compassionate Leadership

'Compassion is the most effective intervention that we have in health care.'
                                              PROFESSOR MICHAEL WEST, VISITING FELLOW, KING'S FUND

One of the core values that the NHS was built upon post World War II was compassion. It is defined as the emotional response to another's pain and suffering, involving an authentic desire to help. To nurture that value, as well as showing compassion in our nursing, we also need to show compassion in our leadership.

The evidence for how compassion can not only help patients but also ease burnout amongst staff is summarised in a revolutionary book by Stephen Trzeciak and Antony Mazzarelli called *Compassionomics: The Revolutionary Scientific Evidence That Caring Makes a Difference.* The authors define compassionomics as the scientific evidence that caring makes a difference to patient outcomes and safety. Some examples include:

- Patients randomly assigned to compassionate palliative care survived 30% longer.
- Compassionate care can enable an 80% improvement in optimal blood sugar control in diabetes.

Not only does compassion make a difference to patients, but it also makes a difference to provider wellbeing, employee engagement and organisational performance. In neuroscience terms, when we experience empathy, the pain centres in our brains light up—we feel the pain of another. But when we focus on compassion—the action of trying to alleviate another's suffering—the reward pathway associated with affiliation and positive emotion lights up. Empathy hurts, but compassion heals. Empathy is feeling; compassion is action (Trzeciak and Mazzarelli 2019).

In 2016, a national framework to guide leadership development was published by NHS Improvement called *Developing People Improving Care*. There are five conditions that the framework stresses are important, one of which is compassionate and inclusive leadership.

There are four behaviours:

- Attending: Being present with those we lead is described as 'listening with fascination'
- Understanding of the challenges that those we lead face
- Empathising with those we lead
- Helping those we lead

In Section 3 we will discuss why compassionate leadership is so important to creating the right culture to deliver high-quality care. We have already discussed empathy, and as you see it is an important part of compassion, but alongside this is the skill of listening.

Listening

'I had a preceptor when I was training to be a nurse practitioner and he said to me once if you listen to the patient long enough he will tell you what's wrong with him.'

BARBARA STILWELL, NURSE, RESEARCHER AND ACADEMIC (TIPS BOX 3.3)

TIPS BOX 3.3

Listening

Just as you listen to your patients to discover what is going on with them, the same is true as a leader when you listen to your team.
- Listen more than you talk.
- Build up a picture of what is happening by asking questions, just like you would when you are trying to do an accurate nursing assessment.
- When you talk to colleagues, listen to what they are telling you.
- Keep your curiosity alive.

Source: Author's interview with Barbara Stilwell 2020.

The Power of Being Listened To

'The greatest compliment that was ever paid me was when someone asked me what I thought and attended to my answer.'

HENRY DAVID THOREAU, AMERICAN WRITER

CASE STUDY 3.2	**Alison Booker, Student Dietician**

As part of the #150Leaders programme Alison Booker, a student dietician, had the opportunity to attend a Health Education England event in London and be on a panel to discuss the future of the recruitment and retention of allied health professionals. She reflected that the event had given her the opportunity to gain insight into key national strategic work that she would never otherwise have had the opportunity to gain. She talked in particular about the power of being listened to and of feeling that her opinion really mattered. It gave her the confidence to believe that she really was a leader. She went on to be selected to be the 2020 student representative of the British Dietetic Association.

The point here is that, as a leader, you can pay attention and really listen to others, and in doing so you will help them to grow.

Summary

Everybody can develop the right skills and behaviours to become a leader. Each of us has preferences in how we lead. It is really important to become self-aware and understand our strengths and skills as well as our weaknesses.

High-profile care failings in the NHS have led to national leaders setting out evidence-based leadership frameworks and self-assessment tools that help existing and future nurse leaders to understand themselves better and gain feedback on their performance.

Rather than a 'command-and-control' style of leadership, modern NHS leaders are encouraged to develop soft skills such as EI, empathy and compassion, and to show their authentic selves. In doing so, nurse leaders can create strong relationships and earn the trust of those they lead.

Good leadership is not about being in charge, but about taking care of the people in our charge.

References

Barrick, M.R., Mount, M.K., 1991. The big five personality dimensions and job performance: a meta analysis. Personnel Psychology 44 (1), 1–26.

Forsey, C., Undated. What's authentic leadership, & how do you practice it. <https://blog.hubspot.com/marketing/authentic-leadership>.

Goleman, D., 1995. Emotional Intelligence. Bloomsbury Publishing Inc., London.

Goleman, D., 1998. Working with Emotional Intelligence. Bloomsbury Publishing Inc., London.

Judge, T., Bono, J., Ilies, R., Gerhardt, M., 2002. Personality and leadership: a qualitative and quantitative review. The Journal of Applied Psychology 87, 765–780.

Lake, C., King, J. 2018. Understanding yourself as leader. In: Swanwick, T., McKimm, J. (Eds.), ABC of Clinical Leadership. Wiley, Chichester.

Long, T., 2020. Effect of authentic leadership on newly qualified nurses: a scoping review. Nursing Management. 27 (3), 28–34.

Mansel, B., Einion, A., 2019. 'It's the relationship you develop with them': emotional intelligence in nurse leadership. A qualitative study. British Journal of Nursing, 28 (21).

McLelland, D.C., 1973. Testing for competence rather than for "intelligence". American Psychologist, 28 (1), 1–14.

NHS Improvement, 2016. Developing People, Improving Care. A national framework for action on improvement and leadership development in NHS-funded services. <https://www.southwestleadership.nhs.uk/wp-content/uploads/2017/11/Developing_People-Improving_Care-010216.pdf>.

Nursing and Midwifery Council, 2018. Future Nurse: Standards of Proficiency for Registered Nurses.

Sinek, S., 2017. Empathy – best speech of all time. TED Talks. <https://www.youtube.com/watch?v=IJyNoJCAuzA>.

Solheim, N.D., 2020. What working with psychopaths taught me about leadership. TEDx Stavanger.

Trzeciak, S., Mazzarelli, D., 2019. Compassionomics: The Revolutionary Scientific Evidence That Caring Makes a Difference. Studer Group, Pensacola.

Managing Yourself

OBJECTIVES

After reading this chapter and completing the activities, you should be able to:
- Identify your strengths as a leader and how they may complement others
- Take steps to manage imposter syndrome and build your confidence
- Develop personal strategies to develop resilience
- Introduce time-management tools
- Practise self-compassion.

Relevance to the Nursing and Midwifery Council (NMC) Code

Promote Professionalism and Trust
Paragraph 20:
Uphold the reputation of your profession at all times
20.1 keep to and uphold the standards and values set out in the Code
20.2 act with honesty and integrity at all times, treating people fairly and without discrimination, bullying or harassment
20.3 be aware at all times of how your behaviour can affect and influence the behaviour of other people
20.5 treat people in a way that does not take advantage of their vulnerability or cause them upset or distress
20.6 stay objective and have clear professional boundaries at all times with people in your care (including those who have been in your care in the past), their families and carers

Managing yourself when you are in a student leadership role, alongside your studies and working on placement, can be tough. The last chapter focused on effective leadership behaviours and started to help you to understand yourself and the people around you. In this chapter we will look at a couple of case studies from student nurses who have gone through such introspection and discuss what they learnt.

We will also take some of the most common issues experienced by student nurses on self-management when in leadership roles. Here you will find plenty of tips from colleagues on how they recognise and address these concerns. Hopefully this will also help you realise that you are not alone in feeling certain ways and quite often what you feel is normal.

CASE STUDY 4.1   Getting to Know Yourself

'You're often faced with so many ethical decisions, so many different people that, if you don't know yourself, then you're not able to deal with others.'

NATALIE ELLIOTT

Natalie Elliott, an adult nursing student at Glasgow Caledonian University, talks candidly about becoming an accountant because it was 'safe and well paid'. Eventually she realised that she was living the life that others expected of her, rather than the one that she herself wanted.

For Natalie, who successfully applied to do the #150Leaders programme for health care students, her challenge was to understand herself better and have the courage to speak up. She felt that others around her were getting these 'great, wonderful awards' and she was 'doing nothing', until she realised that her journey as a leader was more about finding out who she was.

She was particularly keen to combat her negative self-talk and to switch her perceptions of her weaknesses into strengths.

Natalie describes herself as a natural introvert, happier with listening and getting to know people and what makes them tick, rather than offering her own opinions.

She applied for the #150Leaders programme and found herself at a residential event in a room with '50 other loud and extrovert students'. She describes how she does not like to be in the spotlight and remembers feeling deflated that day, feeling like she did not fit in.

What helped was speaking to her coach (an experienced nurse) who supported her during her time on the #150Leaders programme. The coach helped her to explore how she was feeling, and this helped Natalie to decide that she needed to find out who she was.

She concluded that if she wanted to make an impact, she needed to conquer this negative thinking. She decided to speak up at the next #150Leaders event, even if it was just once. She describes over-thinking the situation: that if she spoke up it might be 'wrong'. But even speaking up once felt very empowering and spurred her to think that she could do it more often. She got to know the people in the room and began to think that she was in a safe place in which to speak.

She now knows that her introverted nature is a strength. She describes shadowing an experienced nursing professor and observing him in meetings. She was surprised that he was not 'leading' the meetings. He did not say much but rather sat and listened and drew other people into the conversation. This helped her to shape her leadership style, realising that her strengths are around listening to a team and making them feel valued, and in so doing she has her team behind her.

Natalie recognises that people are reluctant to be honest and say that they do not know everything. But she thinks that to be happy you need to be authentic and true to yourself, know yourself and your values, and show honesty.

For more thoughts from Natalie, visit her blog https://natalieelliott.wordpress.com/2019/10/29/i-cant-be-a-leader-because/.

■ **Time Out**

Reflect on Natalie's experience. Write a few notes in your diary about what might have struck a chord with you. What are your own values and strengths? How true you are to yourself? In what ways might Natalie's words inspire you?

Here are my own reflections: As I am an extrovert, Natalie's words are a reminder to me that I should listen more than I talk. As a senior NHS manager, I had a learning disability nursing colleague who was an introvert. She spoke rarely and quietly and mostly sat and listened, but when she did speak, the room fell silent and the whole world seemed to stop and listen. We were polar opposites, but we had complementary skills. We formed a friendship that took us forward during some difficult leadership times. I learned a great deal from her not only about myself, but about the nature of learning disability nursing and the injustices experienced by people with a learning disability.

Valuing Difference

'Value your difference and think of your vulnerabilities as your strength.'

STACY JOHNSON, MBE,
ASSOCIATE PROFESSOR AT THE UNIVERSITY OF NOTTINGHAM

We sometimes aspire to be just like someone else, or be what others expect us to be. What we actually need is to be able to look into ourselves to see whether this is really what makes us tick and discover our strengths. Natalie has realised that her introversion and her interest in what others have to say are her strengths.

Sometimes we need help from others who may see us more clearly to be able to do this. In the next chapter we will talk about coaching, mentorship and reflection.

Diversity is important in leadership, and it is crucial not to compare yourself and your skills to others. Adele Nightingale, education lead for nursing and allied health professionals at Bolton NHS Foundation Trust, uses the analogy of guests bringing dishes for a party buffet:

'If we all brought bread sticks then no-one would be invited to the party ever again.'

We all have something to give, and it is up to us to develop that self-knowledge and self-belief.

We are naturally drawn to and take comfort in others who share our views and who are like us, but we need to take care that this does not lead to 'group think'—where ideas go unchallenged and new thinking might not be sought.

So, leaders who value difference do what they do best and surround themselves with people who have different skills or may think differently to them. As a result, better decisions can be made because of the diversity of thought that this brings. These ideas reflect the current collective and inclusive leadership approaches in the NHS that we discussed in Chapter 2.

Strengths-Based Leadership

Tom Rath (2007) writes about studies at the well-known pollster organisation Gallup, revealing that people who can focus on using their strengths every day are more than six times as likely to be engaged in their jobs and more than three times as likely to report having an excellent quality of life.

When undertaking personal development reviews we may be used to personal tutors, mentors and managers giving feedback on what we have done well before focusing on helping us to address our weaknesses. Our culture, says Rath, is fixated on helping people to overcome their deficits. Rath's maxim is

'You cannot be anything you want to be—but you can be a lot more of who you already are.'

Strengths-based leadership focuses on achieving significant change and growth potential by focusing on improving strengths rather than fixing weaknesses. The father of strengths psychology was Donald Clifton, who back in 1998 started researching a new language to describe what is right with people rather than what is wrong and needs fixing. He founded Selection Research,

Inc., which later acquired Gallup Inc. Clifton became its chairman, and Gallup went on to develop CliftonStrengths—a series of questions to help people discover their strengths. Clifton published *Now Discover Your Strengths* (2001) with Marcus Buckingham, which became a best-seller. You will find details of where to find the Clifton StrengthsFinder tool and accompanying book in the resources section at the end of this chapter.

The downsides of a strengths-based approach also need to be considered. These include limiting your ambition to try things you have never done before and becoming pigeon-holed as being good only in one area.

■ Time Out

Form a group of five to eight trusted colleagues.
1. Pin a sheet of card to each other's backs.
2. Invite everyone to write on each person's card what that person's key strengths are.
3. Help each other to remove the card from their backs and allow them a few minutes to digest what people have written.
4. In turn, invite each person to talk about what they have learnt:
   - ■ What they already know about their strengths
   - ■ What surprised them
5. Then have a discussion about how this person can further develop their strengths.
6. Once everyone has spoken, consider:
   - ■ What complementary strengths do you have as a group?
   - ■ How might you capitalise on these strengths?

A strengths-based perspective is commonly taught in social work to enable social workers to develop the skills and strengths of their clients. The pioneer of this approach was Dennis Saleeby (2006), an emeritus professor at the University of Kansas. Saleeby suggested that the framing of the core values of a strengths-based perspective pivots around three things: possibility, capacity and reserves (Fig. 4.1).

Saleeby developed a set of seven strengths-based questions that social workers could use with their clients (Box 4.1).

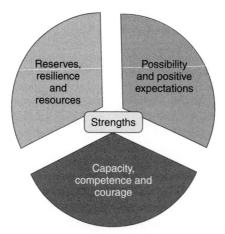

Fig. 4.1 Strengths dynamic. (Adapted from Saleeby, D., (Ed.), 2006. The Strengths Based Perspective in Social Work Practice. Person Education, Inc.)

BOX 4.1 ■ Seven Strengths-Based Questions

1. Survival questions: How have you managed to overcome/survive the challenges that you have faced? What have you learnt about yourself and your world during those struggles?
2. Support questions: Who are the people that you can rely on? Who has made you feel understood, supported or encouraged?
3. Exception questions: When things were going well in life, what was different?
4. Possibility questions: What do you want to accomplish in your life? What are your hopes for your future, or the future of your family?
5. Esteem questions: What makes you proud about yourself? What positive things do people say about you?
6. Perspective questions: What are your ideas about your current situation?
7. Change questions: What do you think is necessary for things to change? What could you do to make that happen?

(Adapted from Saleeby, D., (Ed.), 2006. The Strengths Based Perspective in Social Work Practice. Person Education, Inc.)

■ Time Out

Focusing on a particular issue that you need help with, consider and answer Saleeby's seven questions, writing the answers in your reflective diary. Make some notes about what you have discovered about yourself and your issue under three headings:

1. What possibilities and positive expectations have you uncovered?
2. What capacity, competence and courage can you draw on?
3. What reserves, resilience and resources have you identified?

Many students, for example, express self-doubt, so the esteem question may encourage you to remember and focus on any positive feedback that you have received. I keep a folder of 'positive tweets' and certificates on my wall to remind me on bad days that I should be proud of certain achievements.

Not only are Saleeby's questions useful for when you want to consider your leadership strengths, they are also powerful questions to use with patients or colleagues wanting advice on what to do. It is a good idea to keep these questions in the notes app on your phone, as these are ideal 'coaching' questions to help patients or colleagues discover their own solutions.

Imposter Syndrome

'Some people can't believe in themselves until someone else believes in them first.'
SEAN MCGUIRE, FROM THE FILM *GOOD WILL HUNTING*

Imposter syndrome arises from anxiety or self-doubt about your competence. You may falsely attribute your accomplishments to luck or other external forces. You feel that any second you may be found out as a fraud. If this is you, then you are not alone.

The first thing to say is that it is normal to feel like this. Nearly every student interviewed for this book mentioned imposter syndrome. Case Study 4.2 reflects many student's feelings on being an imposter:

CASE STUDY 4.2 | **Imposter Syndrome Made Me Dread Some of My Lectures**

DOREEN DUBE, SECOND-YEAR, ADULT NURSING, UNIVERSITY OF NORTHAMPTON AND 2020–21 NURSING TIMES STUDENT EDITOR

Being accepted into university was a big achievement. However, after beginning the nursing course I started to have underlying feelings of self-doubt that always made me question whether I deserved to be where I was.

Continued

CASE STUDY 4.2	Imposter Syndrome Made Me Dread Some of My Lectures—cont'd

Many of the students within my cohort had several years of healthcare experience, which made me feel more out of place because I had no experience.

Other changes added to the feeling of not belonging, such as adjusting to life abroad while also adapting to the move from secondary education to higher education.

I was able to put a name to my increasing feelings of self-doubt after remembering an article I had read for my university interview. I was experiencing the imposter syndrome, which has been described as feelings of inadequacy, unworthiness and an inability to accept one's achievements. It thrives off of the discomfort individuals may face when being pushed out of their comfort zone, for example transitioning to a new role. It can also make us compare ourselves to others.

The imposter syndrome can have a negative effect on people, in my case it made me dread some of my lectures in fear of having my inadequacies highlighted and I always questioned my abilities. For others, it may include avoiding new roles that may require increased levels of responsibility.

The thought of being a 'fraud' when experiencing the imposter syndrome is illegitimate; instead it is a result of being unable to accept your accomplishments.

At times the feelings of inadequacy can creep up on us but there are ways to overcome them. Putting a name to how you are feeling is important. Once I identified that I was experiencing the imposter syndrome I was able to research ways to overcome it. The next step is talking to someone that may have gone through a similar experience. One of my lecturers spoke about her nursing journey and to my surprise she mentioned that she had no experience prior to beginning her course. Hearing that an experienced faculty member was once in my shoes was reassuring and it put me at ease. Also, talking to student nurses from the cohort above mine further helped to alleviate the self-doubt I was experiencing.

Learning to reframe my thinking has helped me significantly. Initially I viewed not having experience as something negative, however a piece of advice I received from my lecturer was to treat my lack of experience as an opportunity to learn. I did exactly that going into practice for the first time. I had an open mind ready to absorb all the information I could, asked all the questions I could think of and allowed myself to receive information from different sources within my placement area. This helped me develop my knowledge and build a good rapport with staff members on the ward.

Another important tool for overcoming the imposter syndrome is self-reflection. As mentioned earlier, the imposter syndrome can make us experience false feelings of inadequacy. However, engaging in self-reflection and seeking feedback from peers can highlight legitimate areas for self-improvement. During the reflection process it is useful to remember times where you have successfully handled unfamiliar situations. This provides an opportunity to call on strategies you once used while adjusting to a new role. Lastly, an important aspect of the reflection process is to celebrate your achievements. Doing this helps you appreciate how far you have come and it can be a source of motivation, encouraging you to work towards the next goal.

This blog was previously published in 2020 by *Nursing Times*. It is republished here with their kind permission.

So, as well as remembering that imposter syndrome seems to happen to us all, it is important to recognise that we may be judging ourselves too harshly, that we may be our own worst critic and that we underestimate our achievements. It is also important that we talk about how we are feeling and ask for advice (Tips Box 4.1). By doing so, we can get an outside perspective on our perceptions of capabilities. I say 'we' because I have imposter syndrome too!

TIPS BOX 4.1

Top Tips From Student Nurses on Coping With Imposter Syndrome

- Put a name to what you are feeling. You are not alone—many people experience imposter syndrome. You are not a fraud.
- Accept your accomplishments—it is not luck or a fluke.
- Talk to someone more senior with similar experience. They may tell you that they once felt like you, but yet you see that they have achieved much.

- Learn to reframe how you are feeling: 'no experience' becomes 'an opportunity to learn' or 'anxiety' is really 'excitement'.
- Ask questions and ask others for help, rather than sit and worry.
- Reflect on times when you have successfully handled situations.
- Seek feedback from others to get an external reality check.
- Remember successes and celebrate achievements.
- Think about all your achievements—read positive messages you have been sent.
- Keep positive quotes and positive people around you rather than those who may feed your doubts.
- Remember to give positive feedback to others, for example on Twitter, and say thank you if you receive compliments.

Based on discussions with Rebecca Lennox, adult student nurse; Claire Carmichael, newly registered general practice nurse and blogger Doreen Dube.

'I'm open to challenges. I want to see where it takes me. I'll figure a way out, I always do.'
GLORIA SIKAPITE, THIRD-YEAR ADULT STUDENT NURSE

Social Comparisons

A book called *The Spirit Level* (2009), written by eminent professors and epidemiologists Richard Wilkinson and Kate Pickett, helps us to understand where imposter syndrome might come from. The book demonstrates that for each of 11 different health and social problems—physical health, mental health, drug abuse, education, imprisonment, obesity, social mobility, trust and community life, violence, teenage pregnancies and child wellbeing—outcomes are significantly worse where there are income inequalities between rich and poor (this is controversial and hotly debated). Wilkinson and Pickett explain that these adverse outcomes may happen because of social comparisons: The feeling that everyone around you is better or smarter or richer than you. They call this 'social evaluative threat'.

If you are sat there, waiting for an interview and someone else comes in and says a few words to you, you may be thinking 'They look smart—and what they've just said tells me that they have more experience than me. I have no chance at getting this job,' then this is a social evaluative threat.

In the case of student nurses, you may find people covering up that feeling of threat with outer signals such as expensive clothing, bravado or aggression, or alternatively they may shrink away from situations where they may feel less than others. If you read Natalie's story or Aalijah's quote from Chapter 1 about feeling that they do not have a right to even be somewhere, then you see this in action. Notice that when Natalie gets to know people and realises that they are supportive that her threat level lowers too.

Keep this idea of social comparisons in mind when dealing with not only colleagues, but also more senior nurses who may feel threatened by your questions or may fear that your more recent study may reveal that their knowledge is out of date. Patients too might feel that they are being judged by you, or they may not want to reveal certain information, for example that they cannot read or that they think that they drink too much.

Scarcity

In her book *Daring Greatly* (2013), research professor Brené Brown talks about 'scarcity', by which she means never being enough—smart enough, thin enough, certain enough, etc. Brown explains the three components of scarcity:

- Comparison—the same issue that Wilkinson and Pickett identified
- Shame—a fear of ridicule

- Disengagement—feeling that it is better to stay quiet than offer an opinion or try something new

Vulnerability

'Vulnerability is courage in you and inadequacy in me. I'm drawn to your vulnerability and repelled by mine.'

BRENÉ BROWN

You will remember that part of being authentic is to show your true self and be vulnerable. Vulnerability is also about being able to ask for help. But Brown says that displaying vulnerability is hard because it may be perceived as weakness, when in fact it is an act of courage. Her advice is to disclose appropriately rather than overshare, and to avoid using your vulnerability to get attention or to shock people.

Failure

'I've embraced the idea of failure equals First Attempt In Learning.'

ROBIN WILLIAMS, ACTOR

'You can fail as many times as you like but you don't really fail until you start to blame somebody else.'

ROY LILLEY, NHS COMMENTATOR

Linked to these ideas of shame and vulnerability is fear of failure (Tips Boxes 4.2 and 4.3). Failure is often linked to fault and blame, but the most important thing to do as a leader is to find out what happened and learn from it. To do that, leaders need to create a culture of psychological safety so people know that they will not be blamed. The language used by leaders changes from 'who did it' to 'what happened'.

If someone is afraid of failure they will avoid taking risks and wriggle away from responsibility, and they will not grow as people. By contrast, some of the world's greatest leaders have been shaped by their failures. Before success at Microsoft for example, Bill Gates created a product that analysed traffic data that completely failed.

New ideas can be tested at small scale, and simple adjustments can turn failure into success.

Pushing Through Fear

'The only way to feel better about myself is to go out and do it anyway. Pushing through fear is less frightening than living with the underlying fear that comes from a feeling of helplessness.'

SUSAN JEFFERS, AUTHOR OF *FEEL THE FEAR AND DO IT ANYWAY* (1987)

CASE STUDY 4.3   **Alicia Burnett, Student Midwife**

Most people are afraid of failing and so might not even take the first steps on their leadership journey.

Alicia Burnett's mother was a nurse. Alicia remembers sneaking a look at her mother's anatomy and physiology books, and she would always be drawn to the reproductive system.

Years later, having had the experience of working in a nursery and not knowing what to do when a child in her care became sick, she succeeded in getting a place to train as a children's nurse. Competition for the few training places available was often fierce, but she successfully applied and completed her training.

| CASE STUDY 4.3 | **Alicia Burnett, Student Midwife—cont'd** |

But Alicia had always had it in her mind to become a midwife and thought she could do that at any time, until she discovered that the student bursary to do the training was about to be withdrawn.

So, despite fighting to become a newly registered children's nurse, she decided to apply to become a student midwife—another competitive field. Her colleagues thought that she should work in children's nursing for a while before making such a move. They told her that it was extremely competitive and that she may not succeed. Her thinking was that she had survived her student nurse training and got a job as a staff nurse and that she would succeed again. Some universities turned her application away because she was already a registered nurse, but Alicia had the drive and confidence in herself to succeed. She was accepted as a student midwife in the very last intake to receive the full training bursary.

'You very much have to be your own sunshine, your own motivator. You're not always going to find support in the environment. My parents are very supportive, but they're much more grounded in reality than I am—the dreamer. I'm very much affected by naysayers and negative emotions, so I don't tell them, so it doesn't affect me.'

Alicia uses the mindset of building on one success to achieve another. She consciously surrounds herself with others who are passionate and want to improve the care they give.

In the later chapter on communication, Alicia's story continues as she brings together student midwives from across the world to support each other during the global COVID-19 pandemic in 2020.

TIPS BOX 4.2

Work Through Fear to Take Decisions

1. Adopt a no-lose mindset of 'whatever happens this decision will be an opportunity to learn and grow'.
2. Do your homework on all the alternatives, and talk to people about your plans.
3. Establish your priorities based on the things that will bring you satisfaction rather than doing what other people want you to do.
4. Trust your subconscious, which may make better choices than your conscious, logical mind.
5. Decide that, whatever happens, you will handle it.
6. After making the decision, let go of your focus on 'how it's supposed to be' and just go with the flow.
7. Accept total responsibility for the decision. If it does not work, what have you learnt?
8. Do not protect your plan, correct it. Be flexible and change course.

Adapted from Jeffers (1987).

TIPS BOX 4.3

Getting Out of Your Comfort Zone

- *'I like to just throw myself at something and then if it doesn't work then I'll learn from it. I just embrace the opportunity. If it doesn't work I take the positives from every situation.'* —Alison Booker, student dietician
- *'Put yourself out of your comfort zone and your comfort zone gets bigger'*—Ian Unitt, newly registered learning disability nurse

Fake It Till You Make It

'Our bodies change our minds, and our minds can change our behaviour, and our behaviour can change our outcomes.'

AMY CUDDY, SOCIAL PSYCHOLOGIST

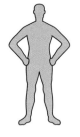 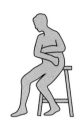

High-power pose   Low-power pose

Fig. 4.2   High- and low-power poses.

There is lots of evidence that our nonverbal communication governs how people think and feel about us. Amy Cuddy (2016), working at Berkley University, took this a step further and tested whether our nonverbal behaviour governs how we think and feel about ourselves. She conducted psychological experiments where some students (Fig. 4.2) were invited to do 'low-power poses' (where their bodies were 'closed'—arms folded/hunched) and other students did high-power poses (shoulders back, head up, standing tall, feet apart, hands on hips). Each student was then subjected to a stressful job interview. What she found was that just 2 minutes of practising a 'power pose' would make students feel more powerful (Tips Box 4.4).

■ **Time Out**

If you are one of the students thinking 'I'm not supposed to be here', practise 2 minutes of power posing somewhere private just before a stressful situation.
Make a conscious decision to show the world who you are and what you have to offer.

TIPS BOX 4.4

Tips From Students on Faking It

- *'When I apply for things I say to myself I'm applying for this because I'm amazing and I think I'm going to get it. But I'm not really thinking that!'*—Rebecca Lennox, adult nursing student
- *'If you wait until you feel you're ready then you're never going to do it, so you may as well pretend like you're ready and it will come.'*—Newly registered therapeutic radiographer Sarah Bradder

Finding Your Body Balance

To feel more confident and grounded before public speaking it may be helpful to find your body balance (Fisher and Kayes 2018). This means feeling the ground under different parts of your feet:
- Stand with the feet shoulder-width apart, preferably with your shoes off.
- Without lifting any part of your feet, shift your weight by leaning forwards and hold for a count of five.
- Shift your weight by leaning backwards slightly. Hold for a count of five.
- Shift onto the outsides of your feet. Hold for a count of five.
- Shift onto the insides of your feet. Hold for a count of five.

- Raise your heels off the floor slightly. Hold for five seconds.
- Go back down. Feel where the parts of the feet touch the floor.
- Lift your big toes and count to five.
  Based on Fisher and Kayes (2018).

Overconfidence

At the other end of the spectrum is tipping over into overconfidence. This is where self-awareness and the ability to reflect carefully is important. Do this either on your own or with a colleague who is prepared to be honest about whether the problem is you or whether others may not be appreciating constructive challenge.

Resilience

Nursing as a profession is known as a vocation, and many nurses are hard-wired to put others before themselves. The stress of leadership plus the emotional nature of nursing (called emotional labour) can lead to burnout.

Resilience is 'a process whereby people bounce back from adversity and go on with their lives' (Dyer and McGuinness 1996). It is much discussed in nursing, with some arguing that to be resilient is to put up with a bad situation and that the focus should be on improving the working life of nurses rather than helping nurses to cope with it.

There are many articles where the focus is on developing resilience with solutions such as mindfulness, seeking support, staying healthy and so on. But Adele Nightingale, education lead for nursing and allied health professionals at Bolton NHS Foundation Trust, uses an approach to resilience called the ABC of resilience (Reivich and Shatté 2002). It emphasises on an ability to focus not on events themselves, but on how you interpret them. This links back to the idea of emotional intelligence and being able to know yourself, understand others and regulate your emotions, so that it is not a knee-jerk reaction.

ABC stands for

A = adversity
B = beliefs
C = consequential feelings

'Not everything is an adversity, not everything's an incident. Actually sometimes they're just obstacles, they're things we need to get over and we just need to look at them differently. This is about learning and leaping forward, not about bouncing back. We don't want you to come back to your current state, we want you to move on and advance.'

ADELE NIGHTINGALE

To illustrate this, Adele tells a typical story of seeing a colleague on the corridor and waving and being completely ignored. This is a low-level example of A—adversity. She then asks her students how they interpret this and gets various answers back such as 'the other person was ignorant' or 'I'd worry that she might not be ok' and so on. One incident can generate differing feelings depending on someone's belief systems. But we don't know what is happening in other people's lives. If for example you think that someone has ignored you, you might feel fed up all day—the C of consequential feelings.

The ABC model is therefore about reflecting on what adversities trigger you most and tune in to your beliefs about how you interpret events and how that makes you feel.

I can think of occasions when I worked as a staff nurse in intensive care. When my colleagues walked on shift, the first thing they would do would be to look for the patient with the most machines and the most theatre greens around them. Some would pray that they were not allocated to care for someone who they perceived as the sickest patient and the most work. That is, their adversity (sick patient) triggered their beliefs (hard work) and their consequential feelings (stressful and demanding).

Other nurses interpreted this differently: they still saw the sickest patient, but their belief was that if they were chosen to look after them then this was a sign that they were skilled and trusted. Consequently, they were happy to be able to demonstrate their skills and proud that they had been chosen. My own response was somewhat in the middle (I was young and I wasn't the best ICU nurse!): I would be flattered if I was chosen, but to cope with the pressure I would say to myself 'this isn't forever. It's just for x hours. I'll do my best, I'll learn something and then it will be over,' and it was!

Adele advises that to become more resilient we need to become more response-able (responsible) and choose how we respond to adversity.

■ Time Out

Set an alarm on your phone for it to beep every hour. When the alarm goes off, focus on your beliefs and record what you believe in your reflective diary. For example, you come home from work and your partner/housemate still has not tidied the living room like they promised. What do you believe? What consequential feelings do you have?

Do this for 2 days every week for as long as it takes to tune into your beliefs without the alarm. Start to consider how you may change your response to trigger events (like your partner's untidiness or being called 'the student' rather than by your name, or, like me, being allocated the most complex patient).

Grit

Grit is described as a special combination of passion and perseverance to achieve long-term goals (Duckworth 2013). This idea has been tested in US junior schools, and the evidence shows that 'grittier' children outperform intelligence (IQ) tests and graduate junior school. Grit is unrelated or inversely related to measures of talent. What really matters is following through on your passions (Tips Box 4.5).

What makes people grittier is still being researched. But one idea that might help is having a 'growth mindset' (Dweck 2014)—the ability to grow your abilities through hard work. Here, people engage with the idea of moving from the 'tyranny of now'—failing an assignment for example and feeling that your abilities are fixed—to the power of 'not yet'—the ability to process poor performance, learn, correct and move forward.

How progress is rewarded is also crucial and needs to focus on praising the process of learning (like perseverance, positive strategies and focus) rather than rewarding intelligence or talent, so that people learn resilience.

TIPS BOX 4.5

- When practising leadership, follow your passion rather than what you think you should do.
- Be as clear as you can on your purpose—the idea that what you do matters to other people.
- Practise, practise, practise!
- Think of how you talk to yourself when striving for something you passionately want—use words like 'not yet' rather than 'I failed'.
- When you do something outside you comfort zone, think of what you have learnt and visualise the neurons in your brain making more connections and believing that over time you will become smarter.
- Based on the strengths perspective mentioned earlier, you may also need to think about choosing which skills and abilities to develop, depending on your strengths.

Based on Duckworth (2013) and Dweck (2014).

Saying No

'Saying yes can become a habit, but when you have eight or nine opportunities you're just going to burn yourself out. So you have to prioritise.'

IAN UNITT, NEWLY REGISTERED LEARNING DISABILITY NURSE

You have the right to set boundaries for yourself. Be honest and clear about why (authentic leadership). You might want to make a counteroffer, such as 'I can't do this right now but can help you in 2 weeks, if that's OK?'

Time Management

Good time management is essential for a leader. It allows us to focus on what we want to do and to achieve our goals. Student nurses have many pressures on their time, often juggling family, study, work and clinical placements, never mind taking on leadership challenges (Tips Box 4.6).

TIPS BOX 4.6

- Most important is to do a simple audit of where your time is currently being spent. To do this, log what you are doing every 15 minutes for a couple of days.
- Review your log and decide:
  - Which tasks could you stop/delegate/do more efficiently?
  - Make a list of meetings and prioritise which are most important. Are there any meetings that could be made shorter/more efficient? Are there any that you could stop attending?
- Break down your leadership project into a rough timeline of tasks—what do you want to achieve the next month/in 6 months/in 12 months (see Chapter 15 on project management for more detail).
- Plan the tasks that you want to achieve this week, including what you want to get out of each meeting.
- Keep a to-do list for each day and tick items off as you do them. Do the most difficult or the most mundane when you have the highest energy, usually at the start of the day.
- Organise your working space so that you have what you need to hand. Throw or give away things you do not use.
- Plan for 'dead' time such as when travelling or waiting; use this time to think, read, catch up on emails or make phone calls.
- Set up an efficient filing system so you can find and file things quickly.
- Plan when to do your emails to keep on top of them. It is a good idea to have just two or three set times each day so you are not tempted to lose concentration by breaking off from tasks to check your emails.
- Use subfolders in your email system to file emails that you need to keep rather than print them out.
- Keep a folder of articles to read to keep up to date. Set time aside weekly to read them. Use scanning to help you get the feel of content by reading the:
  - Title
  - Abstract or executive summary
  - First line of each paragraph
  - Conclusion
- Long hours with no breaks do not increase your productivity. Make time to relax every day, and book regular holidays as far in advance as you can.
- Perfection takes more time. Plan for 'good enough' for that assignment, meeting, etc.

Leadership in Transition

Newly registered nurse leaders interviewed for this book were keen to point out the culture shock from feeling comfortable in a student leadership role to feeling that they are back at square one with their leadership when they became registered nurses. They talked candidly about their confidence being knocked and feeling that they were starting again (Tips Box 4.7).

> 'They feel that they should be bossing being an NQN as much as they were a student. And obviously it's taken them 3–4 years to get to the point where they are as a student, so logically it would take them time [to develop their leadership as registered nurses].'
>
> DANIEL BRANCH,
> CURATOR RCN NEWLY QUALIFIED NURSE PROJECT (HTTPS://WWW.RCN.ORG.UK/GET-INVOLVED/
> FORUMS/NRN-NETWORK) AND NEWLY REGISTERED LEARNING DISABILITY NURSE

TIPS BOX 4.7

Self-Compassion During the Transition to Registered Nurse

- Seek support from within the work environment during your preceptorship.
- Keep a reflective diary, including a log of your emotions, to help you to understand why you are experiencing these emotions.
- Think about your own learning needs, not just those around you and how you can address them.
- Effective leadership is not your sole responsibility. Remember that delegation is important too.
- Invest in and develop others and give recognition and praise.
- Practise collaborative and collective leadership—encouraging the idea that we are all leaders rather than pushing yourself to the front or be pushed forward by the team.
- Practise compassion and empathy not only with patients but with the team too.
- Try not to criticise yourself; talk to yourself as a close friend would.
- Reframe challenges as opportunities to learn.
- Be grateful for what you have and your strengths, rather than focusing on what you do not have.
- Find the right level of generosity, remembering that you also have to be generous to yourself.
- Be mindful—try to stay in the moment and be aware of what is happening right now without judging.
- If you make mistakes, seek feedback from a more senior nurse, reflect on what you have learnt and express your thoughts and emotions during debriefs with the team.

Based on Butler (2017a, b, c).

Summary

It is important as an emerging leader to get to know your strengths, your beliefs, your values and your mindset. Every leader is different, and this is your opportunity to find out more about yourself and how your particular talents may be complemented by others in your team.

Self-doubt, fear of failure and ridicule are all normal feelings in leaders. They push through fear and enlarge their comfort zones. By appropriately sharing vulnerabilities, leaders demonstrate their authenticity, which helps build relationships and trust.

Leaders spend time developing their mindsets; the evidence is that leaders can examine and alter their response to adversity to make them more resilient. They also show grit: persevering to achieve their passions, using the growth mindset of 'not yet' instead of 'I failed'.

The transition to registered nurse is a difficult time in a leader's journey. More than ever at this point nurse leaders need to practise self-compassion, including seeking support from others, avoiding negative self-talk and reflecting on learning.

Resources

There are two ways to do a Clifton StrengthsFinder test. This first is to buy a new copy of Tom Rath's book
   (see references) and find a unique access code. Enter the code into the Clifton StrengthsFinder website and
   complete the assessment. Do not buy a second-hand copy of the book, as the code has a one-time only use.
The second way is to purchase access to the assessment tool online at https://store.gallup.com/h/en-gb.
Branch, D., 2020. The importance of empowerment to my nursing journey. RCN Newly Qualified Nurses.
   <https://www.rcn.org.uk/news-and-events/blogs/empowerment-and-my-nursing-journey>

References

Brown, B., 2013. Daring Greatly. Penguin, London.
Butler, Z., 2017a. My first year as a registered nurse: a crisis of confidence, a shift in perspective. Nursing
   Standard. <https://rcni.com/nursing-standard/students/newly-qualified-nurses/my-first-year-a-registered-
   nurse-a-crisis-of-confidence-a-shift-perspective-121501>.
Butler, Z., 2017b. My first year as a registered nurse: learning how to deal with mistakes. Nursing Standard.
   <https://rcni.com/nursing-standard/students/newly-qualified-nurses/my-first-year-a-registered-nurse-
   learning-how-to-deal-mistakes-123451>.
Butler, Z., 2017c. My first year as a registered nurse: reflecting on what makes an effective leader. Nursing
   Standard. <https://rcni.com/nursing-standard/students/newly-qualified-nurses/my-first-year-a-registered-
   nurse-reflecting-what-makes-effective-leader-122271>.
Cuddy, A., 2016. Fake it till you make it. TED. <https://youtu.be/RVmMeMcGc0Y>.
Dube, D., 2020. Imposter syndrome made me dread some of my lectures. Nursing Times Online, 02.01.20.
Duckworth, A., 2013. Grit: the power of passion and perseverance. TED. <https://youtu.be/H14bBuluwB8>.
Dweck, C., 2014. Developing a growth mind set. TED. <https://youtu.be/hiiEeMN7vbQ>.
Dyer, J.G., McGuinness, T.M., 1996. Resilience: analysis of the concept. Archives of Psychiatric Nursing
   10, 276–282.
Fisher, J., Kayes, G., 2018. This Is a Voice. Wellcome Collection, London.
Jeffers, S., 1987. Feel the Fear and Do It Anyway. Random House, London.
Rath, T., 2007. StengthsFinder 2.0. Gallup Press, New York.
Reivich, K., Shatté, A., 2002. The Resilience Factor: 7 Essential Skills for Overcoming Life's Inevitable
   Obstacles. Broadway Books, New York.
Saleeby, D., (Ed.), 2006. The Strengths Based Perspective in Social Work Practice. Pearson Education, Inc.
   Boston.
Wilkinson, R., Pickett, K., 2009. The Spirit Level: Why More Equal Societies Almost Always Do Better.
   Allen Lane, London.

Using Networks, Coaches and Mentors

OBJECTIVES

After reading this chapter and completing the activities, you should be able to:
- Describe the main differences between coaching, mentoring and supervision
- Network with peers and more experienced leaders, both face to face and virtually
- Practise self-coaching and/or peer coaching
- Explain the benefits of mentoring, reverse mentoring and shadowing
- Identify potential mentors
- Practise positive reframing of difficult experiences using group supervision
- Draw together a summary of who you are and what you value.

Relevance to the Nursing and Midwifery Council (NMC) Code

Paragraph 8:
Work Cooperatively
8.4 work with colleagues to evaluate the quality of your work and that of the team

Paragraph 9:
Share your skills, knowledge and experience for the benefit of people receiving care and your colleagues
9.1 provide honest, accurate and constructive feedback to colleagues
9.2 gather and reflect on feedback from a variety of sources, using it to improve your practice and performance
9.3 deal with differences of professional opinion with colleagues by discussion and informed debate, respecting their views and opinions and behaving in a professional way at all times
9.4 support students' and colleagues' learning to help them develop their professional competence and confidence

---

Relevance to the Nursing and Midwifery Council (NMC) Code—cont'd

---

Promote Professionalism and Trust
Paragraph 20:
Uphold the reputation of your profession at all times
- 20.3 be aware at all times of how your behaviour can affect and influence the behaviour of other people
- 20.8 act as a role model of professional behaviour for students and newly qualified nurses, midwives and nursing associates to aspire to
- 20.10 use all forms of spoken, written and digital communication (including social media and networking sites) responsibly, respecting the right to privacy of others at all times

---

Helpers on Your Leadership Journey

This chapter is all about finding the right people to guide you on your leadership journey and help you to reflect. Some of this 'finding' is about you proactively establishing professional networks. The chapter ends with an exercise to help you to reflect on your personal leadership journey so far.

The Learning and Development Model

> *'Nursing is a very serious delightful thing like life, requiring training, experience, devotion... A power of accumulating, instead of losing, all these things.'*
>
> FLORENCE NIGHTINGALE

You learn to be a leader mostly through accumulating experience and reflecting on it. The learning and development model, born out of qualitative research undertaken by the Center for Creative Leadership in the 1990s, describes how people need to have three types of experience to learn to be a leader, in a ratio of 70:20:10:

- 70% of learning and development takes place in real-life and on-the-job experiences;
- 20% is from ongoing feedback, coaching and from working with role models; and
- 10% occurs in formal off-the-job training.

So, this means that about one-fifth of your leadership development is about reflecting, with the support of others (Gurvis et al. 2016).

From Novice to Expert

Developing your leadership skills follows a similar process to developing your nursing skills: you gather all the experience you have and build it into an expertise. Nursing and leadership are both about dealing with uncertainty, and you get better at addressing this as you become more experienced. As a student, everything is uncertain and so it is important to have supervision and reflect on what has been learnt and what you will do differently next time.

You may have learnt about the concept of 'From Novice to Expert', Patricia Benner's 1984 theory that nurses develop skills and an understanding of patient care over time from a combination of personal experiences alongside a strong educational foundation. She explains that there are five levels of nursing experience: novice, advanced beginner, competent, proficient and expert. As nurses progress through these levels, they start to see recurring patterns, become less reliant upon rules and principles, and develop an awareness of long-term goals. They develop a more holistic understanding of nursing and have a deeper level of understanding to draw on.

The same is true of nursing leadership. However, today's student nurses come with a range of life experience, including leadership experience, so this is a reminder that you may not be starting at 'novice' and to use the leadership expertise that you bring into nursing.

Take Charge of Your Leadership Learning

It is important that you take charge of whom you invite to help you with your lifelong learning to be the best leader that you can be, rather than let your university or your employer dictate it for you. Learning and development are a shared responsibility between individuals and managers (or practice supervisor/personal tutors during preregistration). Remember though that you have agency to form your own relationships and invite people to help you, or conversely to offer help, so you can grow.

■ **Time Out**

Consider the different sorts of people who might help you:
- Role models
- People from different disciplines and different backgrounds
- People outside health and care, who may offer a fresh eye
- Your peer group
- Less experienced students, whom you might help (we look at peer-assisted learning later in this chapter)

Make a list of
- People who already help you to grow as a leader
- Other people who you might like to engage

DEFINITIONS OF LEADERSHIP COACHING, MENTORSHIP AND SUPERVISION

Definitions of preceptorship, practice supervision, clinical supervision, academic assessment and practice assessment are clearly set out by the NMC. However, the definitions used in leadership and management development may mean different things to terms used in nursing. Table 5.1 sets out a broad comparison of the three.

TABLE 5.1 ■ Comparison of Coaching, Mentoring and Supervising in Leadership.

	Coaching	Mentoring	Supervising
Definition	Thinking partner who helps you to unlock your potential	Passes on skills and pushes you forward	Line manager directing actions of employees to improve and achieve organisational goals
When to use	When you are stuck To address a challenge, e.g., making a difficult decision To debrief from or process a situation	To get advice To gain knowledge and skills To get feedback	To improve and evaluate performance To achieve organisational goals To ensure accountability
Key elements	Strengths based Enabling learning rather than teaching or passing on skills Fresh eyes	Mentee is seeking advice and support from a more experienced person.	Supervisor/subordinate relationship Instructions and directions
Background	They may come from any background. Coaches receive specific training. Professional coaches are accredited	More senior leader with a similar professional background	Supervisor or manager
Sounds like	'What do you want to do?' 'What went well?' 'Where next?' 'What's most important to you?'	'Here's a tool I use.' 'In that situation, consider…' 'Let me introduce you to…'	'You are doing well. Try to focus on this target.' 'I expect to see…' 'Next time, do…'

Coaching

'Coaching is unlocking people's potential to maximize their own performance. It is helping them to learn rather than teaching them. ...Coaching is not dependent on a more experienced person passing down their knowledge—in fact, this undermines the building of self-belief which creates sustained performance, as we shall discover. Instead, coaching requires expertise in coaching, not in the subject at hand. That is one of its great strengths. And something that coaching leaders grapple with most— but is key—is to learn when to share their knowledge and experience and when not to.'

JOHN WHITMORE (2002)

A coach will not advise you on what to do, which is probably what students need in the earliest stages of their leadership careers, so it is unlikely (but possible) that you would seek one out.

THREE ELEMENTS OF SUCCESSFUL COACHING

There are three key elements to a successful coaching conversation, so these are what any coach you work with should be doing, or if you are coaching someone else, they can act as a guide:
- Listening—we have already covered the idea of listening with fascination—the sort of deep listening that a coach does to help understand what is happening. But you may also have had the experience of being asked questions and really listened to, and in the process you started to reveal to yourself what you really thought. And the more you talked the more you began to convince yourself of what the answer to your problem might be.
- Powerful questions that can stimulate thought, ignite creativity, surface assumptions and so on.
- Being present—being aware of what is happening right now.

Based on conversations with Zoe Cohen, executive coach.

COACHING IN ACTION

Coaching becomes more common as you become more senior. Some NHS leadership programmes will include the services of a qualified coach. Coachees generally have a specific goal in mind that the coach helps them with, such as developing their skills for a new job, or coping with a tricky work situation.

Mark Radford, chief nurse at Health Education England, uses a strengths-based coaching style with senior nurse leaders using the Clifton StrengthsFinder that we have already discussed. This follows an episode when he was being coached and was told, ...unless you're seriously difficult and a poor leader stop focusing on what you're not good at, play to your strengths.' He chose from then on to navigate his career to fit those strengths and avoid jobs requiring skills that he was not good at. He once surprised an interview panel recruiting for a very senior role by advising them, once he understood the role, that he was not the person they were seeking. The lesson here is not to be seduced into a promotion that you are not suited for.

Finding coaches or key influencers is about recognising that person who inspires you and inviting them to help you, but this can also extend to having compassion for those you admire too. Adele Nightingale, education lead for nursing and allied health professionals at Bolton NHS Foundation Trust, recollects how, when she was a senior lecturer, she reached out to a head of school at a university who was managing the death of a member of the team, inviting her for a coffee and a chat if she needed it.

Another more recent trend in coaching is team coaching. This echoes the idea of collective/collaborative leadership and moves away from the focus on self-development and towards the idea of coaching leaders together for system change.

The GROW Coaching Model

It is helpful to have a structure for a coaching or mentoring conversation. One widely used tool is the GROW model developed by Sir John Whitmore, who is considered the 'father' of coaching. This is a technique for problem solving and goal setting, and it has been used extensively since the late 1980s.

GROW is an acronym for

- **G**oal—help the team member decide where they are going
- Current **R**eality—establish where they currently are—their reality
- **O**ptions—explore various ways to achieve their goal—the options they have
- **W**ill—Ensure your team member is committed to achieving their goal and prepared for the conditions and obstacles they may meet along the way, thus establishing their willingness to follow through on this commitment

■ Time Out

Practise the GROW model yourself by finding a colleague and working through the four GROW questions in turn: goal, reality, options and will. Head over to the resources section to find a written guide.

Self-Coaching and Peer Coaching

It is important to realise that you do not always need external expertise and that you can self-coach or practice coaching as a team of student nurses wanting to tackle an issue where you feel 'stuck'.

There are various tools that can help you to do this.

- Explore the 'thinking environment'. Nancy Kline is the author of *Time to Think* (1999), a bestselling book that helps unlock the knowledge and wisdom that you already have. In the book, Kline identifies the 10 behaviours that help generate the best thinking environment. There is a link in the resources section to the Time to Think website that lists the behaviours, such as removing time pressure to allow 'thinking at ease' and appreciating rather than just challenging what people say.
- Consider Saleeby's seven strengths-based questions that were introduced in the previous chapter and apply them to your own situation.
- Develop you own questions: You can easily search for what are called 'powerful questions' or 'incisive questions' (questions that surface our limiting assumptions) (Tips Boxes 5.1 and 5.2).

■ Time Out

There are two options for this time out. Before you start, search for 'powerful questions' on the internet and choose as many of them as you think will help you and your colleagues with an issue, such as 'what will happen if you do and what will happen if you don't?' or 'what's in the way?'.

Option 1: Peer coaching: Reciprocal deep listening exercises

- Form a team of three.
- Take turns listening to each other talk about an issue that they need help with. Set a timer so everyone has equal time. For each person:
  - The individual spends 5 minutes outlining the issue.

- The other two people take 5 minutes asking clarifying questions so that they understand the issue.
    - They then spend 5 minutes asking powerful questions.
- The individual shares how it went for them and what they discovered for the remaining 5 minutes.
- Roles are then swapped.
- Remember—listen with fascination, do not interrupt, do not offer solutions or advice and be present—no thinking about what to have for tea!

Option 2: Self-coaching

- Find a quiet space where you will not be interrupted in your thinking.
- Outline to yourself what the issue is—this can be spoken out load or written in your reflective journal.
- Ask yourself the powerful or incisive questions that you have prepared, and speak or write your answers.
- Reflect on what you have learnt.

TIPS BOX 5.1

Working With a Coach

- Have a conversation with your prospective coach and decide whether you have the right chemistry to work together.
- Treat it like a partnership of equals.
- Check that they understand that they will not tell you what to do—this person should not be an expert in your field. If you want a person to offer this sort of help, you need to look for a mentor.
- Feel confident enough to give your coach feedback on what is working or not working.
- Expect it to be time limited, and plan for the end of the journey so that you sustain your learning.

Mentoring

Mentors are traditionally more senior leaders who pass on their skills and push you on. Mentors help team members to solve problems, make better decisions, learn new skills and help them progress in their role or career.

Anyone can mentor anyone else, because we all have different experience that we can share. You may be drawn to somebody with different experiences who can give you guidance and connections in areas that you want to know more about. For example, you may choose a local person for the South Asian community as a mentor if you want help to understand how to support people with diabetes locally.

REVERSE MENTORING

CASE STUDY 5.1   **Jessica Sainsbury**

When Jess was a student nurse, she attended an event where she ended up in the same working group as the chief nurse of her trust. In Jess's words, they both 'said it like it was'—they were frank and open in front of each other.

After the event, the chief nurse approached Jess and asked her if she would be interested in a reverse mentorship arrangement.

They discussed what each of them could offer and what each wanted to get out of reverse mentorship. They agreed that their relationship would be open, honest and polite.

Continued

CASE STUDY 5.1   Jessica Sainsbury—cont'd

The chief nurse wanted Jess to help her to use social media better, and in return they collaborated on a project to establish a student council in Hampshire and the Isle of Wight.

They succeeded in establishing the student council, not just for Hampshire and the Isle of Wight, but they were also successful in producing guidance to help roll student councils out across the wider system. By being more inclusive this not only helped students to get their voices heard and profile raised, but it also led to better decision-making.

Jess now has a split role working as a newly registered community mental health nurse for older people and a developing educator in practice.

■ Time Out

What leadership skills and strengths did Jess portray? What type of leader do you think she is? What do you observe to be the main characteristics of the reverse mentoring relationship?

Jess demonstrated authenticity—she was her true self and this attracted the attention of the chief nurse. Jess shows signs of being a transformational leader, going beyond her original goal and galvanising others to amplify the student voice.

Reverse mentoring offers a two-way exchange of skills. Each partner explains what they can give and get from the arrangement and make an agreement about how it will work. It helps boost the confidence of each party and brings fresh eyes and skills to problems. The student partner can act as a change agent, giving honest feedback. The leader can help the student partner to broaden their network.

Reverse mentoring offers leaders the opportunity to return to the shop floor and 'walk the talk'. It can also challenge established hierarchies and inequalities such as those faced by Black and minority ethnic communities. It can build genuine awareness of the barriers faced by such communities.

One criticism of the language of reverse mentoring is that it suggests hierarchy when actually it is about sharing our different experiences.

Finding a Mentor

'There will always be that one mentor, that leader, that shines for you. Remember that moment, how they made you feel, because that will change how you are as a nurse. Remember the bad moments too because that will make you not want to be that person.'

NAOMI BERRY, NEWLY REGISTERED GENERAL PRACTICE NURSE

Let's imagine that either on placement, at university or at a networking event, you become interested in someone who might be a good mentor, but you do not know how to approach them.

What you might do is to start to follow their activities and get to know them at a distance first. Maybe you go to an event specifically because you want to meet them, but you do not have the courage to engage them. One way to tackle this is to ask somebody, maybe a tutor at your university who knows this person, to introduce you. An introduction, especially with a thoughtful comment from your tutor such as 'Can I introduce Jane? She's been studying your work on teams and has a question,' is worth rubies. Of course, you can approach them directly, but do so with a purpose, such as picking up on something that really inspired you, to ask for their help or advice or offer your observations. Do not underestimate that, as a student nurse, you offer a unique insight that may be valuable to that person (Tips Box 5.2).

Shadowing

Another approach is to ask if you might shadow that person for a day so you can get to know them and the way they work more closely. There are other reasons to shadow somebody, for example, you want to raise your profile in an organisation, you want to extend your network or you are thinking of taking a job in a particular discipline.

Before you start, check

- What you both want to get out of it
- What to wear (if you normally wear a uniform)
- Where and what time to turn up and who to report to
- How long you will shadow them for
- If you need anyone's permission, especially if you are working in sensitive work areas

---

TIPS BOX 5.2

Working With a Mentor

- Like with coaching, chemistry is important—if it does not feel right walk away.
- If your mentor offers you advice, show that you value it:
  - Write it down
  - Act on it
- Reflect on your session with your mentor rather than follow what they say by rote—think about how you felt about the guidance given and feed that back to your mentor, even if you found that it did not help you.
- Ask your mentor to help you widen your networks by, for example, introducing you to an editorial board or committee, or help you get an opportunity to speak at an event to help build your experience, influence and credibility.
- This will enable the mentor to vouch for you and write letters of recommendation or references.
- Being a mentor is also good for that person's CV—showing that the mentee has progressed well reflects on the mentor.
- Recognise publicly the help that a mentor has given, at suitable opportunities.
- Be generous and give back by mentoring someone else. Find a co-mentor to develop your skills as a mentor. Helping others will help you to feel good.

Based on Goldmann (2015), Chief Medical and Scientific Officer, Institute for Healthcare Improvement.

Mentor Support and Encouragement

Many students interviewed for this book were encouraged by their tutors to apply for leadership programmes or were put forward for other opportunities. Many of them had not yet recognised their own potential and did not really understand why they had been put forward but went with the flow anyway. The message here is to understand that more senior people may identify your talent before you do, but self-belief may hold you back. Students like Sarah have this advice:

> 'People want to support and help me for a reason—I appreciate that so much. No one can do these things on their own. It always comes off the back of having support, having the platform, having the opportunity. And then it's up to you to say yes really.'
>
> SARAH BRADDER, NEWLY REGISTERED THERAPEUTIC RADIOGRAPHER AND
> STUDENT RADIOGRAPHER OF THE YEAR (2019)

Clinical Supervision

You will recall in the chapter on managing yourself that we looked at how we manage adversity by challenging our beliefs, which can impact our consequential feelings (the ABC model). A linked idea is to practise self-compassion by using clinical supervision to positively reframe how we feel. Here is a case study of how Jo Odell drew on the assistance of peers to reframe how she was feeling:

POSITIVE REFRAMING USING RESILIENCE-BASED CLINICAL SUPERVISION

CASE STUDY 5.2	Jo Odell, Foundation of Nursing Studies Practice Development Facilitator and Inspire Improvement Fellowship Lead

This week my family and I have decided to spend the Christmas period apart. This is for many different reasons, but mainly because we want to keep everyone safe from COVID-19.

Despite making this decision—it will be the first time we have been apart since the start of our family—I was left feeling very bereft. When I shared this with a colleague, she helped me to think differently about how the Christmas holiday period could be. She helped me positively reframe how I was thinking and this helped me feel so much better about the whole situation.

'Positive reframing' is an important element of the Resilience Based Clinical Supervision (RBCS) model along with challenging the 'inner critic' or any negative thinking that we may find ourselves doing. RBCS is a unique model of clinical supervision that is based on a compassionate focused therapy approach and is about being compassionate to ourselves and others. It combines elements of mindfulness with helping people to understand and recognise their emotions, and how strongly our thoughts are connected to our feelings. Positive thoughts give rise to happy, connected emotions whereas negative thoughts result in sad and depressive emotions. Basically, the quality of our thinking affects the emotions we experience and consequently our physical health.

We discovered a website, which has some exercises to download that can help you to practise reframing situations either on your own or with the help of another person.

This exercise talks about taking a four-step approach to reframing:

1. Accept the uncontrollable
2. Focus on the controllable
3. Acknowledge and apply your strengths
4. Find/use positives

Another gives examples of how to positively reframe such as:

'There is too much to do and not enough time'

Reframe: 'If I take a deep breath and write a list and tackle one thing at a time'

This is how my colleague helped me reframe the Christmas situation:

My thoughts: 'I can't see my family'

Reframing: 'Let's think about it as some time off work, to take some walks in the countryside and by the sea'

This reframing also takes me through the four-step approach:

- I can't control the COVID pandemic
- I can control my behaviour to keep people safe
- I live in a beautiful part of the UK
- Some time out and spending time in nature is an opportunity

■ **Time Out**

Jo is referring to The Children's Hospital Philadelphia's –'four steps to reframing':
1. **Accept the uncontrollable.**
   – What parts of the problem are not in your control?
   – What are you willing to give up?
2. **Focus on the controllable.**
   – Even though you may not be able control the problem, what can you control?
   – Which of your thoughts, feelings and behaviours can you control?
3. **Acknowledge and apply your strengths.**
   – What personal strengths can you bring to the situation?
   – What are you good at?
4. **Find/use the positives.**
   – Using your strengths, how can you make the situation better in the short term?
   – Are there any other positives you can find?
   Think about a problem that is bothering you. You may welcome having a partner to help you think through each step.
   Reflect on what you have learnt—have you managed to find any positives in your situation?

The Foundation of Nursing Studies has now incorporated positive reframing into a wider RBCS model (see resources).

Peer-Assisted Learning

'We encourage them to be leaders of their learning. Our experience, to them, is a bit more comforting because we are students, so we are relatable and we know the ups and downs.'
REBECCA HOLLOBONE, STUDENT CHILDREN'S NURSE AND SENIOR PAL
LEADER, UNIVERSITY OF PLYMOUTH

Peer-assisted learning, or PAL, has been a feature at several universities and is an opportunity for students further on with their training to share self-help tips to support more inexperienced students. This is a support method, rather than formal teaching, with the topics identified by students themselves.

The University of Plymouth has not only introduced but researched the benefits of PAL (Carey et al. 2018). Students in their second and third years apply for a paid role to become a PAL leader. Although the payment recognises their efforts, for the student leaders it is much more about giving back knowledge and supporting colleagues.

The students then undertake 2 days of training and are paired across fields, for example an adult nursing student may work alongside a student mental health nurse.

The PAL leaders support a group of about 20 first-year students across the fields of adult, child and mental health nursing. PAL leaders meet with groups of students in mutually convenient ways and offer generic academic support and placement support, focusing on subjects such as drug calculations, essay structure, revision techniques and referencing.

When students first meet with PAL leaders they spend some time getting to know each other. Activities focus on active rather than passive learning and often test the ingenuity of the leaders. One leader, for example, invented an icebreaker game—bouncing table tennis balls into cups that have questions in them. This is just one of many other creative examples used by PAL leaders. These are discussed further in the chapter on creativity.

Leaders such as Rebecca Hollobone show their emotional intelligence and expose their vulnerabilities and failures, and in this way they become more relatable. They can empathise with more inexperienced students, and this helps them to relax.

PAL leaders usually meet their groups at a frequency convenient to them such as fortnightly. In between they communicate using a variety of ways. The leaders meet as a group with their academic PAL co-coordinators to debrief and discuss what went well and not so well, and they also learn from each other.

BENEFITS OF PEER-ASSISTED LEARNING TO STUDENT LEADERS' DEVELOPMENT

These include:

- Improving confidence
- Practising ways of making themselves more approachable
- Developing their listening skills
- Developing their flexibility and responsiveness to peer's needs
- Improving self-awareness (e.g., if they are having a bad day, knowing how their mood affects their tone of voice)
- Being able to read the room—things such as identifying who is quiet, noticing body language and testing ways to involve them: 'If we give up, they give up'
- Feeling that they are making a difference and giving them sense of achievement
- Helping develop their creativity, for example, the PAL leaders arrive in uniform—one correct and one incorrect—and students try to spot the mistakes
- Gaining opportunities for revision and to learn from those around them, including the first years
- Practising enabling and empowering students so they lead themselves

Based on conversations with PAL leaders.

'We're leading them into believing in themselves. One of the biggest pieces of advice that I would give is that this is your journey, this is your degree. Don't ever compare yourself to others.'
ELLIE LOOKER, STUDENT CHILDREN'S NURSE AND SENIOR PAL LEADER,
UNIVERSITY OF PLYMOUTH

Networking

Having looked at coaching, mentoring, supervision and peer-assisted learning, we now turn to networking. It can be hard for student nurses to have the confidence to network and to approach people with a view to widening their network and finding a mentor, so this chapter offers some practical tips (Tips Box 5.3).

TIPS BOX 5.3

Networking Face to Face

One nonthreatening way to start is by networking with fellow students—to approach people who you do not know very well and start a conversation, maybe about what you have just heard or with a question that you have been pondering.

The next step is to ask to go to events that offer wider opportunities to network and to continue to practise introducing yourself to people who you do not know and talking to them. Some may fear that they do not know enough to engage other people, but the way to combat this is to first of all smile and greet them warmly, and then to remember their name and use it while speaking to them. A useful tip to help you to remember names is to either connect their name to some memorable feature (e.g., my name is Heather and the flower heather is purple/pink and at the moment so is my hair!). Another way is to use alliteration—like 'happy Heather'—or rhyme—'Heather in leather'.

Make a good impression on everyone that you meet. Say hello and thank you to everybody, including any waiting staff, cleaners, technical staff etc. If you can help someone by taking their coat while they juggle bags for example, that will be noticed.

Even starting a conversation with a stranger when you are a novice networker can be a trial. Good places are in queues, in event rooms and at shared tables at lunch. Encourage people to talk about themselves and their interests, and genuinely listen to what the other person has to say rather than focus on what you think or know.

What you do not want to do is stick like glue to your friend—you can always arrange to meet them for a debrief at an opportune time. Of course, be explicit about your plans or you may upset them!

One useful way to engage others and hear what they think is to practise reflection at the same time:

- This is what I heard.
- This is what I liked.
- This is what it means to me.
- What did you think?

You also want to practise speaking up. When the chair or facilitator says 'does anyone have any questions?' this is the moment to screw up all your courage and ask the best question that you can (and maybe even a powerful one). Make the question short and do not use the opportunity to make speeches, as this can be irritating.

NETWORKING BRINGS OPPORTUNITIES

CASE STUDY 5.3	Naomi Berry

Naomi, a newly registered general practice nurse (GPN) who spent 12 years as a health care assistant in general practice before qualifying, is passionate about encouraging students to work in primary care.

When attending a GPN conference she was approached to become part of a GPN student nurse network whose purpose is to support student placements in primary care. She was offered training by her local Primary Care Training Hub to help her to do this and now has a notional budget of £5,000 to commission GPN training in her area. Before the COVID-19 pandemic she went into universities and spoke to students about general practice. Naomi is also part of the Twitter team @GPNSNN (student nurse network), encouraging and supporting newly registered nurses to work in general practices.

Her advice is 'If an opportunity knocks at your door, you give it a go'. The exposure that she had at a networking event led to a major opportunity to follow her passion.

WIDENING YOUR NETWORK USING TWITTER

One of the most frequently mentioned ways of developing your network mentioned by nursing students is via social media, particularly Twitter. Over the last few years more and more student nurses have embraced Twitter, with some universities having dedicated programmes to support students to view Twitter as a way to enhance their learning. Other universities have focused on advising students about the NMC guidance on the appropriate use of Twitter, including some of the dangers, and this has had the effect of putting some students off. However, as well as being an opportunity to engage in tweet chats, Twitter is a way to broaden your networks by being able to engage with those involved in health and care worldwide.

A specific way that some students have widened their networks and developed their leadership capabilities is by taking up internship opportunities with more experienced students or registered nurses and helping to curate and develop Twitter accounts. Examples include @WeLDNurses, @WeStudentNurses, @RCNStudents, @UNISONStudentNN, @GPNSNN and @RCNNQN. The role often involves being part of a team, managing the account on a rota and researching, developing and running tweet chats. Sometimes teams produce podcasts to cover particular topics or explain more about their field of nursing.

Many development opportunities are also advertised on Twitter, such as the opportunity to write blogs for nursing journals' student nurse sections. Roles often last for a year and then a handover is arranged to pass on skills and support new interns.

'I've got such a massive circle of contacts. There's always someone I can go to and ask I'm thinking about doing this, what do you think?'

IAN UNITT, NEWLY REGISTERED LEARNING DISABILITY NURSE, TALKING ABOUT HIS INTERNSHIP WITH @WeLDN (LEARNING DISABILITY NURSE NETWORK ON TWITTER)

Reflecting on Your Leadership Journey

There are various ways to reflect on what you have learnt about yourself and how you are developing as a leader. Here, one student leader reflects on a trip to London:

CASE STUDY 5.4   **Nathan Harrison**

Nathan Harrison, an adult student nurse at the University of Salford, had already done some work though his university's nursing society around improving the student experience. He then got the opportunity to speak to a national NHS body that was looking for advice on further developing a tool to survey students about their experiences and also to encourage a better response to the survey.

He recalls arriving outside the building 'proper job interview nervous'. He reflected on what his nerves were all about: his feeling of being very 'other' because the group had already formed and done some work and he was worried about whether he would be able to break into the discussion.

The group knew each other and seemed to him to consist of 'people in uniforms indicating that they were more senior than me'. He thought some of the materials presented at the meeting were poor and he was worried about how his feedback might be taken.

He reflected afterwards on how well he had managed to communicate his ideas and contribute to the discussions and that his contributions had been well accepted. He felt much more confident having been pushed so far out of his comfort zone.

Writing is great way to slow down your thinking and allow for the processing of what has happened. Here is one example:

'I'd take the night bus home and write anonymously in my little diary. Thinking about what upset me from the day and what felt good from the day and why it felt that way.'

AALIJAH BUTTIMER, ADULT STUDENT NURSE

Unlike just thinking about things, which may be random, writing allows you to process and consciously examine a train of thought. It may help you to weigh up and carefully select what you say. Writing lets you take a bird's eye view of the situation and reflect on what you have written.

REFLECTION USING BLOGS

'A friend once challenged me when I asserted that we learn through experience. No, he said, we learn through reflection on experience.'

KATHRYN PERRERA, DIRECTOR AT NHS HORIZONS

Many student nurses take to blogging to share their reflections. The Student Empowerment Group at the University of Chester has set up a series of blogs called 'My First of Everything', where students blog about the first time they have experienced something, such as experiencing a patient's death.

But as well as helping students process their thinking, blogging is an opportunity to share your knowledge with perhaps less experienced students. This in itself is a leadership activity.

Your Reflections So Far

You have now had the opportunity to undertake a range of exercises and use a range of assessment tools (see Chapter 3) to gain a better understanding of yourself:

- Healthcare leadership model self-assessment tool,
- Big Five dimensions of personality: OCEAN,
- Myers Briggs assessment, and
- Time out reflections on emotional intelligence.

You may also have studied a range of models for reflection, such as Gibbs (1988), Kolb (1984) and Johns (1993), that can be used to reflect on your clinical practice. This is now your opportunity to reflect on what you have learnt about yourself, not in terms of clinical practice but rather your leadership strengths, skills and preferences.

■ Time Out

Crafting Your Leadership Story and Narrative

Look back now at your reflective diary and revisit your notes and the feedback that you have received from the assessment tools that you completed. This is your opportunity to draw together a summary of who you are and what you value.

Swansea Leadership Academy has developed a workbook to help you to do this using the mnemonic HEARTS: honesty, emotional intelligence, authenticity, resilience, true connections, self-awareness. It is reproduced here, with the permission of the authors Beryl Mansel, Samuel Richards, Angharad Colinese and the Swansea Leadership Academy advisory panel.

The reflection tool used is the 'What? So what? Now what?' reflective model developed by Rolfe and colleagues in 2001.

The exercise works on three phases:

- Understanding the event (**What?**)
- Making sense of the facts and implications (**So, What?**)
- Identifying the course of action or new solutions (**Now What?**)

Complete the tool now and summarise your leadership goals and actions.

H Honesty: Being honest

- What are my personal values and what really matters to me?
- So what am I learning about myself?
- Now what will I do with this information?

_____

_____

_____

_____

_____

E Emotional Intelligence: The role of self-confidence in emotional intelligence

- What barriers have I overcome to improve my self-confidence?
- So what positive attitudes have I used to overcome these barriers?

Continued

- Now what have I achieved?

_____
_____
_____
_____
_____

A Authenticity: Being genuine
- What would those who know me best tell me about myself if I invited them to really say what it is they see?
- So what am I learning about myself?
- Now what will I do with this information?

_____
_____
_____
_____
_____

R Resilience: Ability to bounce back
- What mental, physical, spiritual and emotional activities/skills have I used to recover quickly from difficult conditions?
- So what have I learnt from challenges and mistakes?
- Now what can I do to develop my resilience further?

_____
_____
_____
_____
_____

T True connections: Make the effort to connect with the right people
- What connections have supported my leadership journey?
- So what are the ways these have helped me?
- Now what will I do to build upon these connections?
- What is my networking goal?
- So what will I do to achieve this goal?
- Now what were the benefits of this connection?

_____
_____
_____
_____
_____

S Self-awareness: Ability to monitor our inner thoughts and emotions
- What are my strengths and what do I like doing?
- So what does that tell me about myself?
- Now what will I do to build on my strengths?
- What would I like to improve about myself?
- So what will I change?
- Now what positive changes have I made?

_____
_____

HEARTS	MY GOALS	ACTIONS
Honesty		
Emotional Intelligence-Self-confidence		
Authenticity		
Resilience		
True Connections		
Self-awareness		

Source: Reproduced with permission from Mansel, B., Richards, S., Colinese, A., and the Swansea Leadership Academy advisory panel. HEART workbook (online). Swansea Leadership Academy.

At this point, you may also want to check out the requirements that the NMC sets out, which include five written reflections on your continuing professional development, plus a reflective discussion with another registrant. This will help you to understand the process that you will go through every 3 years, once you register, to maintain your clinical practice. To do this, visit the NMC website, which is currently accessible at http://revalidation.nmc.org.uk/.

Summary

You are in charge of your own leadership journey. Coaches, mentors, supervisors and peers are there to help you along the way. Networking is a way to meet and get to know a wide range of such people. This can be done face to face and virtually. Sometimes it is helpful to engage in coaching, mentorship and supervision with fellow nurses, and sometimes you can reach out to other disciplines and other sectors to broaden your knowledge and experience.

There are a wide range of coaching, mentoring and supervisory techniques, a few of which are described here. It is important that you reflect on what you learn when working with others. Thinking time is important, as is having someone to be present and 'listen to you with fascination'. Writing your thoughts down can help you to assimilate your learning and plan where you want to go next.

Resources

Foundation of Nursing Studies, Clinical supervision resources. <https://www.fons.org/learning-zone/clinical-supervision-resources/clinical-supervision>.

Hirdle, J., Humphries, B., 2020. Training in coaching to help qualified staff support student nurses. Nursing Times 116 (11), 37–39.

Nancy Kline's Ten components of the thinking environment. <https://www.timetothink.com/thinking-environment/the-ten-components/>.

The GROW Model Guide, Performance consults. <https://www.performanceconsultants.com/document/GROW-Model-Guide.pdf>.

The University of Edinburgh Reflection Toolkit. <https://www.ed.ac.uk/reflection/reflectors-toolkit/producing-reflections/ways-reflecting>.

References

Benner, P., 1984. From Novice to Expert. Addison-Wesley, California.

Carey, M.C., Kent, B., Latour, J.M., 2018. Experiences of undergraduate nursing students in peer assisted learning in clinical practice: a qualitative systematic review. JBI Database of Systematic Reviews and Implementation Reports 16 (5), 1190–1219.

Gibbs, G., 1988. Learning by Doing: A Guide to Teaching and Learning Methods. Further Education Unit. Oxford Polytechnic, Oxford.

Goldmann, D., 2015. Don Goldmann on mentoring. YouTube. <https://youtu.be/T12wrbtPN0k>.

Gurvis, J., McCauley, C., Swofford, M., 2016. Putting experience at the center of talent management. Center for Creative Leadership. <https://cclinnovation.org/wp-content/uploads/2020/03/talentmanagement.e-1.pdf>.

Johns, C., 1993. Achieving effective work as a professional activity. In: Schober, J.E., Hinchliff, S.M. (Eds.), Towards Advanced Nursing Practice (1995). Edward Arnold, London (Chapter 11).

Kline, N., 1999. Time to Think: Listening to Ignite the Human Mind. Ward Lock, London.

Kolb, D.A., 1984. Experiential Learning: Experience as the Source of Learning and Development. Prentice-Hall, Englewood Cliffs.

Rolfe, G., Freshwater, D., Jasper, M., 2001. Critical Reflection in Nursing and the Helping Professions: A User's Guide. Palgrave Macmillan, Basingstoke.

The Children's Hospital Philadelphia. Four steps to reframing worksheet (Adapted from Surviving Cancer Competently Intervention Program (SCCIP-ND) manual). Division of Oncology. Contact cpts@chop.edu for more information.

Whitmore, J., 2002. Coaching for Performance. Nicholas Brealey Publishing, London.

Working With Others

Working in Teams

OBJECTIVES

After reading this chapter and completing the activities, you should be able to:
- Explain the essential characteristics of teams and pseudo teams
- Describe the importance of diversity in teams
- Describe the basic conditions for effective teamwork
- Identify the ABC of wellbeing and motivation in nursing and midwifery teams
- Describe the life cycles of teams
- List the trends in future team development.

Relevance to the Nursing and Midwifery Council (NMC) Code

Prioritise People
Paragraph 1:
Treat people as individuals and uphold their dignity
   1.1 treat people with kindness, respect and compassion
Paragraph 2:
Listen to people and respond to their preferences and concerns
   2.1 work in partnership with people to make sure you deliver care effectively
   2.2 recognise and respect the contribution that people can make to their own health and wellbeing

Practise Effectively
Paragraph 8:
Work cooperatively
   8.1 respect the skills, expertise and contributions of your colleagues, referring matters to them when appropriate
   8.2 maintain effective communication with colleagues
   8.3 keep colleagues informed when you are sharing the care of individuals with other health and care professionals and staff
   8.4 work with colleagues to evaluate the quality of your work and that of the team
   8.5 work with colleagues to preserve the safety of those receiving care
   8.6 share information to identify and reduce risk

Continued

Relevance to the Nursing and Midwifery Council (NMC) Code—cont'd

---

8.7 be supportive of colleagues who are encountering health or performance problems. However, this
   support must never compromise or be at the expense of patient or public safety

Paragraph 9:

Share your skills, knowledge and experience for the benefit of people receiving care and your colleagues

9.1 provide honest, accurate and constructive feedback to colleagues

9.2 gather and reflect on feedback from a variety of sources, using it to improve your practice and
   performance

9.3 deal with differences of professional opinion with colleagues by discussion and informed debate,
   respecting their views and opinions and behaving in a professional way at all times

Paragraph 11:

Be accountable for your decisions to delegate tasks and duties to other people

11.1 only delegate tasks and duties that are within the other person's scope of competence, making
   sure that they fully understand your instructions

11.2 make sure that everyone you delegate tasks to is adequately supervised and supported so they
   can provide safe and compassionate care

11.3 confirm that the outcome of any task you have delegated to someone else meets the required standard

Promote Professionalism and Trust

Paragraph 20:

Uphold the reputation of your profession at all times

20.2 act with honesty and integrity at all times, treating people fairly and without discrimination, bullying
   or harassment

20.8 act as a role model of professional behaviour for students and newly qualified nurses, midwives
   and nursing associates to aspire to

Section 1 of this book has been about knowing yourself as a leader. We now turn to examine how leaders work with others in teams.

As a student nurse, you may already be involved in teamwork or may be leading teams in situations such as:

- practising management skills in clinical allocations,
- organising study groups,
- leading small university projects,
- coordinating nursing societies,
- coordinating peer-support Twitter accounts, and
- being part of a student representative body within your university or trade union.

Once registered, you will similarly be involved in:

- teams of peers, such as district nursing;
- multidisciplinary and multiagency teams, such as discharge planning;
- specialities, such as infection control teams; and
- improvement teams, such as finding ways to accelerate wound-healing rates.

Healthy teams have been shown to lead to better outcomes for patients, families and communities, as well as our organisations (Borrill et al, 2000). There are effective ways to support teamwork, with national policies and strategies across the United Kingdom to help improve teamworking and improve the welfare of team members.

What Is a Team?

A team is any group of people organised to work together, both interdependently and cooperatively, to accomplish a purpose or a goal.

Essentially there are three basic dimensions of teamworking:

1. shared objectives,
2. interdependence, and
3. holding meetings to review progress.

This definition helps us to work out whether a group of people is really working as a team or if, in fact, they are acting as a 'pseudo team'.

The Effectiveness of Real Teams and Pseudo Teams

Even from the days when humans worked cooperatively towards the common goal of hunting for antelope, teamwork has been important. They still reviewed what went right or wrong with the hunt and discussed whether the objectives (sustaining members) were being achieved.

Every year an NHS staff survey is carried out that includes the question 'Do you work in a team?' and about 90% of staff say yes, which seems encouraging. Three follow-up questions are asked:

- Does your team have clear objectives?
- Do you work closely together to achieve these objectives?
- Do you meet regularly to review your performance and how it can be improved?

About 50% of NHS staff reply 'no' to these questions and are described as working in 'pseudo teams'. They are important because the more pseudo teams that there are in an organisation, the higher the levels of staff absenteeism, staff injuries, errors, violent assaults, bullying, harassment and abuse (West and Lyubovnikova 2013).

Having more 'real' teams is associated with lower patient mortality. If the number of real teams rises by just 5% in a hospital, that would decrease deaths by 3.3%, or 40 deaths on average, a year (West 2012).

Multidisciplinary and interdisciplinary teamwork is related to improved patient safety, higher quality care and more innovation (World Health Organisation 2009; Borril et al. 2000)

The reasons why teamwork is linked to positive outcomes is because cooperating and sharing skills and knowledge to achieve valued outcomes are needed to manage the complexity of health care.

Multidisciplinary Working

'A basic knowledge of what we all do in our different fields is hugely important and could help us to break down barriers, reduce health inequalities and, ultimately, improve the quality of care we provide.'

IAN UNITT, NEWLY REGISTERED LEARNING DISABILITY NURSE

Multidisciplinary and interdisciplinary teamwork is related to improved patient safety, higher quality care and more innovation (World Health Organisation 2009; Borril et al. 2000).

Senior lecturer Anne Marie Dodson describes a manager she knew and how she went about appointing staff. For this manager, who was aware that sometimes leaders may feel threatened by team members who may be more knowledgeable or skilled in certain areas, it was all about diversity. She uses the metaphor of gathering all the ingredients together to bake a cake, choosing people with different and complementary skills.

■ Time Out

Identify a member of the team on your current or next placement whose role is not fully clear to you, such as a speech and language therapist or a community mental health nurse. Invite them for coffee and find out more about what they do.

Reflect on what you learnt and how that additional knowledge may improve your effectiveness within the team. For example, you may discover that speech and language therapists undertake swallowing assessments and can help you to identify signs that such an assessment is needed.

Diversity in Teams

'Just because someone is different why do we automatically stay away from them? That shouldn't be the case. We should be cherishing; we should be embracing differences because that's what makes a really great society.'

NATALIE ELLIOTT, STUDENT NURSE, TALKING ABOUT BLACK LIVES MATTER

It is against the law to discriminate against someone because of their age, disability, gender reassignment, marriage and civil partnership status, pregnancy and maternity, race, religion or belief, or sex. These are the 'protected characteristics' enshrined in the Equality Act 2010 that protect individuals from discrimination.

Just as you need different disciplines in your team, you also need diversity of experience, of culture and of thought. However, the NHS sometimes struggles to achieve this diversity. Well-known examples of this include a lack of Black and minority ethnic nurses in senior nursing positions and the discrimination, bullying and harassment they face. Various views exist about how men in nursing are perceived and how we might encourage men to join the profession.

Sexuality is also a pressure point; with one student interviewed for this book—who identifies as nonbinary—reporting the stress of being expected to use a shared changing room whilst being fitted for their very first uniform.

'Don't treat us as different, stop labelling us. We all want the same things.'

RUTH OSHIKANLU, INDEPENDENT NURSE ENTREPRENEUR

Nurses like Ruth are keen to point out that Black and Brown nurses say that they are not one group—they are many cultures, each to be individually appreciated.

This is reflected similarly by Mark Radford, chief nurse at Health Education England, in relation to the role of men in nursing. Men are already disproportionately represented in leadership positions but not in overall numbers. He wants the debate to be about lifting up the entire nursing profession without disproportionately focusing on men. He describes the widespread societal debate in Israel about gender issues in the military as well as in nursing: Israel developed nursing into a graduate profession, and now 25% of nurses are male. It did not do that by targeting men to join the profession but achieved it by raising the profile of the entire profession. Without having nursing as a graduate profession, Mark believes that it will be seen as less worthy and less technical than other health and care professions.

Basic Conditions for Effective Teamwork

■ **Time Out**

Think of a team that you are part of now—at work or at home—that works well. Why does it work? Conversely, think of a dysfunctional team that you belong to. What stops it from being effective?

Fig. 6.1 summarises the evidence for what makes a team effective. Too big a team and it becomes a 'group' and the connections between members weakens. Too small and you may not have the right capacity and skills. The ideal size of a team is about six to eight people and no more than 15. Membership is stable and there needs to be a task that binds the team together. The purpose is clear to members and they set out achievable objectives. The team includes the right skills and the right roles for the task.

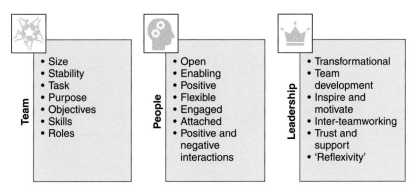

Fig. 6.1 Basic conditions for effective teamwork. (Adapted from West, M.A., 2012. Effective Teamwork: Practical Lessons from Organisational Research, third ed. BPS Blackwell-Wiley, Chichester.)

Effective team members enable work to happen rather than derailing or undermining it. They are attached and engaged in what the team is doing and are flexible about how it is done. There are both positive and negative interactions so that members can challenge each other constructively. And they are open and appreciative of each other and back each other up when times are tough.

Effective teams are led by transformational leaders who can inspire and motivate others. They are interested in the team's development and can enable trusting, supportive relationships, not just within the team but between teams, so that members feel connected and involved in what the wider organisation is doing.

Reflexive Teams

Successful teams are 'reflexive'. This means that they:
- reflect and adapt to change,
- review their objectives in the light of changing circumstances,
- consider how well the team is functioning and can be creative and adaptable,
- have high tolerance to uncertainty, and
- value difference.

Teams function well when both the task and the members are respected. Feeling valued and supported is just as important as getting the job done. Positive emotions are related to team flexibility and openness. They see challenges as opportunities, can control their behaviours better, and are more helpful and generous (Frederickson 2009).

■ Time Out

Having read what helps makes teams effective, reflect on what you may have learnt and how you may be able to implement changes in a team you are in. For example, you may want to have a 10-minute time out after your next meeting to reflect on how the team is working or whether your objectives are clear or still relevant.

Team Creativity

Teams who take time out to be reflexive and think about what they are trying to achieve are more innovative than teams that do not, and their organisation's mortality rates are lower (West et al. 2017).

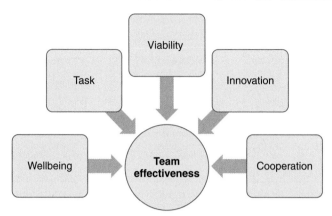

Fig. 6.2   The five main components of team effectiveness. (Adapted from West, M.A., 2012. Effective Teamwork: Practical Lessons from Organisational Research, third ed. BPS Blackwell-Wiley, Chichester.)

Team Effectiveness

There are five main components of team effectiveness (Fig. 6.2). Teams need to be able to achieve their task. Their wellbeing is considered, including their emotional wellbeing and their opportunities for growth and development. They are viable and able to carry on working. They develop in innovative ways, and they are able to cooperate with other teams.

■ Time Out

Consider your current or last placement. Using the five components of team effectiveness, how well do you consider that the team is able to be effective? What is helping or hindering them?

One of the most common issues that you may have written down that currently negatively affects the wellbeing of the team are staff shortages. However, you may also see attitudes such as 'we've always done it this way' and you may see that the team is short on equipment or has had little opportunity for personal development. Maybe you consider that there is a poor working relationship with another department, perhaps because they do not communicate with each other well.

Maybe you see a thriving team, where they take time out to check how they are all doing and share new ideas.

The Patient's Role in Teamwork

If a team is defined as a group of people working towards a common purpose, then it is important to consider when and where patients become part of the team. The NMC Code (2018) states that nurses must:

- work in partnership with people to make sure they deliver care effectively,
- recognise and respect the contribution that people can make to their own health and wellbeing,
- encourage and empower people to share decisions about their treatment and care, and
- respect the level at which people receiving care want to be involved in decisions about their own health, wellbeing and care.

Patients and their carers can be involved at several levels:
- In their own care
- In the development of services—see the next chapter on codesign
- In the development of policy and strategy at local and national levels

Maintaining and Improving the Wellbeing and Motivation of Teams Under Stress

During the COVID-19 pandemic the NHS was under unprecedented pressure, leaving many nurses broken and exhausted. The King's Fund was commissioned by the RCN Foundation to review the causes and consequences of poor mental health and wellbeing among nurses and midwives. It sought to identify solutions to these issues and examples of good practice (West et al. 2020). Here, the focus was on addressing the causes rather than dealing with the consequences.

The King's Fund identified what it called the ABC of the core needs of nurses and midwives:
- Autonomy—the need to have control over their work lives, and to be able to act consistently with their values
- Belonging—the need to be connected to, cared for by, and caring of colleagues, and to feel valued, respected and supported
- Contribution—the need to experience effectiveness in what they do and deliver valued outcomes

West and colleagues (2020) made eight recommendations to NHS leaders to support compassionate leadership (Fig. 6.3).

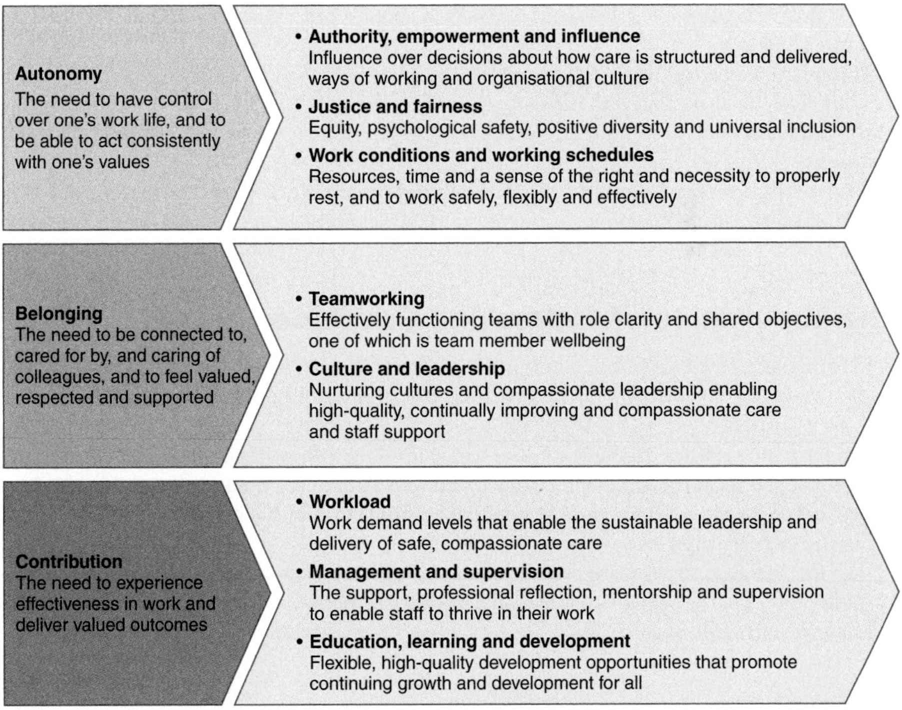

Autonomy
The need to have control over one's work life, and to be able to act consistently with one's values

- **Authority, empowerment and influence**
  Influence over decisions about how care is structured and delivered, ways of working and organisational culture
- **Justice and fairness**
  Equity, psychological safety, positive diversity and universal inclusion
- **Work conditions and working schedules**
  Resources, time and a sense of the right and necessity to properly rest, and to work safely, flexibly and effectively

Belonging
The need to be connected to, cared for by, and caring of colleagues, and to feel valued, respected and supported

- **Teamworking**
  Effectively functioning teams with role clarity and shared objectives, one of which is team member wellbeing
- **Culture and leadership**
  Nurturing cultures and compassionate leadership enabling high-quality, continually improving and compassionate care and staff support

Contribution
The need to experience effectiveness in work and deliver valued outcomes

- **Workload**
  Work demand levels that enable the sustainable leadership and delivery of safe, compassionate care
- **Management and supervision**
  The support, professional reflection, mentorship and supervision to enable staff to thrive in their work
- **Education, learning and development**
  Flexible, high-quality development opportunities that promote continuing growth and development for all

Fig. 6.3 The ABC framework of nurses' and midwives' core work needs. (West, M.A., Bailey, S., Williams, E., 2020. The Courage of Compassion. King's Fund. <https://www.kingsfund.org.uk/publications/courage-compassion-supporting-nurses-midwives>.

■ **Time Out**

Read the report 'The Courage of Compassion' (2020) on the King's Fund website (full reference at the end of this chapter).
Reflect and make notes on how far the student teams that you are part of feel that they can:
- exert autonomy,
- feel valued respected and supported, and
- experience conditions that enable them to feel effective.

What would help?

Your Team's Reputation

'It takes 20 years to build a reputation and 5 minutes to ruin it. If you think about that, you'll do things differently.'

WARREN BUFFETT, BUSINESS TYCOON

■ **Time Out**

Think about how you find out what to expect from your next placement: do you ask your peers what to expect before you go? What do you and they focus on?

Your peers will probably start by telling you about the people and the culture. The evidence from a report by Dimensional Research (2013) on the customer satisfaction of 1046 people showed that 95% of people tell at least one person about a bad experience, and 54% will tell at least five people.

If you have had a bad day with your placement supervisor or senior staff nurse, you might be far more likely to share this with others compared to if it was a good day. And social networks used by students such as WhatsApp make it easy to share how you feel about leadership in a placement.

Worse still, a report from the pollsters Gallup showed that disengaged workers had 37% higher absenteeism, 49% more accidents and 60% more errors and defects (Sorenson 2013).

The Importance of Expressing Gratitude

'The deepest principle in human nature is the craving to be appreciated.'
WILLIAM JAMES, AMERICAN PHILOSOPHER AND PSYCHOLOGIST

When a patient expresses gratitude for your care, how does this make you feel? The chances are, you feel like the work you are doing is valued and worthwhile. We need to extend this idea into our leadership practices. Gratitude is an important attitude to cultivate in both yourself as a leader and in the team that you lead.

The first action is to practise gratitude in our daily lives. By focusing on what we are grateful for, rather than what is wrong in our lives, the evidence is that we will feel more positive and this will improve our wellbeing.

■ **Time Out**

Write a list of the things you are grateful for. Put it on the bathroom mirror to remind yourself.

In the light of this, what does good leadership look like? Good leaders take actions to engender the gratitude of their employees. A landmark academic study by Fehr and colleagues (2017) called *The Grateful Workplace* identified the following as important:

- giving people feedback on how they are doing;
- offering opportunities for staff to meet the beneficiaries of their work, so they feel a sense of pride; and
- establishing employee appreciation programmes such as employee-of-the-month schemes.

In 2014, a US organisation that provides employee surveys called TINYpulse (www.tinypulse. com) produced a report on key trends impacting the workplace. The results of a survey on 30,000 employees indicated that barely a fifth of employees feel strongly valued at work.

The TINYpulse survey also stressed the importance of developing camaraderie at work and the importance of having a friend in the workplace. Methods to encourage socialisation in teams, such as eating together, are also important.

Saying 'thank you' and 'well done' is a strong signal that you appreciate the efforts of your team. This helps people feel that they have support and recognition, which encourages them to go above and beyond for the team, collaborate better and spread the word about how great their organisations are.

One of the barriers to leaders expressing gratitude to their employees, according to *The Grateful Workplace* report, is that leaders are too hesitant to express gratitude for fear of being perceived as weak, soft or incompetent because they are seeking help.

■ Time Out

If you are leading a team at the moment, how might you recognise and thank team members, based on the good practice identified earlier?

The Dynamics of Team Development

How do teams start and what is their life cycle? This was explored in 1965 by Bruce Tuckman and is an enduring reflection of the life of teams. He suggested that teams move through four stages: forming, storming, norming and performing, with performing being the most productive stage. Later, other writers introduced the concept of teams 'adjourning' after performing (see Fig. 6.4).

Originally this was thought to be a linear progression, but today we can think of team development as cyclical, as the 'performing' stage is unlikely to last forever as circumstances change, such as the promotion of a respected leader or the development of the services that the teams provide.

■ Time Out

Tuckman's model gives student leaders a tool to help them and their teams to take time out. They can then reflect on the stage that they are at and what they need to do to, for example progress to the next stage, stay as a 'performing' team or, if they have achieved the team's purpose, to adjourn.

Thinking of a student team that you are in now (a study group, curating a Twitter account, an advocacy project etc.), consider:

- What stage your team has reached
- How you might move the team to the next stage, or keep it performing well
  - Look back at Figs. 6.1, 6.2 and 6.3 to remind yourself of the factors that make teams effective. For example, are roles and responsibilities clear? Do team members need any further training? Have you thanked them recently? Is there unresolved conflict in your team?

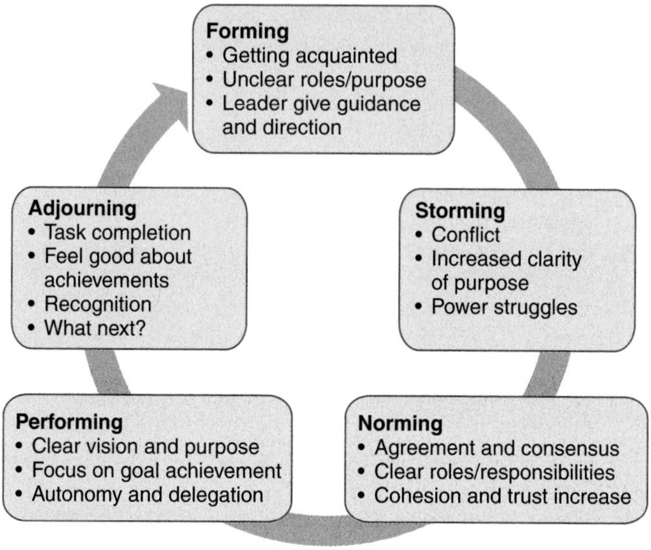

Fig. 6.4 Tuckman's stages of team development. (Adapted from Tuckman, B.W., 1965. Developmental sequence in small groups. Psychological Bulletin. 63 (6), 384–399.)

Creating a Leadership Culture of Team-Based Working

Part of teamwork is the ability to work across boundaries, but in practice we know how difficult this is because the number of organisations that health care providers work with has increased, and so it has become too complex to do. In complex situations heroic leadership becomes unrealistic and so modern NHS leadership is about collective leadership, where everyone in the organisation feels part of achieving the outcome. This is analogous to the person who sweeps the floor at the space agency NASA saying that it is their job to get man on the moon.

So, for organisations it is not just that individual teams are working well, it is about the collective of teams being able to work across boundaries to achieve a common goal. The role of organisational leaders is therefore to set the culture of the organisation for this to happen. We shall discover more about leading within systems and how leaders influence organisational culture in Section 3.

■ **Time Out**

Student nurses do not just work in a team, they work in an organisation that connects teams together, such as ward teams and theatre teams. Organisations like NHS trusts also have essential relationships with other organisations, such as social care. What sort of leadership model do today's organisations need to create effective teams? Why?

Search for 'Michael West: Why Teams? Creating Collective Leadership' on YouTube and jot down a few notes.

Communicating With Your Team

'I had this senior nurse... but her manner in speaking to people was awful. And when I approached my mentor about it, she said oh, she just likes you to know where her place is and that you're below that place.'

'You're not a doctor, you're not a nurse, you're not an HCA, you're not a receptionist, you're not a practice manager: you're a team and you've got to work together to get things to gel.'
NAOMI BERRY, NEWLY REGISTERED GENERAL PRACTICE
NURSE AND FORMER HEALTH CARE ASSISTANT (HCA)

As we discussed in previous chapters, leadership is everyone's responsibility; everyone can be a role model; and outdated, hierarchical approaches such as the one Naomi describes are unacceptable. Communication amongst team members is critical to success. We shall discuss managing interpersonal and team conflict further in this section when we talk about courageous conversations. Good leaders need to be approachable and easy to talk to, so you can discover what is happening and take action early.

What helps is having a good understanding of your own role and the role of others and who is responsible for what. As has been discussed, the goals of the team need to be clear to everyone, whether this may be to hit the 4-hour waiting time in accident and emergency or enabling all the postoperative open heart surgery patients to be extubated and into high dependency before noon. Active listening and asking questions or clarifying information are crucial, as is keeping others briefed, keeping good communication records and sharing information appropriately. Barriers to effective communication may arise from having different cultures and different backgrounds, and different levels of understanding and hierarchies within the team. These issues are summarised in Fig. 6.5.

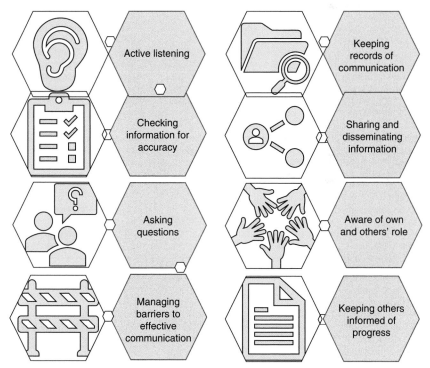

Fig. 6.5 Qualities of good communication in effective teamwork. (Adapted from Rowlands, S., Callen, J., 2013. A qualitative analysis of communication between members of a hospital-based multidisciplinary lung cancer team. European Journal of Cancer Care 22 (1), 20–31; Thomson, K., Outram, S., Gilligan, C., Levett-Jones, T., 2015. Interprofessional experiences of recent healthcare graduates: a social psychology perspective on the barriers to effective communication, teamwork, and patient-centred care. Journal of Interprofessional Care 29 (6), 634–640; and Pettit, A., Duffy, J., 2015. Patient safety: creating a culture change to support communication and teamwork. Journal of Legal Nurse Consulting 26, (4) 23–26.)

CASE STUDY 6.1   Simon James, Student Nurse, Swansea University

'It's the drive we can have when we all work together and use our voice to make change.'

Simon had held many jobs before coming into nursing, from police officer to working in a nightclub to mortgage adviser.

He had been told in the past that he had 'a face that didn't fit' and that it would be impossible for him to succeed. Still, he reflected that he had a range of skills from his various roles, including training others, and wanted to further develop his leadership skills.

As a student nurse, he successfully applied to the Swansea Student Leadership Academy (SWANSLA). This gave him the opportunity to give presentations on behalf of the academy at the South West Regional Student Leadership Conference alongside a fellow student. He delivered promotional talks to new cohorts and at interview selection days. He was also invited to be part of the SWANSLA advisory panel alongside lecturers and fellow students, and he helped choose the next SWANSLA cohort. The academy gave him the push he needed to apply to become a buddy for nursing students in the SWANSLA 2020 intake.

From there, Simon applied to go on the national #150Leaders programme. As part of this he had a leadership project to complete, so he decided to develop the work he started in recruiting future cohorts of students to the SWANSLA programme. By this time, the COVID-19 pandemic had struck and he was unable to attend lectures and events as he once had, so he had to think of another way to promote his university's leadership academy and recruit future student leaders. Simon approached his peers to generate enthusiasm for the idea of developing a promotional video for SWANSLA's leadership academy.

He approached the director of the leadership academy with the idea, who was supportive, and then canvassed several fellow students who agreed to talk on camera about their experience of the leadership programme and what it had done for them.

He established a small project team to help him. His first stop was an old friend who is head of film studies at another university to ask his advice on creating a promotional video that could be shared in various ways, such as via online study groups and on social media. His friend advised that what he needed to do was to create a storyboard showing the various shots that would be filmed. Simon went away to think about what he wanted to achieve—a 5-minute promotional video—and draw his stick figures on his story board to show the various scenes that he wanted to shoot. He engaged the media team at the university who agreed to do the filming and editing. He had ongoing discussions with the filming team to work out timings and locations. Due to COVID-19 restrictions, together they recognised the need to stagger the arrival times of the people who were to be filmed, and he communicated with each person about the plan.

'All the students were excited to be involved and followed the guidelines. We only had a window of about 4 hours due to the unpredictable Swansea weather, so I had to take control when we needed to change scenes around. This required me to change my laid-back leadership style and focus more on man management and organisation.'

SIMON JAMES

He achieved his aim of producing an excellent short promotional video that has been shared widely on social media to showcase the SWANSLA leadership academy.

You can watch the completed video on YouTube using the URL https://youtu.be/gXtbg4YZxd8 or search for 'Student Leadership Academy' at the 'College of Human Health Sciences, Swansea University'.

■ Time Out

Which qualities of effective team communication (see Fig. 6.5) are exhibited in Simon's story?

Simon knew that the social distancing resulting from the pandemic meant that he needed to find different ways to communicate with his audience—the potential nursing students. He asked questions of and listened to his friend to discover what he needed to do. He then shared what he had learnt with the academy director and his fellow students—and listened to their feedback. He drew out his storyboard so that both he and everyone in the team agreed what the final video would look like. He engaged the media team and got them on board. Everyone's roles were clear, and everyone played their part.

How to Delegate

If we are aiming for leadership at every level and collective and collaborative leadership rather than a heroic leadership model, then it is important that we learn to delegate. Delegation is about giving another person authority and responsibility for a task and should be viewed as part of their development, rather than being about dumping work on them (Tips Box 6.1).

TIPS BOX 6.1

Delegating

- Tasks can be stretching, but do not delegate a task to someone if it is beyond their capabilities or if a task is mission critical and failure would cause you big problems.
- Brief the team member on what you want them to do. A written brief is advisable if the team member is new to the task.
- Identify if they need additional training or support.
- Give them appropriate resources and authority for the task.
- Agree on timescales.
- Invite them to come back to you with any questions or concerns, so you can resolve issues quickly and early.
- Give praise and feedback to help them to learn from the process.

Leading Teams by Example

'If I told people that I was a HCA prior, I'd get a lot of jealousy back [from nurses and HCAs]...I don't understand it, I'm not going to overtake them, we're all trying to get to the same position. I'm not going to undermine them or anything.'

'We get told at university to ask questions; ask why they're doing it, but sometimes if you ask, they don't like it. And I don't know if it's that they think I'm trying to tell them how to do their job, I'm not, I don't understand. There's a definite hierarchy when you go in as a student nurse.'

'They're [students] our future nurses, we should be mentoring them. Protecting them as much as we can to mould them into a good nurse. But if you treat them like that in their first or second year, they're not going to be like that [a good nurse] because they've seen bad behaviour.'

NAOMI BERRY, NEWLY QUALIFIED GENERAL PRACTICE NURSE AND FORMER HCA, SPEAKING ABOUT HER EXPERIENCE AS A STUDENT ON A PLACEMENT

Maybe you have had similar experiences to Naomi, but as student leaders you can be role models and avoid passing on poor behaviours such as these.

Role Modelling Team Leadership

Anne Marie Dodson, senior lecturer at Birmingham City University, talks about how she leads by example. She has high standards for herself and her team, and she finds that role modelling those standards is more powerful than telling people off.

She learnt from another leader in education that it was important to always have your door open, be compassionate, get to know the individuals that you are working with, know their strengths and know their limitations. It is also important to know their family situation, like you would with a patient, so it puts what is happening into context and makes it easier to work with them in a team.

'You can't be what you can't see.'

ATTRIBUTED TO MARIAN WRIGHT EDELMAN, AMERICAN CIVIL RIGHTS ACTIVIST, AND OTHERS

Leaders from minority groups and those with protected characteristics need to be visible as role models so that others can aspire. The culture and systems of an organisation can put more hurdles in place, however, so it is important for aspiring student nurse leaders who may be subject to potential discrimination to connect and support each other, be visible and to seek out empathetic mentors and coaches.

Confidence may be an issue, and so fellow students have a role in giving positive feedback to peers whenever possible and to engage and encourage nurses from minority groups who have potential to put themselves forward.

The Future for Teamworking in the NHS

▣ Time Out

Do a search on the internet for the most recent national NHS strategy on workforce development for your country (see resources section). What are the key developments and trends that will affect the future of teams?

Across the four nations of the UK, some of the themes you might have read about are listed in Box 6.1.

Summary

The three essential features of a team are that they have shared objectives, are interdependent and they reflect and adapt to changing circumstances. Well-functioning, motivated teams are essential, not just for the wellbeing of the team itself, but for the organisation and for the quality of patient care given.

BOX 6.1 ▣ Future Trends in Teamworking

- Compassionate leadership and delivery—this is a theme we have already discussed in Section 1.
- An increased focus on creating a culture of staff wellbeing rather than supporting staff after their wellbeing has been compromised—prevent rather than cure.
- Inclusivity—teams need to embrace diversity in all its forms, which this will encourage a sense of belonging. Challenges and tensions from the perspectives of different people enable teams to make decisions that better reflect the needs of both teams and local people. The focus on inclusivity also means addressing deep-rooted inequalities among staff groups. Inclusivity also means working across sectors with NHS contractors such as general practices, social care, local authorities and the voluntary and social enterprise sector.
- Changing ways of working—the COVID-19 pandemic led to step changes in ways of working. Teams now need to work flexibly, including using technology to enable more remote working and technical care. This includes remote multidisciplinary team meetings, case presentations, handovers and teaching sessions, as well as a move to remote consultations. The campaign 'every nurse an e-nurse' (Royal College of Nursing 2018) highlights the need for teams to access electronic health care records to share information and coordinate care. Data from different sources aids the detection of trends and new insights into what is happening in both individuals and populations. Patient apps help with self-care.
- Changing roles—teams will increasingly include both new staff and returners, volunteers and flexible, innovative new roles. Research teams, including nurses, are becoming an increasing priority to rapidly investigate some of the urgent health needs of the 21st century.

Organisational leaders are crucial in determining the culture of the teams within their organisations, encouraging collective leadership and cooperation between teams and between partner organisations such as with social care organisations.

Team members' wellbeing is dependent upon their ability to exert autonomy, have a sense of belonging and feel that they are contributing to their organisations. Taking time out to reflect is more likely to lead to innovation. Effective communication is essential and includes features such as listening, asking questions, and checking and sharing information.

The future for teams is centred around inclusivity and flexibility within a culture characterised by collectivism, compassion and belonging.

Resources

Department of Health Northern Ireland, 2017. Health and Wellbeing 2026 – Delivering Together.

Health Education and Improvement Wales and Social Care Wales, 2020. A Healthier Wales: Our Workforce Strategy for Health and Social Care.

NHS England, 2020. We Are the NHS: People Plan for 2020/2021 – Action for Us All.

Rosengarten, L., 2019. Teamwork in nursing: essential elements for practice. Nursing Management. doi: 10.7748/nm.2019.e1850.

Scottish Government, 2017. Everyone Matters: 2020 Workforce Vision Implementation Plan 2018-2020.

References

Borrill, C., West, M., Shapiro, D., Rees, A., 2000. Team working and effectiveness in health care. British Journal of Health Care Management 6 (8), 364–371.

Borrill, C.S., Carletta, J., Carter, A.J., Dawson, J.F., 2000. The Effectiveness of Healthcare Teams in the NHS. Department of Health, London.

Dimensional Research, 2013. Customer Service and Business Results: A Survey of Customer Service from Mid-Sized Companies. <http://cdn.zendesk.com/resources/whitepapers/Zendesk_WP_Customer_Service_and_Business_Results.pdf> (accessed 04/03/2021).

Fehr, R., Fulmer, A., Awtrey, E., 2017. The grateful workplace: a multilevel model of gratitude in organizations. Academy of Management Review 42 (2), 361–381.

Frederickson, B., 2009. Positivity. Random House, New York.

HM Government, 2010. The Equality Act.

Pettit, A., Duffy, J., 2015. Patient safety: creating a culture change to support communication and teamwork. Journal of Legal Nurse Consulting 26 (4), 23–26.

Rowlands, S., Callen, J., 2013. A qualitative analysis of communication between members of a hospital-based multidisciplinary lung cancer team. European Journal of Cancer Care 22 (1), 20–31.

Royal College of Nursing, 2018. Every Nurse an E-nurse Campaign - A Cognitive Whiteboard Animation. YouTube. <https://www.youtube.com/watch?v=Ii3ScK_T8Fg> (accessed 16/12/2021).

Sorenson, S., 2013. How Employee Engagement Drives Growth. Gallup. <https://www.gallup.com/workplace/236927/employee-engagement-drives-growth.aspx> (accessed 04/03/2021).

Thomson, K., Outram, S., Gilligan, C., Levett-Jones, T., 2015. Interprofessional experiences of recent healthcare graduates: a social psychology perspective on the barriers to effective communication, teamwork, and patient-centred care. Journal of Interprofessional Care 29 (6), 634–640.

TINYpulse, 2014. Employee Engagement & Organizational Culture Report. <https://www.tinypulse.com/landing-page-2014-employee-engagement-organizational-culture-report> (accessed 04/03/2021).

Tuckman, B.W., 1965. Developmental sequence in small groups. Psychological Bulletin 63 (6), 384–399.

Unitt, I., 2018. Learning Disability Nursing Is Everybody's Field. Student Nursing Times. <https://www.nursingtimes.net/students/learning-disability-nursing-is-everybodys-field-12-11-2018/> (accessed 26/02/2021).

West, M.A., 2012. Effective Teamwork: Practical Lessons from Organisational Research, third ed. BPS Blackwell-Wiley, Chichester.

West, M.A., Bailey, S., Williams, E., 2020. The Courage of Compassion. King's Fund, London. <https://www.kingsfund.org.uk/publications/courage-compassion-supporting-nurses-midwives> (accessed 02/03/2021).

West, M.A., Eckert, R., Collins, B., Chowla, R., 2017. Caring to Change: How Compassionate Leadership Can Stimulate Innovation in Health Care. King's Fund, London.

West, M.A., Lyubovnikova, J., 2013. Illusions of team working in health care. Journal of Health Organisation and Management 27 (1), 134–142.

World Health Organisation, 2009. Framework for Action on Interprofessional Education and Collaborative Practice. World Health Organisation, Geneva.

Engaging Others in Cocreation

OBJECTIVES

After reading this chapter and completing the activities, you should be able to:
- Identify the level of participation in any given initiative
- Describe the benefits of person-centred care
- List multiple ways to gather data and information about the patient experience
- Describe the benefits of listening to patient stories
- Be able to distinguish the assets that people possess from their needs
- Describe the attributes of leaders who advocate for others.

Relevance to the Nursing and Midwifery Council (NMC) Code

Prioritise People:
1. Treat people as individuals and uphold their dignity
2. Listen to people and respond to their preferences and concerns
3. Make sure that people's physical, social and psychological needs are assessed and responded to
4. Act in the best interests of people at all times
5. Respect people's right to privacy and confidentiality

Introduction

As a student, you come into health and care settings with a range of life experiences and arrive at your universities and placements with fresh eyes. You may be motivated to cocreate initiatives both by your past experiences as well as be inspired by what you see and perceive could be different, if you work with others. This is an ideal opportunity to work alongside patients, families and communities and with your teams to cocreate better ways to meet needs and practise some leadership skills along the way.

Coproduction, Codesign and Cocreation

These terms are used interchangeably sometimes, which is confusing!
- Codesign is an attempt to define a problem and then define a solution.
- Coproduction is the attempt to implement the proposed solution.
- Cocreation is the process by which people do both.

(McDougall 2012)

So, we can think of designing the best way to keep ourselves warm by building a fire as a codesign activity, and gathering the kindling and firewood together and arranging it in a fire pit as coproduction. The fire that we then light is an example of cocreation!

Ladder of Participation

When we lead, we must think about how participation affects the redistribution of power and how various stakeholders might feel about this. Giving up some power can be hard for some.

'The idea of citizen participation is a little like eating spinach: no one is against it in principle because it is good for you.'

SHERRY ARNSTEIN

We will be discussing more about power in Chapter 9, but for now we need to understand what is called the ladder of participation (Fig. 7.1), which was first described by Sherry Arnstein in 1969.

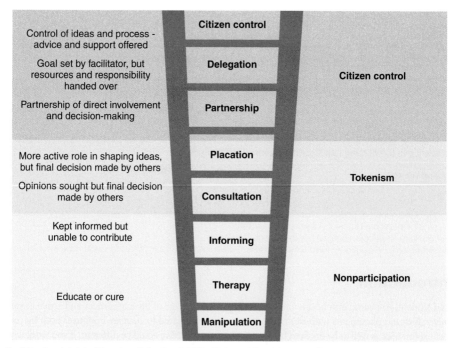

Fig. 7.1 Arnstein's ladder of participation (1969). (Adapted from Arnstein, S., 1969. A ladder of citizen participation. Journal of the American Planning Association 35 (4), 216–224.)

In nursing terms, it is not always easy to involve colleagues, partner organisations, patients and the public in our leadership activities. We should always consider asking people whether or how they would like to be involved. Nor would it always be appropriate, for example in urgent or emergency situations when stuff just must get done! Sometimes it is difficult to ensure involvement across a broad demographic that is representative of the population served who might not come forward, such as marginalised or stigmatised groups, like sex workers.

Criticisms have been raised nationally that patient and public involvement (or PPI as it is often called) has been tokenistic and that the expertise required to involve people meaningfully is often lacking (Ocloo and Matthews 2016).

▨ Time Out

As you read about the various ways of enabling participation presented in this chapter, think about where on Arnstein's ladder each approach represents.

Are solutions codesigned, coproduced or cocreated?

Compare your thoughts to those in the summary section at the end of the chapter.

Person-Centred Care

One of the 2019 NHS Long Term Plan's priorities is 'person-centred care': enabling people to have more choice and control of their own health and care. This means creating genuine partnerships between people and the health professionals and others who support them to understand what matters to them rather than what is the matter with them. This chapter gives some examples of how nurses and health care students have developed this relationship with patients and with each other.

Quite often, health and care services focus on providing services to or for people, rather than working alongside people to offer dignified, compassionate and respectful care. And because health and care organisations are huge and complex, sometimes people end up fitting into the system and the whole experience is not tailored to their wants and needs. Goals are often described in organisational terms, such as clinical outcomes, rather than what the person might see as a goal for themselves. Decisions may be taken without reference to the person and/or their family.

In person-centred care, the health and care professional works alongside the person to develop the knowledge, skills and confidence that they need to more effectively manage and make informed decisions about their own health and health care. It is coordinated and tailored to the needs of the individual, and, crucially, it ensures that people are always treated with dignity, compassion and respect.

Improving the Patient Experience

Right from the very first contact through to the very last, such as in end-of-life care, the experience of the patient, carer and family is now seen by health and care organisations as central. Improving patient experience requires not only good leadership, but a receptive culture, a focus on how the system of care is organised, a way to collect and analyse patient feedback, and then a way to use that information to improve care (Tips Box 7.1).

▨ Time Out

On your current or next placement, find out how the organisation collects and monitors information about the patient experience.

What feedback did they get and what changed as a result?

TIPS BOX 7.1

Leading With Patient Experience

- If you are working on an assignment or project, consider different ways of gathering information on patient experience.
- A good leader will be actively listening not just to patients and families, but also to staff who are in daily contact with them.
- Think of how you might use digital storytelling to share stories that illustrate how person-centred care might be improved.
- Think about who you do not see as well as who you do see. For example, is your team seeing homeless people? If not, why?
- If patients are not engaging with you, ask them why that might be. Check and challenge your assumptions about people: Can they read? Do they have transport? Have you ignored them or discriminated in some way?

There are many ways that organisations collect patient feedback:

- Complaints procedures: the right to complain is written into the NHS constitution
- Inspections by the Care Quality Commission (CQC)
- Adult Inpatient Survey: an annual survey conducted by the CQC
- Independent feedback services such as Care Opinion, which allow patients to record their stories of care in an anonymised and moderated way
- National patient and staff surveys managed by NHS England, including
  - Friends and family test: an anonymous survey asking 'Overall, how was your experience of our service?'
  - GP patient survey: an annual survey of patients in primary care conducted by Ipsos Mori
- Patient stories: often, the boards of NHS organisations listen to stories to understand what care is like from a patient or carer perspective
- Cards, letters and verbal feedback from patients

The Importance of Storytelling

'Stories are data with a soul.'

BRENÉ BROWN, AUTHOR AND ACADEMIC

Stories are an essential tool as you develop as a leader. Listening to patients tell their stories in the way that they want to will enable you to understand how your nursing care is perceived by others. It may help you to understand how your role fits with the wider organisation of care given to that patient—the care pathway—and whether or not the health care piece of the puzzle fits with other parts of the patient's life, such as housing or transport.

■ Time Out

Think of a time when someone told you their story about their experience of health or care services. In what ways does this differ from data collected in other ways?

CASE STUDY 7.1	The Experience of Working-Class Men

A community nurse, well known in the community in which she works, walks into a local pub to be greeted by the news that the local health improvement worker has visited and conducted a fun quiz with the men on their drinking habits. The men laugh as they tell the nurse the story 'We didn't tell her the truth; we just told her that we drank to recommended limits.'

Unlike surveys, quizzes and questionnaires, storytelling is a way to discover what really matters to people and can reveal unexpected information or in the case study above, perhaps more truthful accounts. It may, as in the men's story, lead to the need to ask more questions.

As she continues to get to know the regulars, the nurse discovers that there is a culture of heavy drinking in this particular community, often masking emotional problems in the men's lives (Henry 2017). Some of the men are fathers and, with her support, decide to set up a community bicycle recycling project that also runs family cycle rides. This helps refocus some of the men on meaningful activities and away from drinking.

From the author's own case study, based on a project called 'Dadly Does It' (Robertson et al. 2015).

Stories can be a tool for helping us to improve the quality of our care and can prompt us to consider where we need to move from improvement to innovation.

Patient experience and person-centred care focus on finding out what matters to the patient and their family and then taking action to make that even better. There are a wide variety of ways that health and care organisations get feedback on their services. Some of it is standardised data collection, which allows comparison over time and between different organisations, while some rely on visits and asking questions. Complaints tell us much about what is not going right but may miss out on what is going well.

So, storytelling is a way to uncover and share the human factors in health care. Often, patients and families will simply tell you what they think, while others prefer to do so anonymously using online services such as Care Opinion. But we can also use something called digital storytelling—using pictures video and audio—to give us a richer insight.

Perhaps the most well-known project that does this in health care is one called Patient Voices, which was established by Pip Hardy and Tony Sumner in 2003. Enabling people to speak for themselves in a sincere and authentic way and to share their experiences enables an emotional connection. The story focuses on people, rather than the more abstract: the services they receive.

The Patient Voices programme was initially set up by Pip and Tony with two main aims:

- to give patients a voice and a chance to influence decision-makers by helping them to realise the effects of their actions and decisions; and
- to provide a freely accessible bank of stories to help anyone who might want to improve health and care services.

You might want to watch a few stories in a clinical area that you have worked in/will be working on at the Patient Voices website to help you to understand the experience of patients in more detail.

Storytelling: Marginalised Communities

Digital storytelling has been used to great effect to help the most marginalised become more visible, including communities such as Gypsy Romany Travellers (GRTs) and the homeless.

■ **Time Out**

Search YouTube for the term 'We took it to the European Court', a video created by the Friends, Families and Travellers (FFT) Project. This is the story of Jim Connors, who was evicted from a Traveller site in Leeds. Jim took his case to the European Court of Human Rights.

Reflect on how you felt as Jim told his story. What was it about this story that affected you the most? What was the impact on his health?

How might you use what you learnt to work differently in the future with people from Gypsy Romany Traveller communities?

Jim's story illustrates the marginalisation that is still experienced by GRTs, whose average age of death is between 50 and 68 years old. Experiences such as Jim's have led to the establishment of advocacy groups such as the FFT and Leeds Gypsy and Traveller Exchange (Leeds GATE).

Nurses and, in particular, health visitors have been intimately connected with these communities for many decades. But in the case of Leeds GATE, for example, rather than educating these communities about how to interact with NHS services, health leaders have cocreated services with Leeds GATE based on the unique culture of the communities themselves. This has led to the development of an outreach nurse role.

'The success of this project lies in the joint support and leadership from Leeds Gypsy and Traveller Exchange (Leeds GATE), Leeds Clinical Commissioning Group (CCG) and Leeds Community Healthcare. Find mentors, work closely with community groups: they may know more than you do.'
LIZ KEAT, OUTREACH NURSE FOR THE GYPSY
ROMANY TRAVELLER COMMUNITY IN LEEDS

Following several exploratory workshops involving GRT communities and the people who support them, Leeds GATE (2020) took to video to explain the blockages that GRT communities experience in accessing health and care. They used the analogy of roads, bridges and tunnels (2020) and they designed their video around this analogy, using the story of a typical Gypsy family called the Lee family.

Roads represent the route that the majority of people use to access services—they are built to be accessible to as many people as possible. The Lee family experience a 'roadblock' when trying to access GP services. Because their nomadic life means that they have no fixed address, they are refused GP registration.

None of the family can read and write, so they could not access the information that the surgery gave them. This delayed access to needed treatment and, eventually in desperation, the family sought help from a friend who lives in a house to temporarily use their address to register with a GP. This is called a 'tunnel': a community-led solution to getting around a block in the road that is often underground and innovative. These tunnels can often be unseen, hazardous and misunderstood.

Bridges are sometimes built by services who recognise a difficulty and design a solution with the involvement of the community. In the Lee family example, they access the support of a health advocate funded by the NHS to access ongoing care and continuing GP support.

The problem with a bridge, however, is that sometimes it takes away the motivation to fix the road. Marginalised communities can become the responsibility of bridge builders rather than road builders, and the road block will remain for other travelling families.

Services sometimes see marginalised communities as hard to reach rather than understanding that there is a road block to be fixed. Leeds GATE members explain that what they really need is to have the road widened so that there are multiple ways to travel.

We shall look more into how student nurses might use digital stories to communicate as a leader later. We will also learn more about the evidence base and structure of stories in general.

Let us look now at building on data and stories that enable health and care services to make improvements and think about taking action to involving the patient themselves in improvement.

Experienced-Based Codesign

Experience-based codesign (EBCD) is an eight-step process developed by the Point of Care Foundation that has been run in organisations across the world. It enables staff and service users to work in equal partnership to codesign services and care pathways.

The process starts with observing clinical areas before filming interviews with staff, patients and families. The films are edited together and screened at staff and patient feedback events. Areas for improvement are jointly agreed and improvement groups are set up where staff, patients and families jointly work on improvements (Tips Box 7.2).

TIPS BOX 7.2

Using EBCD

- Focus on experience and emotion rather than opinions or attitudes.
- Identify opportunities for improvement.
- Empower patients, families and staff to make positive changes.
- Emphasise realistic goals that will benefit both staff and patients.
- Encourage learning about how patients and staff can work together.

Note: A complete EBCD process can last 12 months and requires organisational buy-in by senior leaders. It is probably not one to try as a student, but you could ask to observe.

Asset-Based and Strengths-Based Approaches

More recently, the concept of asset-based nursing has started to come forward (Henry and Howarth 2018). Nursing has traditionally sought to assess needs and deliver services to meet those needs, but increasingly it is being acknowledged that good nursing care is a balance of:

- providing nursing care to and for people, based on their *needs* (such as a nurse in A&E administering a nebuliser to a child with acute asthma) and
- working a partnership with people to develop the best outcomes based on their *strengths* (such as the nurse supporting pub regulars to develop a community cycling project).

In the second example, the nurse sees the men around her as assets: people who know what might help them to improve their wellbeing. The analogy often used in asset-based thinking is that of a glass half full (Fig. 7.2).

People and communities have needs or deficiencies to be solved by delivering services for people.

People and communities have skills and talents that can be complementary to the skills and talents of staff. Solutions are coproduced.

Fig. 7.2   Needs-based and asset-based thinking.

An asset-based approach works best when problems stem from social and cultural determinants, rather than simply clinical ones. You would not, for example, use it if someone needed immediate postoperative care for an appendicectomy. The men in the case study 7.1, for example, told the nurse about things like family breakdown, posttraumatic stress from active service in the army and bereavement. Men viewed the pub as somewhere to go to have a laugh, forget their worries and avoid being alone. But in this community, many people also enjoyed cycling and some of the men knew how to fix bikes.

Student nurse leaders can learn to switch between a glass half empty and focus on meeting needs, and a glass half full and focus on seeing people as part of the solution to their own problems.

The assets or gifts that people can share with us can be thought of in three ways:

1. Assets of the head: what people know
2. Assets of the heart: what motivates people, what they value and appreciate
3. Assets of the hand: physical skills that they may be able to share

(Rippon and Hopkins 2015)

■ **Time Out**

Next time you have the opportunity, talk to a patient and discover their assets of head, heart and hand. Can any of these assets help them in their recovery or help other patients in the same position?

Example: One of the men in the Dadly Does It case study was off sick with work-related depression and stress. He had experience with mending bikes and taking his wife and three small children on family cycle rides. The nurse enabled him to access funding from Cycling UK to gain a qualification so he could learn to repair bikes properly and sell them cheaply to local people, and in the process his depression improved. He cofounded a community interest company with another local man skilled in bike repair. Eventually he stood for election to be a ward councillor and is now representing his ward, leaving behind a career that he felt had made him ill.

Now do the same exercise with your student cohort and university—maybe you have a problem with timetabling your studies or you want to set up a new society with the help of the student union. What assets can you see around you that can help?

Students as Assets in Cocreation

In 2018 when the NMC introduced its new standards of proficiency in preregistration nursing programmes, the University of Chester programme planning team (PPT) reached out to its students to invite them to give their input into the design of a new syllabus. The process reflected the standards for education and training, which stress the importance of empowerment for nurses and midwives.

A student empowerment group (SEG) was set up, cochaired by two student nurses: Daniel Branch, a learning disability student and Rose James, an adult nursing student. The SEG reached out to students across the different fields to gather their views on the ideas coming out of the PPT. Daniel and Rose then liaised between the PPT and the SEG to give input into the curriculum design. The process took 18 months, culminating in a presentation to the NMC of the new syllabus on validation day.

Behind this initiative were a number of key concepts to enable this empowerment, which are shown in Fig. 7.3. The leadership shown by Daniel and Rose and their fellow members of the SEG was recognised by them winning the Student Nursing Times award 2020 in the category

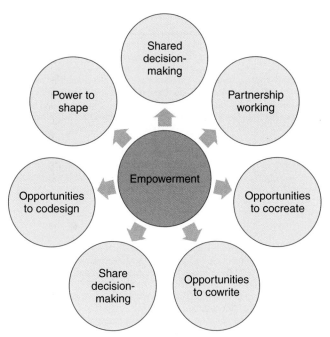

Fig. 7.3 Key concepts in empowerment of student nurses. (Branch, D., James, R., 2020. Presentation as part of the RCNi Student Nurse Award, Student Empowerment Group, University of Chester.)

of 'outstanding contribution to student affairs'. In their presentation for the award, they referred to the global Nursing Now campaign, which between 2018 and 2020 raised the profile of nursing and midwifery and its role in improving health. The campaign sought to empower nurses to use their knowledge, skills and expertise and to take their place at the heart of tackling the health challenges of the 21st century.

Daniel remarked that the development of his empowerment was a gradual process. What helped was having an 'official' role and title, which enabled him to develop his confidence to engage with stakeholders such as senior placement representatives across health and care and, because the work was cross field, to develop his understanding of the different fields of nursing. He is a strong advocate for universities empowering student nurses so that they are able to challenge appropriately when on placement. The skills he developed while part of the PPT meetings were transferrable to, for example, his involvement in multidisciplinary team meetings as a newly registered nurse in terms of his ability to prepare appropriately and have the confidence to engage with people from a range of different backgrounds.

Leadership Through Advocacy

Leading from the last activity, let us look at how to lead through advocating for others. Advocacy is defined as 'active support for an idea or cause'.

> 'Were there none who were discontent with what they have, the world would never reach anything better.'

> FLORENCE NIGHTINGALE

CASE STUDY 7.2

In 2020, Joy O'Gorman was a student on the adult branch at the University of Plymouth. She was also one of the students participating in the #150Leaders programme run by the Council of Deans of Health. As part of the programme, each student was invited to undertake a leadership project. This became a trickier task due to the COVID-19 pandemic. Joy proposed that she and fellow students from nursing, allied health professions and midwifery could work together to raise the profile of the contribution of students who had volunteered to work during the pandemic. Student dietician Olivia Mason, radiographer Ismat Khan, paramedic Ashleigh Sayers, midwife Abbie Rich, nursing associate Ian Costello and fellow student nurse Natalie Elliott joined Joy in doing video diaries of their COVID-19 placement experiences.

Joy had previous experience of working with the media, when she had appeared on the Victoria Derbyshire programme advocating that the assessment meetings with personal independent payment claimants should be recorded in disputed cases. She successfully re-engaged the journalist whom she had worked with on that programme to see if the BBC would be interested in BBC TV news airing their pandemic video diaries.

She hosted a webinar with the six other students about the idea and quickly realised how much each discipline was contributing during the crisis and what could be learnt more widely. For instance, the student paramedic revealed that 90% of her calls were related to mental health during lockdown; a notable change to normal practice.

Joy followed this up with a webinar for fellow student leaders with the Council of Deans of Health who were running the #150Leaders programme. The seven students, acting as panel members, talked of their COVID-19 experiences and busted some myths, such as student radiographers did much more than just pressing a button. They talked about how their placements had affected them and what they had observed during the pandemic. This inadvertently enabled these students to act as role models for fellow students who many have been anxious about what a COVID-19 placement experience was like and how their safety was being managed.

Collaboration extended to each student's university and placement, and each gave their support and permission to be involved.

In sharing their video diaries, Joy and her colleagues had the following aims:
- to raise the profile of undergraduate health care students and their contribution during the pandemic;
- in doing so, demonstrate to the wider workforce that they were not just 'the student';
- to showcase the value and diversity of the whole multidisciplinary team, including some whose role was not always well understood, like radiographers; and
- to promote understanding of their fellow students of the value of interdisciplinary working.

'Diet is a key part of rehabilitation. If a patient is not fed well and doesn't have the energy for things like physio, it's going to be more difficult to get them home, so I work very closely with the physiotherapists and others to help patients recover.'
                                        STUDENT DIETICIAN OLIVIA MASON, UNIVERSITY OF PLYMOUTH

Joy persuaded the journalist of the public interest inherent in their stories: how legislation was changing to allow students to work as part of nursing care teams in a delegated framework that meant the removal of their supernumerary status but not of the student status and the need to optimise their learning (NMC 2020/21).

The journalist recorded a joint webinar with all seven students and received all their video diaries to provide an overview of their COVID-19 experiences. Then, on July 20th the BBC broadcast the diaries throughout the day, offering a unique insight into life on the NHS 'front line' at the height of the pandemic.

Joy was careful to recognise the emotions of fellow student nurses who had not volunteered and draw attention to the work of all students throughout their studies:

'For many different reasons not everyone was able to go straight into a clinical environment, and I applaud all my peers, both those who chose to pursue extended placements, and those who took the difficult decision not to, due to personal circumstances. This must have weighed heavily on them as the nation celebrated its 'NHS heroes'. I would love therefore for BBC viewers to recognise these diaries are just a small glimpse into the great work students usually do up and down the country during our degree years.'

■ Time Out

What sort of leadership skills did Joy and her colleagues display?
Who were the key stakeholders and how did she engage them?
What will be the benefit of students understanding other professions?
What were the barriers and how did she overcome them?

The core values of leaders who advocate are:
- concern for fellow human beings,
- a keen sense of justice, and
- an emphasis on the common good (Tips Box 7.3).

TIPS BOX 7.3

Advocacy

- Choose to serve first and lead second.
- Do not try to lead a community but serve the collective will.
- Understand where the power lies and be sensitive to underlying power shifts.

The students articulated a range of concerns in their aims around raising the profile of health students and explaining clearly what each discipline can contribute.

The skills of a successful advocate include collaboration, influence, problem solving and communication. Joy reports that 2 months of hard work went in at the start to ensure buy-in from students, their universities, the BBC and NHS Trusts, supported by the Council of Deans of Health. The students needed good communication skills to ensure that everyone's concerns and doubts were identified and addressed. The group set up a WhatsApp group to coordinate the work and offer mutual support. A key concern for many was the media angle that the BBC would take. This risk was reduced by the students sharing this worry with the journalist and negotiating the angle that would be taken.

Some of the benefits to be gained by students increasing their understanding of other disciplines are that in the future they will be better able to engage and involve them as leaders and it will improve their ability to offer person-centred care by meeting needs holistically.

Joy and her colleagues were successful in anticipating what the difficulties may be, such as allaying the concerns of NHS Trusts and universities, and gaining permission for them to be involved and to allow filming. Joy also considered the feelings of those students who chose a 'theory only' route and did not volunteer to nurse during the COVID-19 crisis. This enabled the public to understand the hard work put in by all students over the course of their degree. The result was a real win-win: universities and trusts used the diaries to promote themselves, the role of students was highlighted and the BBC got an excellent interest story.

Summary

Staff, patient and public involvement is at the heart of health and care. This chapter has been about engaging others in our leadership to enable the best outcome for patients, citizens and colleagues. Arnstein reminds us that there are eight steps on the ladder of participation and at each step forward, more power is shared, which is difficult for some, leading to tokenism.

At the nonparticipation end of the ladder is education and delivering services to and for people, which is appropriate in many circumstances. In asset-based nursing terms, this is needs-based or deficit-based care. Further up the ladder we begin to see patient experience, where we start to get feedback in various ways and use that information to lead.

Person-centred care starts to shift us further up the ladder, offering people more choice and control over their lives, and experience-based codesign leads us onto the next rung of the ladder with partnership working.

An example of partnership was when health care students used their digital stories during the COVID-19 pandemic to advocate for fellow students in a powerful way. Stories are a great way to understand the human factors in health and care. And when the NHS partnered with Leeds GATE, they formed a powerful alliance to tackle the health inequalities experienced by GRTs.

Lecturers at the University of Chester partnered with student nurses to develop a new curriculum and at the same time empowered the students to take ownership of their learning.

At the top of the ladder is citizen control, as shown in the Dadly Does It project, where men are viewed as assets and enabled to use their strengths and skills to find their own solutions.

As you travel on your leadership journey, think through what rung on the ladder of participation you need to be on. Think about whether you are codesigning, coproducing or both. Consider the benefits of sharing power with your stakeholders, how you will do it and how you might manage the reaction of others who may lose power and influence as a result. Will you lead from the front or become an enabler or facilitator of change? Can you think through who will be an asset and how to draw out their strengths? Can you enable others to take credit for something that you have initiated?

True cocreation takes time, courage, humility, plenty of listening, an ability to engage with diverse groups and views and an ability to negotiate successfully. It is likely that you will make mistakes and it is important that you do, so you can learn from them.

Resources

Patient Voices. <www.patientvoices.org.uk>.
Point of Care Foundation. <www.pointofcarefoundation.org.uk>.

References

Arnstein, S., 1969. A ladder of citizen participation. Journal of the American Planning Association 35 (4), 216–224.
Covid Video Diaries. <https://www.bbc.co.uk/news/av/health-53451153>.
Health Education England, 2017. Bitesize Case Study: Dadly Does It. <http://www.ewin.nhs.uk/sites/de-fault/files/eWIN%20BiteSize%20Case%20Study%20-%20LM%20Dadly%20Does%20It.pdf>.
Henry, H., 2017. Pub Nurse. <https://www.linkedin.com/pulse/pub-nurse-heather-henry/>.
Henry, H., Howarth, M., 2018. An overview of using an asset based approach to nursing. Journal of General Practice Nursing 4 (4), 61–66.
Leeds GATE, 2020. Roads, Bridges and Tunnels. Vimeo. <https://vimeo.com/425444661>.
McDougall, S., 2012. Co-production, Co-design and Co-creation: What Is the Difference? Stakeholder Design. <https://www.stakeholderdesign.com/co-production-versus-co-design-what-is-the-difference/>.
NHS England, Involvement Hub. <https://www.england.nhs.uk/participation/>.
NHS Plan, 2019. Department of Health. <www.longtermplan.nhs.uk/>.
Nursing and Midwifery Council, 2020/21. Current Emergency and Recovery Programme Standards. <https://www.nmc.org.uk/standards-for-education-and-training/emergency-education-standards/>.
Ocloo, J., Matthews, R., 2016. From tokenism to empowerment: progressing patient and public involvement in healthcare improvement. British Medical Journal Quality and Safety 25 (8), 626–632.
Rippon, S., Hopkins, T., 2015. Head, Hands and Heart: Asset-based Approaches in Health Care. Health Foundation.
Robertson, S., Woodall, J., Hanna, E., Rowlands, S., Long, T., Livesley, J., 2015. Salford Dadz: Year 2 External Evaluation. Project Report. Unlimited Potential. <https://eprints.leedsbeckett.ac.uk/id/eprint/1728/>.

CHAPTER 8

Being Assertive and Courageous

Having Difficult and Courageous Conversations

Leading by Positively Disrupting

Understanding a Student's Role in Serious Care Failures

OBJECTIVES

After reading this chapter and completing the activities, you should be able to:
- Demonstrate assertiveness techniques
- Make a conscious choice about how you interpret and respond to interpersonal conflict situations
- Ask for what you want
- Describe how to raise a concern about poor care.

Relevance to the Nursing and Midwifery Council (NMC) Code

Practise Effectively
Paragraph 9:
Share your skills, knowledge and experience for the benefit of people receiving care and your colleagues
- 9.1 provide honest, accurate and constructive feedback to colleagues
- 9.2 gather and reflect on feedback from a variety of sources, using it to improve your practice and performance
- 9.3 deal with differences of professional opinion with colleagues by discussion and informed debate, respecting their views and opinions and behaving in a professional way at all times
- 9.4 support students' and colleagues' learning to help them develop their professional competence and confidence

Preserve Safety
Paragraph 14:
- 14 Be open and candid with all service users about all aspects of care and treatment, including when any mistakes or harm have taken place
- 14.1 act immediately to put right the situation if someone has suffered actual harm for any reason or an incident has happened which had the potential for harm
- 14.2 explain fully and promptly what has happened, including the likely effects, and apologise to the person affected and, where appropriate, their advocate, family or carers
- 14.3 document all these events formally and take further action (escalate) if appropriate so they can be dealt with quickly

Being a student nurse can be a challenge. Every day you are learning new things, are in new situations and have to respond with confidence to the people around you: patients, colleagues, clinical staff and university faculty members. NHS organisations and universities are large and complex, and work is emotionally and physically demanding, with teams often competing for resources. Patients and families are often under stress, or they may hold challenging views. So, it is not surprising that conflict arises. Students are predominantly trained in clinical issues, so they are rarely prepared with tools to manage conflict.

This chapter is about how you as a student leader, working in a team, can be assertive and courageous. Although some of this subject matter may be considered as management skills rather than leadership, student leaders interviewed for this book found conflict difficult and so it has been included. In addition, if leaders do not air the problem, then the team members are left confused and the issue remains unresolved, leading to escalation and unnecessary frustration for all involved.

Student nurses find themselves in several different types of situations where they may have to be assertive and courageous in their leadership. Students may:

- experience bullying and harassment from patients and staff;
- have difficulty speaking up about the way clinical issues are managed;
- face abuse from staff and patients about protected characteristics such as their gender assignment or race in contravention of the Equality Act 2020;
- have their opinions and ideas overlooked or rejected; and
- have to manage interpersonal or team conflict.

This chapter is about giving you some basic tools as a leader to help you to manage these situations. We shall then go on to introduce ideas on how you can also be positively disruptive—in a safe way—a concept known as rebel leadership.

This chapter does not cover managing situations involving patients because these are likely to be covered in your degree course. You will find references in the Resources section to articles that will help you here. Each organisation will have zero tolerance, bullying and harassment, managing violent incidents and antidiscrimination policies for you to consult, alongside in-house training programmes.

Let us start with some common situations where student nurses need courage.

Being Courageous on Your First Day in Placement

A common issue for students is when they turn up for their first day at a new placement and nobody is expecting them. It really helps if you know in advance the way to the placement, can find where to put your belongings and where you can make a drink.

Student nurse Gloria Sikapite's way to deal with this is to visit or phone the placement a week in advance and introduce herself to a staff member, so that she feels that she has already made a contact there. If she arrives and is still not expected she can mention the visit/call and the name of the contact, which makes her feel more confident and addresses her 'first-day jitters'.

Build Courage Before Interviews or Presentations

This same technique works when you are doing a big presentation or you have a job interview: do a 'dummy run' to find out which bus to take or where to park. Visit the room that you will be presenting in/being interviewed in. Introduce yourself to staff. If you are using technology to present, check where the electrical sockets are and whether devices are compatible. Will you be asked to use a lapel microphone? If so, then think about what clothes you wear: clothing without pockets may mean you having to hold a battery pack. Look at the layout of the room and of the screen and think about where you stand so that people can see the screen.

Always have a plan B–so if the technology fails, for example (and does it not always go on the blink in high-stress situations?), then have a hard copy of your presentation and talk through the presentation instead. In interviews you can hand out hard copies to the interviewers so that they can follow along.

If you have emailed a presentation in advice, check that the right people have received it and that it works at their end, but always bring the presentation in at least two ways—a hard copy and maybe a way to download it through cloud storage.

Courageous Conversations

The term 'courageous conversation' has emerged over the last few years, and it is generally defined as being about how to broach difficult subjects with those close to you at home and at work such as your partner, child, manager or patient.

CASE STUDY 8.1 | **Choosing How to Think About a Challenging Situation**

RACISM

Gloria Sikapite is an adult student nurse at the University of Hertfordshire who has experienced racism from patients. This is how she processes her emotions:

'If you see my colour and you feel you don't want to be around me, that's a "you" problem not a "me" problem.'
'I got slapped by somebody's son ... I decided that it was up to me to decide how that would affect me and I decided that I won't force myself on anyone but I'll let them know what they're missing out on.'
'A few patients have made comments and what I always say is if you feel my colour will affect in any way my care for you, let me know, and we will try and find somebody who you feel can give you the care that you need. But I should let you know that I don't think you can get a better person to care for you.'

(Note that NHS Trusts and universities have zero-tolerance policies on racism and experiences like Gloria's should always be reported—see Mitchell 2019.)

Gloria makes a conscious choice about how she will interpret a highly charged situation (Case Study 8.1). She shows great self-belief, something she says was instilled in her by her parents and that she now passes on to her own children.

Viktor Frankl, the Austrian psychotherapist who wrote the famous book *Man's Search for Meaning* (1959) following his internment in a concentration camp in the Second World War, declared that the final freedom that a person has is the freedom to be able to choose their attitude to conditions in their life. This freedom became a basic tenet of 'logotherapy', Frankl's psychotherapeutic approach based on the idea that a person's primary motivational force is to find meaning in their life.

■ Time Out

Think about a challenging situation that you have faced recently at home or at work. How did you feel? In what way could you have chosen to adopt a more positive way to think about it?

Staying Under the Radar

Many student nurses may say that it is better to stay under the radar and not speak up, as it will only cause trouble for them if they do. But there is a price to pay in terms of the growing feeling that you are taken for granted/disrespected/abused or that people in your care or colleagues may be harmed. Resentment may rise and this may lead to disengagement and further affect relationships at work and even the way care is provided.

Being an undergraduate is often a difficult position, but it is also an opportunity to try things out and maybe learn by getting things wrong. This means exposing yourself to vulnerability (Brown 2010), which is part of being authentic. This is the time that you can learn from experience and prepare yourself for life as a registered nurse.

Problems With Speaking Truth to Power

'We need to stop trying to "fix the silenced" and rather "fix the system". This requires us to focus more time and resources on enabling those who are in perceived positions of power to skilfully invite those silenced to speak and then in turn listen up themselves.'

REITZ AND HIGGINS (2020)

Reitz and Higgins undertook research into why health workers did not speak out about problems in their organisations. Their surveys found that 40% of UK health care respondents claimed they knew, or may know something important that, if known about, could negatively impact their organisations. Forty-three percent of these respondents had not spoken up formally about their concerns.

Power imbalance is at the bottom of this. The top reasons for not speaking up are that the person will be perceived negatively followed by the fear of upsetting or embarrassing another person.

Unsurprisingly, they discovered that the more junior you are, the less likely you are to speak up and that there is a 'superiority illusion': that people think that it is not them that is the problem—it is everyone else. They also discovered that leaders believe that people speak up more often than they do, and that the more senior you are (and especially if you are male), the more you believe that there will be positive consequences from speaking up.

The advice that Reitz and Higgins gives is that it is up to the leaders of the system to change how they operate:

- Assume that they are scarier than they think they are and listen, not just in formal meetings, but use a variety of forums and situations to listen.
- Question who they listen to, and look out for unconscious bias by noticing how they respond to different voices.
- Watch their body language to avoid inadvertently sending out 'shut up' messages such as raising an eyebrow or looking bored.

The message here for student nurses is that leaders will underestimate the problems associated with speaking up safely in the organisations that you study or work in. As you become more senior you need to be on the lookout for unconscious bias and find ways to make it less intimidating for others to speak up.

Be a Role Model

'If you are treating somebody like that, it's your choice. But you've also influenced that person. They won't come back and work with you.'

GLORIA SIKAPITE, ADULT STUDENT NURSE, TALKING
ABOUT HER EXPERIENCE OF POOR LEADERSHIP

If you are developing your leadership skills to lead a team, the first thing is to be able to role model some basic behaviours, such as:

- managing your expectations;
- being assertive; and
- managing your own behaviours by using your emotional intelligence (being aware of your own feelings and managing them).

As well as role modelling, you can also watch out for peers or members of your team who may need support to manage conflict and pass on these skills. Let us take these one by one.

Manage Your Expectations

You cannot change people's basic personality, but you can influence them to change their behaviour (Jay 2001). So, if you are an organised person working with someone who is laid back and slightly disorganised, then you must accept that they will never be like you. It is your expectations of the person that will disappoint you rather than the person, and this can cause resentments and frustrations (Tips Box 8.1).

Sort Out Your Ego

Your ego can get in the way of being objective, and you will focus on being right instead of being true. The conversation will focus on your frustration or anger towards the other person, who will feel attacked and fight back, making resolution harder to achieve (Sandford online).

TIPS BOX 8.1

Building Cooperation

- Helping people feel understood and respected in this way will build cooperation.
- Lower your expectations. Say 'I know that sometimes you struggle with time-keeping (you might want to add a mitigation that you know of, such as coping with a young baby or travelling on the bus) but when we meet next week it would really help if you could arrive on time'.
- Be specific with your requests, and limit the number of specific requests at a time to two or three.

Be Assertive

If you feel that people overlook you, lose their temper to get their own way, criticise you (Case Study 8.2), get impatient when you do not grasp concepts quickly, or beg favours and make it hard to say no, then the chances are that you need to develop your skills of assertiveness.

Being assertive is about treating others as equals and expecting the same in return. Practising assertiveness will mean that you are treated with more respect, although it will not be a cure-all for more difficult personalities (Tips Box 8.2).

TIPS BOX 8.2

Be Assertive

- Express your feelings. Start the conversation by saying 'I feel…' rather than attacking the behaviour directly by saying something like 'I really hate it when you' or 'Please don't.' So for example, you may say 'I feel angry when you don't allow me to express my views.'
- Be honest, but not rude. 'I disagree' is quite confrontational for example, compared to 'I have reservations about this, and I think it needs rethinking.'
- Stand your ground and do not be intimidated. So for example, if a colleague is trying to get you to support an idea that you think is truly dreadful, say 'I'm sorry I can't support it.' If they insist, keep saying 'I'm sorry, I'd like to be able to support it, but I can't.'
- If people ask you to do something that you do not want to, then say no and add a simple explanation such as 'I'm sorry, I can't. I have an assignment due in 2 days.' If you feel guilty you might say 'David's good at that, why not ask him?' but take care to choose someone who is assertive enough to say no too!
- Start with being assertive over minor points with colleagues who are easier to handle before tackling really difficult people over more emotive issues!

Adapted from Jay (2001).

CASE STUDY 8.2	Managing Conflict With Emotional Intelligence

BEING BULLIED

Tom (not his real name) was in his first role as a newly registered learning disability nurse. On the unit was a female band 6 nurse who had worked in the prison service. In the first couple of weeks, on three occasions when he was speaking, she put her hand up in front of him to stop him speaking. He asked a colleague about it, and he said that 'She does that to everyone' but Tom thought it was so rude.

He admits that he, a grown man, felt like crying with frustration and he knew that he had to sort it out because it had made him feel so weak. He kept beating himself up thinking 'You should have said this, you should have said that' but he realised that if he had spoken in that moment, he might not have been able to control himself and would have regretted it.

Having thought it over, he emailed her, giving the dates of the three occasions that she put up her hand and gave the names of staff who had witnessed it. He explained what he was trying to achieve and how her actions had made him feel.

He offered her opportunity to meet and clear the air. In his mind he knew that what he was doing was making it clear to her that he had a trail of evidence and was making efforts to solve the problem between them early and informally.

The nurse replied by email saying that she was really sorry that she had made him feel like that and promised that they would sit down together. But they did not meet and the behaviour stopped. Tom thought he did not need the meeting because she had realised what she would done. His confidence improved as he realised how well he had handled things.

But several weeks later Tom came across a patient who was becoming very aggressive—punching and kicking. Tom decided that the best approach was to defuse the situation by inviting the patient to go with him for a cup of tea and talk it over, in a safe area. The same nurse came along and told Tom to restrain the patient, but Tom thought that this escalation was not needed and indeed his approach had demonstrated that he had successfully calmed the situation.

When he left the patient, the nurse challenged him in front of staff, saying that he had not done as she had said. As a junior member of staff Tom felt very uncomfortable in responding to her publicly, so he invited her to talk about it away from the ward. They exchanged their points of view, and Tom explained that he was the first person there and his assessment of the situation was that he thought that the patient did not need restraining. He made reference to the trust's policy, which was to take the least restrictive approach. He invited her, as someone who had been doing the job for a long time and had experience, to take this forward if she was unhappy with his actions.

■ **Time Out**

What techniques did Tom use to assertively challenge the nurse?
What thought processes helped?

We covered leading with emotional intelligence in Section 1. In conflict situations, our emotions can run riot and we may respond uncharacteristically in the moment.

Tom was aware of emotions and kept them in check. He knew that he needed to challenge the behaviour and to do so in private. He talked about how the nurse's behaviour made him feel rather than complaining or labelling her a bully. He gave clear instances of her behaviour and he explained his own actions, with reference to organisational policy. He gave her space to reply. See Tips Box 8.3 for more advice on how to manage conflict.

TIPS BOX 8.3

Manage Conflict

• Show integrity. Have difficult conversations in private and face to face. Email, text or WhatsApp conflicts rarely resolve anything and can escalate. Tom used email as a tool for invitation but not discussion.

- Be mindful. Conflict can make us feel sad, angry or frustrated. Take a look at what is happening to your emotions before you respond.
- Decide in advance (if you can) the key points that you want to make. Avoid exaggerations 'You're always talking over me', labels 'You're such a moaner' or judgements 'You're hopeless with data'.
- Focus on yourself and not them. A good sentence structure might be:

  When you ____ I feel ____ because ____. It would be great if _____. If you take for example the common problem of being called 'the student', the sentence might be 'When you refer to me as "the student" I feel like I have no value because it indicates that the team doesn't see me as an individual. It would be great if you could call me Jane.'
- Focus on how they behave, not how they (in your view) are, and be able to give actual instances. For example, 'I've been working here for 4 weeks and I've not been called Jane or "student nurse" McGregor once.'
- Now let the other person have their say. Part of compassionate leadership is listening, so do not get so wrapped up in your emotions and what you are going to say that you forget to listen to other people's point of view.
- Remain open and avoid judging, especially in the heat of the moment.
- Stay calm and think before you speak. Do not get carried away and say something that you may regret.
- Some may find staying calm harder than others, so if you feel that you cannot stay calm, then remove yourself from the situation.
- If you are too emotional to express your feelings, then do not speak at all. Say something like 'I don't feel happy about this, I'll talk to you later'.
- Stick to the facts. Do not become defensive or apportion blame.
- Suggest a solution and see how the other person feels. For example, 'Putting my name on the board when I am on shift rather than "student" will help people to remember my name, because I know people are really busy and may forget.'
- Ask for help if needed. A colleague or placement supervisor can support you or act as a mediator as long as they are unbiased, can set ground rules and can help you to identify what you both want out of it.
- Reflect on what you learnt.
- If the situation continues after your informal attempts to resolve it do not work, consult your organisation's bullying and harassment policy and involve the human resources (HR) team from the beginning.

Adapted from Jay (2001).

Giving Feedback Assertively

We discussed delegation in the chapter on teamwork but how, perhaps as part of a management assessment, do you assertively give feedback (Tips Box 8.4) to a team member who has not performed as you wished, as well as stand up for yourself? One of the biggest issues mentioned by students participating in the book was handling health care assistants who had high standing in the clinical team but just did not respect them.

TIPS BOX 8.4

Giving Feedback

- Collect all of the facts and speak to them in a place that you will not be overheard.
- Focus on the problem, not the person.

Continued

- State the problem objectively using 'I' statements rather than 'you'. Do not bring emotion, blame or shame into it. For example, 'Sharon, I asked you to help Mrs Smith, Simmonds and Ali to get washed and dressed, but they aren't ready.'
- State what you need and expect. 'I asked you to do this so that they would be ready for their X ray appointments at 10.30.'
- Ask if anything is wrong that you should be aware of and listen with empathy if the conversation looks like there may be underlying issues.
- If they say something sarcastic like 'nothing is wrong with me' then you must be strong and point out that this is not what you see. Let them know that their behaviour is not acceptable.
- Stay calm and show that you have listened to what they have said by recapping the conversation. 'I'm sorry to hear that Mrs Gartside was being sick and you had to deal with this first. What I suggest is that if you are running short on time that you let me know and we can get you help.'
- Point out their strengths and give examples of where their performance has been good. 'You're a really thoughtful person and I can see that Mrs Gartside looks settled now.'
- State how you see the issue being resolved. 'But next time you're running behind please let me know in good time.'
- Make notes on what you did and said in case they challenge what you did later.
- Do not share what you discussed unless requested by the ward manager or your practice supervisor.

Being Assertive in Team Meetings and Situations

There are quite a few tools that can be used to raise concerns in team meetings and enable discussion. One of these is about enabling your team to 'cus', which generally is not a good thing(!) but in this instance may be vital.

CUS stands for:

- Concerned
- Uncomfortable
- Safety

If a team member says 'I am concerned about...', then this is a trigger word to direct the team's attention and encourage members to listen closely to what the team member is concerned about.

If the issue is not resolved and the team member then says 'I am uncomfortable because...', then this is a further trigger to escalate and flag the matter, which may have been missed or overlooked that may turn into an error or dangerous situation. (Notice again that these are both sentences starting with 'I' rather than bringing in any personalities.)

Finally, if a team member says 'This is a safety issue', then the team must stop and evaluate what is happening.

Managing Conflict in Teams

It is the responsibility of the team leader to set the tone and ensure that the team is well run. Poorly run teams are more likely to experience conflicts. This means returning to the chapter on the basic features of effective teams and ensuring that:

- the aim and objectives of the team are understood by all;
- roles are well defined and understood, and team members are interdependent;
- constructive challenge is welcomed and understood; and
- the team takes time out to reflect.

In addition, it is important to identify any personal issues that might be troubling a team member by being open and approachable.

If you discover early on that there are allegations of violence and aggression, bullying, harassment or discrimination, you may want to stop at this point and consult your organisation's HR team, look up your organisation's policy and seek help.

One of the most common reasons for conflict in teams is personality clashes, and in this situation it is wise to offer to act as mediator (with their agreement) to bring the two parties together. If you see them separately, they may wonder what you said to the other or they may misrepresent what you said to them.

Mediation and Negotiation

Mediation and negotiation are both methods to resolve issues between parties and gain agreement. Sometimes the terms are used interchangeably, but they mean different things; to draw out some of the main differences and similarities, refer to Table 8.1; refer to Tips Box 8.5 for mediation guidance.

TABLE 8.1 ■ The Main Differences Between Mediation and Negotiation.

Mediation Example: Resolving Differences Between Two Team Members	Negotiation Example: Nursing Union Negotiations for a Pay Rise
This is a facilitation of a discussion between partners in dispute.	Parties agree to meet directly with each other—no intermediary.
Mediator is neutral and impartial, not involved in any decisions or agreement.	Parties seek common ground to reach agreement.
Mediator can meet each side separately and/or meet with both.	Parties in a disagreement meet directly with each other.
Primary goal is to gain understanding of the other parties' perspective, which may lead to a longer-lasting resolution.	Primary goal is to reach a compromise and agreement.
It is more likely to reach a win:win agreement.	It is more likely to reach a win:lose agreement.

TIPS BOX 8.5

Mediation Between Two People

- Collect all of the facts (including any personal issues) in advance and speak to them in a place that you will not be overheard.
- Create a relaxed, informal atmosphere when nobody feels under any time pressure.
- Explain that your role is to ensure harmony in the team to enable it to achieve its objectives. Your role is to focus on addressing the issues to get the team back on track, without allocating blame. Do not offer any opinions, even if you think someone is being unreasonably difficult.
- Invite them, in turn, to use the same assertive feedback techniques covered earlier:
  - Allow each other to finish.
  - Focus on the problem, not the person.
  - State the problem objectively using 'I' statements rather 'you'.
  - Do not bring emotion, blame or shame into it.
  - State what they need and expect—the other listens.
  - Show that they have listened to what the other person has said by recapping the conversation.

Continued

- Do not finish the meeting until the participants make an agreement about how issues will be resolved.
- Agreements should be mutual. Be on the lookout for one party making more concessions than the other. If one party is coerced, they are unlikely to follow the agreement.
- Be cooperative if you are asked to help with aspects such as reassigning tasks, reviewing priorities or setting timescales.
- Make a follow-up date to review progress. At this meeting thank them for any progress made.

Based on Jay (2001).

NEGOTIATION

Nurses negotiate every day with their patients, with families, with colleagues and with other departments and teams. When a nurse tries to help somebody to give up smoking or stick to their medication regimes, this is negotiation, so it is really important as a student nurse leader to understand the basics of negotiating (Tips Box 8.6) (Case Study 8.3).

CASE STUDY 8.3   **Barbara Stilwell, Nurse, Researcher and Academic**

'When I first went to WHO [World Health Organisation] 28 years ago I was incredibly intimidated because everybody was a doctor, everybody was a man and nobody wanted to listen to a nurse. They were actually quite rude sometimes. But I discovered that I had a superpower which nobody else had in WHO, and my superpower was listening. I had been trained for my entire career both in nursing and psychology to listen to what people were saying because it provides clues to making a plan.

So I would sit and listen because that was the one thing I knew that I could do really well. When we got to the end of meetings and there had been conflict and stuff going on I would say "Well it sounds like there are three things going on here. Here they are and how about doing this to resolve this thing." Everybody would go "How did you do that, it's amazing!"

WHO said would you like to train as a negotiator for us? So they sent me on the negotiation course at Harvard [University], and it was only because I listened. And I went on this course like other people who negotiated things like peace in the Middle East went on, and I qualified as a negotiator.

I would say if anybody has an opportunity to go on a formal negotiation course they should do it, because it really teaches you how to look for people's vested interests and what they want.

And I would say to student nurses that you are coming from a position of powerlessness, but in another way you are very powerful because you are the workforce of the future and it's in the interests of the NHS to keep you as a student and to keep you as a nurse.'

TIPS BOX 8.6

Develop Your Negotiation Skills

- Nursing, as Barbara says, is all about listening. We have looked at this already, but when you are in the middle of a difficult discussion and maybe you strongly believe that you are right, then you may forget.
- Consider your alternatives. In negotiating parlance, this is called a BATNA (best alternative to a negotiated agreement). This is defined as the most advantageous alternative if the agreement that you are looking for fails. This is a common negotiating tactic that is considered before the negotiation begins. At the national level, you may see nursing unions discuss their BATNA before going into pay negotiations. They will discuss internally the minimum percentage increase in salary that they think their members will accept, after which they may, for example, ballot on industrial action. If you want to negotiate a development in a student-led

initiative, such as the development of a Twitter account that you are involved in and it fails, you have to think about the alternative, which may for example be that you walk away. Consider too what the other party wants and needs and what their BATNA may be.

- Do your homework. Find out as much as you can about the other party. So, if you want to negotiate a role on a particular committee and you need to convince the other party that you are the best person, then research on what they do, identify who is on the committee, read their reports and so on.
- Break the negotiation down if there are several issues to be resolved. For example, your first job offer in another part of the country may need a negotiation about relocation expenses, courses that can be offered and so on.
- Avoid issuing ultimatums, such as 'If you don't lose weight we will have to...' This makes people feel that they are being backed into a corner.
- Paraphrase the other person's words. This helps to show that you are listening and checks that you heard them correctly. It also helps to correct any misunderstandings and it gives you time to think.
- Be curious and ask questions about the other person's position such as 'What is concerning you here?' or 'Why is this so important to you?'. This will help uncover the other person's values and beliefs.
- Focus on facts rather than persuasion, such as '70% of student nurses say that not knowing their shifts in advance is causing them stress, and 30% are considering leaving their courses,' rather than 'We really need our shifts 3 weeks in advance.'
- Find common grounds where you agree. So, for instance, you may both agree on the importance of student welfare, in the example of knowing shift patterns.
- Skilled negotiators are polite. Beginning a negotiation on a negative will encourage the other party to be negative. Use your emotional intelligence to read the emotions of the other party and manage your own emotions. This helps to build your relationship.
- Be honest and show integrity. This will help to build the relationship.
- Timing is important. For example, when applying for a job as a health care assistant do not try to negotiate for a higher hourly rate until you have been offered the job.

Based on Principles and Tactics of Negotiation (2007).

Asking for What You Want

'Yes is the destination; no is how you get there.'
RICHARD FENTON AND ANDREA WALTZ, AUTHORS OF *GO OR NO GO*

▨ Time Out

On a scale of 1 (impossible) to 10 (very easy), how easy is it for you to ask for what you want? How do you react when your requests are rejected or ignored?

Maybe you have responded that it is hard for you to ask for things and that you are afraid that people will say no and that you will feel rejected. This is the topic of a book called *Go for No* (2010) written by Fenton and Waltz, which follows the story of a fictional salesman called Eric Bratton.

Student participants on the #150Leaders programme talked repeatedly about 'putting their hand up' for opportunities to develop themselves as leaders or asking for help, but asking for what you want could be alien to you. Alternatively, you may be confused about what you could potentially ask for (such as 'Will you mentor me? Can I go to this event? Can I arrange a placement here?') and whether you, as a student nurse, could ask for it.

This may be part of the self-concept of seeing yourself as 'just a student' or perhaps an uncertainty about how the system works. But as we have seen, putting yourself outside your comfort zone as a leader can make your comfort zone larger, as you gain more confidence and broaden your network of connections.

'Going for no' is a selling technique where the idea is that the more times you successfully survive a rejection, the more you will 'numb' yourself to the emotional sting. This is about developing the right mindset to handle and respond to rejection and build your courage and confidence. Eventually the more you ask, the more you will succeed.

This is reminiscent of Frankl's idea of choosing how you respond to situations and developing a 'winning mindset'.

The Rise of Radical and Rebel Leadership

Over the last few years, several books have been published about being a radical or a rebel leader. Some have transformed into social movements both in and around the NHS, and so it is helpful for student nurse leaders to have some awareness of what they are and their history, especially if you identify as someone who wants to disrupt the status quo.

The School for Organisational Radicals was set up in the NHS in 2004 based on the realisation that radical change was rarely achieved by top-down leadership and that it was more about empowering change from the ground up. It offered grass roots activists 1-day courses on the tools and techniques needed to undertake various improvements. The focus was on sharing knowledge about improvement methods and how to create social movements.

In 2014 the school changed its name to the School for Health and Care Radicals (SHCR) to acknowledge the importance of health and social care working better together. The school was delivered as a massive open online course (MOOC) open to anyone in the world. Members were encouraged to become organisational radicals by developing the capability to 'rock the boat and stay in it' to understand how organisations work and to learn how to create change using well-known theories of change.

Rebels at Work

The work of the SHCR was heavily influenced by a book called *Rebels at Work* (2015) by Kelly and Medina, in which they share their own experience of being rebels at work and give practical advice to others.

'Rebel' is often synonymous with troublemaking, so Kelly and Medina are keen to point out that there is a difference between good and bad rebels (Box 8.1), so we shall start here because it is very important that student leaders who are keen for change do it to create new and better ways to do things rather than just rail against the system.

■ **Time Out**

Think of someone who is good at getting new ideas adopted. Look at the characteristics of good and bad rebels listed in Box 8.1 and think how they apply to that person. What can you learn from them?

Not everyone will identify themselves as a 'rebel'—they may simply care deeply about their organisation, their peers or their patients, and may feel compelled to act when their concerns reach a tipping point. Rebel actions may be large or small—or may start out small and often accidental and explode: you will remember that Brian Dolan just sent one tweet about his frustrations about pyjamas being a patient's uniform and this grew into the social movement called #EndPJParalysis.

Case Study 8.4 is an example from one student nurse leader who took the initiative during the COVID-19 pandemic in 2020.

BOX 8.1 ■ The Characteristics of Good and Bad Rebels

Bad Rebels	Good Rebels
■ Complain	■ Create
■ 'Me' focused	■ Mission focused
■ Pessimist	■ Optimist
■ Anger	■ Passion
■ Energy sapping	■ Energy generating
■ Alienate	■ Attract
■ Problems	■ Possibilities
■ Vocalise problems	■ Socialise opportunities
■ Worry that...	■ Wonder if...
■ Point fingers	■ Pinpoint causes
■ Obsessed	■ Reluctant
■ Lecture	■ Listen

Kelly, L., Medina, C., 2015. Rebels at Work. O'Reilly Media Inc., Sebastapol.

CASE STUDY 8.4 Think Theory

During the 2020/2021 COVID-19 pandemic, student nurses across the United Kingdom had their studies and clinical placements interrupted as they waited to find out what would happen. Universities scrambled to develop online study capabilities, almost 'going into meltdown' according to one tutor, to get this done in a timely manner.

At the start of the pandemic, second- and third-year student nurses in the last 6 months of their training in the United Kingdom were given the option to go through emergency registration with the NMC and be paid to work in clinical areas or remain on a 'theory-only' route, meaning that they focused on their studies and did not go on their clinical placements.

The messages about which students would be called forward kept changing, and some students reported that communication from universities about when and how they would continue with their lectures was poor.

Many students battled during this time to work through their choices and their feelings. Some grieved for the interruption in their studies on courses that they had often fought hard to gain. Others expressed concern about how they would make up for lost time. Students fretted over whether to work in a clinical setting if they had an underlying long-term condition and risked infecting either themselves or vulnerable family members. Feelings of guilt about not being able to help out were common.

Brian Webster, a student on the adult pathway at the University of Dundee, decided to take the initiative to support those who chose the theory-only route. He set up the website https://thinktheory19. wixsite.com/website and a Twitter account called @ThinkTheory19. Brian was mentored by a senior nurse who helped and supported him to deliver the Think Theory project as a support network for those students that chose the online theory route. Brian described it as 'a place to connect students from across the UK, share skills and experiences and make lifelong relationships'.

Brian created a short survey on the Think Theory website (Webster 2020) to ascertain the pressures on students in making their decisions and how students felt in taking their decisions. Brian said, 'The feedback I got was, with the focus on the students opting in, that those who hadn't had been forgotten about. Students felt glad to be noticed again.'

The answers indicated that most expressed guilt about not opting to work, and they felt anxious and unsupported. Students appreciated these surveys because they allowed them to feel that they were not alone in feeling as they did.

The website included prerecorded vlogs from nursing leaders that included messages emphasising that no choice was the 'wrong' choice. Brian adds 'The students really took a lot from the nurse leaders' messages. It was ok their friends and families saying "don't worry, it's your choice", but hearing that from the likes of the chief executive of the Nursing and Midwifery Council and world-recognised professors really gave them the confidence in their choice and alleviated some of the worries and fears they had.'

Brian did have some pushback on the design of his survey from one commentator who said it was biased towards encouraging negative feedback and did not allow students to fully express their views. They added that everyone involved in supporting the students was going through an unprecedented time and this should be taken into account. Brian's response was one of openness, publishing not only the criticism but also all of the free-text responses to his questionnaire.

How do you know that you are a rebel? Kelly and Medina suggest that rebels have three common tendencies (Kelly and Medina 2015):

1. They are future thinkers and are energised by creating possibilities rather than achieving certainty.
2. They see emerging trends early and think further ahead.
3. They come from different backgrounds or cultures, and so bring different ways of thinking.

Persuading Senior People About Your Ideas

The key to successfully presenting your ideas is to understand the organisation and its goals, build supporters and understand risks (Tips Box 8.7).

TIPS BOX 8.7

Persuading Tactics

The key to successfully presenting your ideas is to understand the organisation and its goals, build supporters and understand risks:

- Show how your idea supports the organisation's values, objectives, policy, etc. rather than your own. For example, students' ability to self-roster will aid retention rates and save staff time (rather than just focusing on supporting student wellbeing).
- Be open about risks (we shall address how to do a risk assessment of projects in Section 3). Find out about what most concerns the person/department that you are speaking to first so that you can address them in your risk assessment. For example, if budgetary control is a concern and you want to introduce a more expensive wound dressing to the formulary, then present data on how wound-healing rates will increase, reducing the need for frequent dressing changes and staff time.
- Seek to understand the perspective of others by talking it through with them early and understanding the likelihood of your idea succeeding. This can save lots of wasted time and energy.
- Find out how decisions are made and who you might approach to get on the agenda so you can access those who make these decisions. For example, in general practice you might speak to the practice manager who tells you that there is a monthly meeting and that agenda items need to be submitted to them a week in advance.
- Understand business planning cycles. In the NHS, planning cycles usually start around December ready for the start of the financial year on 1st April. The last 3 months of the financial year (January to March) are the time, if you need funding, that any budgetary underspends are addressed.
- Plan what you are going to say in meetings and have a goal in mind.
- If you are a future thinker, outlining the whole plan may confuse or scare people. It might be best to summarise your ideas and present the safe first step.
- Never criticise senior people who have concerns about your ideas.
- Never go over their heads.
- Ask direct questions like 'I sense that this idea isn't a priority for you. What could I do to make it one?'
- Build a rebel alliance. Sharing ideas and taking on board suggestions can make your case stronger. If your colleagues do not support the idea, then you may have to rethink it. A group presenting a case is stronger than an individual, and you will be taken more seriously. Rebel alliances can be formed by just inviting colleagues for coffee, through to setting up tweet chats and Google hangouts, introducing an item at your university nursing society or via your professional body's forum.
- Act in a trustworthy way by doing what you say you will, admitting mistakes and being respectful.

(Kelly and Medina 2015)

Be More Pirate

Be More Pirate: Or How to Take on the World and Win (Coniffe 2019) is a book that uses the analogy of pirate leadership and presents their traits as inspiration for entrepreneurs working in the 21st century. The author compares the pirate's traits with those of the cooperation movement, where disaffected communities rebelled against injustices by cooperating under a democratic 'pirate code'. Both pirates and cooperatives, Coniffe claims, challenge and express their political discontent to the establishment to create a more equal society. Modern-day cooperatives express their rebelliousness by challenging the 'normal' way of conducting business and seeking to offer a more socially focused alternative.

Nesta, a UK innovation foundation, had championed the Be More Pirate movement that has emerged following reports of readers breaking rules. Nesta sees the approach as a way of making social change by tackling health inequalities, shifting the balance of power in the workplace and increasing organisational sustainability (Alli and Lloyd 2019).

The approach is about knowing which rules to break, rewriting the rules, creating agile and dynamic systems that respond quickly and redistributing the power to avoid its abuse.

Of course, there is a long tradition of students breaking rules; perhaps the most famous being the 1989 Tiananmen Square protests, which were student-led demonstrations calling for democracy, free speech and a free press in China. However, clinical rules usually have a good evidence base and should not be broken without expert supervision.

Nonviolent Struggle

If you are part of a student union or trade union, you may be interested in learning more about nonviolent protest. One of the best resources around is *Blueprint for Revolution* (2015) by Srdja Popovic, who was a Serbian activist and a member of Otpor!, a student movement that helped to topple Serbian president Slobodan Milošević. This fascinating book gives real-life case studies illustrating creative ways to undertake nonviolent struggle based on the work of American political scientist Gene Sharp (1973), who identified 198 methods of nonviolent action. I have added a link that lists these methods in the resources section.

One example is how an Israeli insurance salesman called Itzig Alrov took on the fight against the rising cost of living by starting a cottage cheese protest on Facebook. Once the Israeli government withdrew a national subsidy for this basic and important part of the Israeli diet, the cost soared from 4 to 8 shekels. Alrov chose the price of cottage cheese as a symbol of capitalism and started a national boycott, resulting in cheese going mouldy on supermarket shelves. Eventually the manufacturers, forced with falling profits, relented and reduced the price to 5 shekels.

After seeing this small battle won, Israeli students were emboldened to launch their own Facebook page to start a campaign against the high cost of housing. They took their tents and pitched them in one of Tel Aviv's loveliest suburbs to say that they would live on the streets until rents were made affordable. Hundreds of thousands of people joined in the demonstrations. Eventually the government capitulated, and recommendations about affordable rents were signed into law.

This book and Sharp's methods may provide inspiration for your own nonviolent protests.

▦ Time Out

Investigate the nonviolent protests that are currently going on in your community and compare them to the list of Sharp's methods in the resources section. Which are being used? Are they working? What other methods could they use?

In my own community, the most obvious one that I can see is about redeveloping a local green spot into housing and industrial developments and the knock-on concern about air quality. The methods used petitions, protests, banners, posters and lobbying, meaning plenty of scope for more entrepreneurial ideas!

Leadership and Learning From High-Profile Failures

'Far better it is to dare mighty things, to win glorious triumphs, even though checkered by failure, than to take rank with those poor spirits who neither enjoy much nor suffer much, because they live in the grey twilight that knows not victory nor defeat.'

THEODORE ROOSEVELT

Reviews of high-profile failures in care, such as those at Bristol Royal Infirmary and the North Staffordshire NHS Foundation Trust, point towards problems in terms of leadership, resulting in cultures and systems that allow poor care. A summary of some of the reasons behind care failures is given in Box 8.2.

BOX 8.2 ■ Commonly Identified Causes of Care Failings

- Disconnection between clinical leaders and boards
- Lack of visible leadership and supervision of more junior staff
- Boards failing to proactively seek assurance and proactively plan services
- A focus on achieving targets at the expense of patient care, with associated bullying cultures to achieve targets
- Poor accountability and decision-making structures
- Staff shortages and an inappropriate skill mix
- The issues above leading to poor morale and motivation, leading to:
  - Falling standards of care
  - Poor communication with patients and families
  - Inadequate complaints handling
  - Inhibition of whistleblowing

Based on Academy of Medical Royal Colleges and Faculties in Scotland (Scottish Academy) (2015).

Trzeciak and Mazzarelli (2019) identified three hallmarks of burnout:
- A lack of personal accomplishment (the feeling that one can make a difference);
- Emotional exhaustion (being emotionally depleted and overextended); and
- Depersonalisation (an inability to make a personal connection).

When depersonalisation is combined with emotional exhaustion, it culminates in 'compassion fatigue'—literally running out of compassion for patients (Trzeciak and Mazzarelli 2019). We shall discuss more on the culture of compassion in leadership—and the lack thereof—in the chapter on systems and culture, but it seems clear that failing organisations tend to lack compassion for their people, which has a knock-on effect on how staff then care for their patients because they may have run out of compassion.

Anne-Marie Dodson, a senior lecturer at Birmingham City University, teaches her students about what was learnt from the Francis inquiry into failures in care at North Staffordshire NHS Foundation Trust. She explains that after the trust and the unions were investigated, the investigation moved onto the local universities and the students, who were asked what they had seen and whether they raised concerns. This illustrates that students are a powerful resource for asking questions when they may see poor standards of care. Robert Francis made several recommendations about ensuring that the focus of student nurses' interest in nursing was on compassionate, hands-on care. These include:

- Recruiting students to nursing courses based on their values, attitudes and behaviours;
- An ability to demonstrate a passion for nursing and a caring nature;
- A minimum requirement of 3 months spent in direct patient care under the supervision of a registered nurse before applying; and
- An aptitude test to ensure that a potential student nurse was willing to undertake hands-on care rather than just the technical aspects.

Based on Entwistle (2013).

Raising Concerns as Student Nurses

Student nurses can be powerful when they share concerns, because when concerns are shared and collated, they form a pattern that can be acted upon.

Anne-Marie shared an example of a student from her university who did speak up about standards of care that she had witnessed on placement, which resulted in the chief nurse suspending staff pending investigation, the ward being closed and students being moved out.

As a result of the Francis report, in 2015 the NMC updated its code to take account of some of the findings and recommendations. The new code includes a focus on delivering the fundamentals of care, a duty of candour (being open and honest when things go wrong), responsible social media use and the requirement for all nurses to raise concerns about patient safety and to act on concerns.

The NMC also updated its guidelines on how to raise concerns.

■ Time Out

These NMC guidelines on how to raise a concern outline the actions that student nurses should take if they identify a concern.

Find the publication on the NMC website by searching for 'Raising concerns: Guidance for nurses, midwives and nursing associates'.

Make a note of the actions that student nurses should take: who to inform, who to seek help from and where to get advice.

Section 8 of the guidance states:

8.1 Inform your mentor, tutor or lecturer immediately if you believe that you, a colleague or anyone else may be putting someone at risk of harm.

8.2 Seek help immediately from an appropriately qualified professional if someone for whom you are providing care has suffered harm for any reason.

8.3 Seek help from your mentor, tutor or lecturer if people indicate that they are unhappy about their care or treatment.

The most important thing is that you find someone to talk to in either your placement, university or professional body or trade union. There is also a whistleblowing charity called Protect (https://protect-advice.org.uk/).

The Public Interest Disclosure Act 1998 enables nurses and midwives to make protected disclosures to the NMC and other organisations, protecting them from retaliation or victimisation when they raise concerns (Case Study 8.5). As of 6 April 2015, this protection was extended to student nurses and midwives.

CASE STUDY 8.5   **Helene Donnelly**

'As nurses and midwives, let's unite as a body of professionals who do care. And by doing so, we will expose those who do not.'

HELENE DONNELLY, ambassador for cultural change at Staffordshire and Stoke-On-Trent Partnership NHS Trust

As a newly registered nurse she raised concerns at Mid Staffordshire Hospital around failures in care. She was instrumental in the instigation of the Francis Enquiry and the NMC's subsequent publication of guidance on raising concerns.

▣ Time Out

Conduct a search on NMC's website (https://www.nmc.org.uk/) to discover Helene's story and how she was able to influence the nursing and midwifery profession. Make a note of the leadership skills that she demonstrates.

How have current local leaders responded to her story?

Helene's story displays compassion, bravery and communication skills, both written and verbal. It describes how she observed what was happening, listened to fellow nurses and pieced together an understanding of how what she was witnessing related to the culture and the system that she and others were working in. Helene showed concern for patients and colleagues and a values-based dogged determination to see through what she identified as a cover-up, even when she had left the hospital.

The leaders in the trust that she now works in could have perceived her as a troublemaker, but instead they have recognised her strength and skills. They offered her an appointment as an ambassador for cultural change within her trust, with an ability to go anywhere and speak to anyone (Tips Box 8.8).

TIPS BOX 8.8

Build a Learning Culture

- Accept and acknowledge that mistakes will be made—build trust and value honesty.
- Learn first, then take actions to improve and then share your learning with others. Do not apportion blame or cover your own back.
- Maintain hope and optimism when communicating, and be honest when you do not know the answer.
- Remember everyone is trying their best. Role model empathy and understanding.

Adapted from Allen (2020).

Summary

It is difficult for student nurses, in the early stages of their leadership careers, to have courageous conversations with peers and colleagues in teams. There is a price to pay, however, for those who choose to stay under the radar, where resentment and disengagement can grow and affect not only you but those around you and in your care. It is the responsibility of organisational leaders, however, to help staff to speak up safely and avoid trying to fix the staff before fixing the system.

Courageous conversations involve managing your expectations of others, practising your ability to be assertive and showing emotional intelligence, particularly about how you choose to think about situations. They start with expressing how you feel and why, and then listening to what the other person or people say and seeing if you can come to agreement. You can also become courageous in asking for what you want and managing your fear of rejection by 'going for no' and considering it as the pathway to yes.

Some of you may see yourselves as wanting to positively disrupt what you observe around you. There is a long history of fostering the talents of the rebel leader in the NHS, but there is a big difference between doing this from the position of disaffection and alienation versus those who strive optimistically for possibilities.

Visionary leaders can learn to align their ideas to those of their organisations, seek out the perspectives of others and start to plan for risks early. What also helps is developing a cooperative movement that can work together to change some outmoded rules using entrepreneurial methods, which can often start out as small wins.

Student nurses have a role to play in identifying and disclosing poor care. They are protected from retaliation and victimisation by an act of law. The NMC offers written guidance on what student nurses must do in this event.

Resources

Academy of Medical Royal Colleges and Faculties in Scotland (Scottish Academy), Short-Life Working Group on Hospital Reports, 2015. Learning from Serious Failings in Care.

Ali, M., 2018. Communication skills 6: difficult and challenging conversations. Nursing Times 114 (4), 51–53.

Stone, D., Patton, B., Heen, S., 2000. Difficult Conversations: How to Discuss What Matters Most. Penguin, London.

War Resisters International. Gene Sharp's 198 Methods of Nonviolent Action. <https://wri-irg.org/en/resources/2008/gene-sharps-198-methods-nonviolent-action>.

References

Allen, S., 2020. Creating space for compassion, empathy and learning. The King's Fund. <https://www.kingsfund.org.uk/publications/creating-space-compassion-empathy-learning>.

Alli, A., Lloyd, J., 2019. Does our Economy Need More Pirates? Nesta. <https://www.nesta.org.uk/blog/does-our-economy-need-more-pirates/>.

America Society for Clinical Oncology. Principles and tactics of negotiation, 2007. Journal of Oncology Practice, 3 (2), 102–105.

Brown, B., 2010. The Power of Vulnerability. TEDeX Houston. <https://www.ted.com/talks/brene_brown_the_power_of_vulnerability?utm_campaign=tedspread&utm_medium=referral&utm_source=tedcomshare>.

Coniffe, A., 2018. Be More Pirate: Or How to Take On the World and Win. Penguin, London.

Entwistle, F., 2013. Recommendations on student nurse training. Nursing Times 109 (13), 23.

Fenton, R., Waltz, A., 2010. Go for No. Courage Crafters, Orlando.

Frankl, V., 1959. Man's Search for Meaning. Beacon Press, Boston.

Jay, R., 2001. Fast Thinking: Difficult People. Pearson Education Limited, Harlow.

Kelly, L., Medina, C., 2015. Rebels at Work. O'Reilly Media Inc., Sebastapol.

Mitchell, G., 2019. Cut racism out of NHS patient contract, urges diversity champion. Nursing Times. <https://www.nursingtimes.net/news/policies-and-guidance/exclusive-cut-racism-out-of-nhs-patient-contract-urges-diversity-champion-08-11-2019/>.

Popovic, S., Miller, M., 2015. Blueprint for Revolution. Scribe Publications, London.

Reitz, M., Higgins, J., 2020. Speaking truth to power: why leaders cannot hear what they need to hear. British Medical Journal Leader. doi: 10.1136/leader-2020-000394.

Sandford, K., 7 Keys to Having a Courageous Conversation With Anyone. Lifehack. <https://www.lifehack.org/articles/productivity/7-keys-having-courageous-conversation-with-anyone.html>.

Trzeciak, S., Mazzarelli, D., 2019. Compassionomics: The Revolutionary Scientific Evidence That Caring Makes a Difference. Studer Group, Pensacola.

UK Government, 1998. Public Interest Disclosure Act 1998.

Webster, B., 2020. Survey Results. <https://thinktheory19.wixsite.com/website/post/survey-results>.

Using Power and Influence

OBJECTIVES

After reading this chapter and completing the activities, you should be able to:

- Define power and influence
- Describe different forms of power
- Differentiate between what you can influence and what you can control
- Utilise a range of influencing tactics
- Describe successful lobbying tactics
- Compare old and new power tactics and state when each might be appropriate
- Describe the three main roles in tipping point leadership
- Engage and support followers.

Relevance to the Nursing and Midwifery Council (NMC) Code

Promote Professionalism and Trust

Paragraph 25:

Provide leadership to make sure people's wellbeing is protected and to improve their experiences of the health and care system

Throughout their career, all our registrants will have opportunities to demonstrate leadership qualities, regardless of whether or not they occupy formal leadership positions.

This chapter is about understanding the sources of power and influence that student nurses can use when working with others.

The way that power and influence is used today is changing, and we shall discuss these ideas of 'old power' and 'new power' and when to use them. We shall investigate the types of people to look out for who can help us to be successful in influencing others, and we shall look at the importance of followership.

What Is Power and Influence?

Several definitions of power have been used in nursing. Power has been defined as having control, influence or domination over something or someone (Chandler 1992). Others define power as 'the ability to get things done, to mobilize resources, to get and use whatever it is that a person needs for the goals he or she is attempting to meet' (Kanter 1993). Power is the *capacity to* influence others to change someone's attitude or behaviour to get things done. Influence refers to any behaviour that attempts to alter someone's attitudes. Influence is therefore effectively 'power in motion'.

American social scientist and writer Rosabeth Moss Kanter has some words to say about powerlessness that may help students to understand certain behaviours that they may see:

> *'It is powerlessness that often creates ineffective, desultory management and petty, dictatorial, rules-minded managerial styles. Accountability without power—responsibility for results without the resources to get them—creates frustration and failure. People who see themselves as weak and powerless and find their subordinates resisting or discounting them tend to use more punishing forms of influence. If organisational power can "ennoble", then, recent research shows, organisational powerlessness can (with apologies to Lord Acton) "corrupt".'*

ROSABETH MOSS KANTER (1979)

Being Aware of What You Can Influence

Before we go much further, we need to discuss the difference between what we are concerned about, what we can influence and what we can control (Case Study 9.1).

Craig is obviously a very driven person who has reflected on his passion for nursing. He has recognised that it is not wise for him to spread himself too thinly. He has begun, with the help of his senior charge nurse, to differentiate between three things (Fig. 9.1) to help him to focus his efforts and manage his own wellbeing.

The first is his circle of concern: Craig is the sort of nurse who thinks very broadly about all the things that concern him but has realised that he cannot do anything about them.

Next comes the circle of influence: things that Craig could do something about, but he does not necessarily have control over. Craig mentions health inequity here.

CASE STUDY 9.1   **Circles of Influence**

Craig Davidson is a newly registered public health community staff nurse in an Asylum Health Bridging Team. Prior to this he worked on an infectious diseases ward. With his colleague and friend Clare Manley he records a regular podcast called *Retaining the Passion: Journeys Through Nursing*, where they discuss their journeys through nursing and shine a light on key issues affecting the nursing profession and wider society by speaking to various guests about their lived experiences. In one episode, he candidly discussed his thoughts on what he feels that he can influence:

'I'm not sure that I create a perfect work life balance for myself. There're so many things I want to change in the world, so I looked up circle of concern, influence and control. I think what I'm going to really spend time focusing on is ... looking less at my circle of concern. I will still have the things that I am passionate about ... one of which is our podcast and retaining the passion of nursing. One is advocating for health equity; be that LGBT+, BAME or women's rights, and the intersectionality between them. But I'm going to have a real focus on my circle of control: what is it that I can do in my daily practice as a nurse; what can I really achieve in my first preceptorship year. Otherwise, my focus gets a bit too split.

I'll be honest, I worry that I might end up burning myself out... I had that chat with my senior charge nurse this week and she was like "it's so obvious you're so passionate Craig and you've got a great relationship with your patients and this is something we love about you in this team. But we want you to have a long, sustained career and we don't want you to burn out." It was a lovely, nourishing, flourishing conversation.'

LGBT+: lesbian, gay, bisexual and transgender (often used to encompass any sexual orientations or gender identities that do not correspond to heterosexual norms); *BAME*: black and minority ethnic.

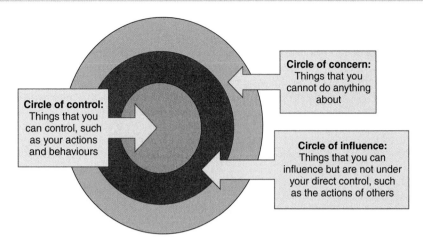

Fig. 9.1 Circles of concern, influence and control. (Based on Covey, S., 1989. The Seven Habits of Highly Effective People. Simon and Schuster, New York.)

Craig ultimately recognises that this is his preceptorship year and he has to be pragmatic about what he can achieve while setting into life as a newly registered nurse. He has narrowed down his circle of influence to things within his direct control, which he defines as establishing his own good nursing practice.

Focusing your thinking in this way helps to avoid rumination and inaction over things that concern you but that you cannot do anything about. Proactively focusing on issues that you can directly control and can also *realistically* influence helps you to do a few things well and achieve them. This will help you to grow in confidence as a leader.

▩ Time Out

Set some time aside to think about all the issues that concern you as a student leader. Draw a circle of concern on a big sheet of paper. Draw a smaller circle of influence inside the circle of concern and a circle of control within that, as per Fig. 9.1.

Write all of your leadership concerns (things that you would like to do something about) down on separate Post-it notes and set them to one side. This list might include things like:

- Patient safety issues
- Service improvements that you have been thinking about
- Your own wellbeing issues
- The funding of student nurse education
- The quality of your learning
- Research priorities that you consider to be important
- The rights of certain groups

Taking each Post-it note at a time, consider whether you can really influence that issue. Self-limiting beliefs might come into play here, so really challenge yourself to see what is outside your control or influence, taking into account the people around you who could help you and stretch you.

Place the Post-its that you think are outside your influence in the circle of concern, such as improving the funding of student nurse education. Then look at the remaining Post-it notes and think about what is in your direct control, such as your own wellbeing: maybe you want to see friends more or get fit. Place those in the circle of control. The remaining Post-its can then be placed in the circle of influence.

Now consider the two to three issues that you truly have energy to tackle, that are in your control or that you can influence. Take the decision to be more proactive on those issues for the next 12 months and put aside those that you cannot change or do not have time for.

Influencing Tactics Through the Ages

One of the most memorable texts through the ages has been Dale Carnegie's book *How to Win Friends and Influence People*, first published in 1936. The business magnate Warren Buffet is quoted as saying that 'Carnegie changed my life'. Much of what Carnegie advises (which is still very much worth reading) is now part of the modern health and care leadership training and has already been mentioned in this book. Things like:

- be a good listener—we talked about 'listening with fascination';
- give honest and sincere appreciation—this is part of compassionate leadership;
- remember and use the other person's name—something that students say is lacking;
- talk in terms of the other person's interests, become genuinely interested in people, make the other person feel important and do this sincerely—nursing is now very much focused on person-centredness, both with patients and with colleagues; and
- talk about your own mistakes before criticising the other person—today we might associate this openness with authenticity. Carnegie does not recommend directly criticising poor performance but to draw attention in a more indirect way. An example might be a way to discourage fellow students who may be wearing their uniform incorrectly. You might talk about how you forgot to take your rings off before duty and noticed at lunchtime that you were still wearing them. You might add how terrible you felt: that you might be setting a bad example to a first-year student or give the wrong impression to a patient that you did not care about infection control.

There are also other things that he said are helpful, such as:

- 'Arouse in people an eager want'—by this he means talking to people in terms of what they need, rather than what you need. A recent example was a student nurse who wanted her local trust to allow students to self-roster. She talked in terms of the hardship faced by students who could not manage their family life because they did not get their shift patterns until they started a placement. She described in detail the effect on the mental health of her colleagues. Instead of focusing on how this would be better for the student, she would get a better response by selling the idea in terms of how self-rostering would be better for the trust or for the university, or both: would it save staff time? Would it engender goodwill so that newly registered nurses would apply for roles at the trust? Would it reduce the number of students who drop out of their courses?
- Let the other person feel that the idea is theirs. Carnegie talks about planting a seed in a person's mind and then leaving them to come up with an idea themselves. In that way the person feels that they own the idea and is more likely to be committed to it.
- Show respect for other people's opinions: never say 'You're wrong'. By winning an argument, you lose your opponent's goodwill and you are unlikely to change their minds. Instead, Carnegie cautions that you listen, consider whether the other person may have a point and maybe even allow them to feel important, if you think this is what they are seeking.

Why Nurses Need to Develop Their Skills of Using Power and Influence

There are some compelling reasons why nursing at both undergraduate and postgraduate level needs power and influence. One of the main reasons of course is that we can advocate for our patients, carers, families and communities. We are close to them and can present our ideas for improving care and improving the systems that deliver that care. We can also use power and influence to help prevent nurses from being overlooked or marginalised. Undergraduate nursing students often talk about their perceived lack of power, but remember that you are large in number and capable of organising yourselves to be a powerful force.

As we saw in the chapter on courage and assertiveness, lessons from major care scandals tell us that poor leadership leads to a feeling of powerlessness in staff. This can affect nurses' job satisfaction, can lead to burnout and can engender the sort of disaffection that can end up with nurses losing their compassion and depersonalising the care they give.

Many of the issues of power in nursing hail from our history, as nursing has historically been seen as women's work undertaken behind closed doors (Wuest 1994). The persistent invisibility of the work of nurses has been cited as one of the reasons for the lower status of nursing in the health care hierarchy (Benner 2001; Wolf 1989).

> *'The gendered construction of nursing leaves a legacy which continues to feed the current crisis, including suppressing wages and downgrading working conditions. Historic perceptions that care is a naturally feminine skill or characteristic sit in direct opposition to the high level of skills and professionalisation required in contemporary nursing.'*
>
> CLAYTON-HATHWAY ET AL. (2020)

Nurses may be more reluctant than most to discuss power because, although there are more men in nursing now, the majority are still women (Spratley et al. 2000), and women have not traditionally exerted their power (Rafael 1996). Historically nurses have had difficulty acknowledging their own power (Rafael 1996). This reluctance to discuss and use power may be one explanation for nurses' inability to control their practice. Over recent years, however, we have seen some major strides globally to empower nursing and market its potential.

The Nursing Now Campaign and the Triple Impact

In 2018 a global campaign, Nursing Now, was launched, involving 30 countries. It grew to have a presence in 126 countries with over 700 worldwide groups active in raising the status and profile of nurses. This project originally arose from the All-Party Parliamentary Group (APPG) on Global Health, which is a group of members of both the House of Commons and House of Lords with a common interest in global health. Their 2016 report stressed that 'universal health coverage cannot possibly be achieved without strengthening nursing globally'. Part of this was about increasing the number of nurses globally, but also it was—and is—about ensuring that the contribution of nurses is properly understood and that they are enabled to work to their full potential.

By increasing nursing numbers and developing their role, the APPG report described a wider triple impact (Box 9.1).

The Nursing Now campaign (https://www.nursingnow.org/) operationalised the recommendations in the APPG report and sought to empower nurses to take their place at the heart of tackling 21st century health challenges and maximise their contribution to achieving Universal Health Coverage. It was funded by the Burdett Trust for Nurses in collaboration with the World Health Organisation and the International Council of Nurses.

The campaign ran for 3 years until May 2021 and focused on five core areas:
1. Ensuring that nurses and midwives have a more prominent voice in health policy-making
2. Encouraging greater investment in the nursing workforce
3. Recruiting more nurses into leadership positions
4. Conducting research that helps determine where nurses can have the greatest impact
5. Sharing of best nursing practices

Each of these five core areas had programmes of work attached, including the Nursing Now Challenge (formerly the Nightingale Challenge). This challenge attracted employers of nurses and midwives globally to provide leadership development opportunities for young nurses and midwives. Over 31,000 nurses and midwives from 806 employers in 79 countries accepted the

---

BOX 9.1 ■ The Triple Impact of Nursing

1. **Better health:** By this the APPG meant that nurses are the most numerous health professional and in, say, the developing world they may be the only professional who people see. Nurses undertake a very wide range of roles; they often come from the communities they serve and therefore understand the culture and possess creativity and imagination to meet the needs of people.
2. **Improving gender equality:** The APPG argued that nursing should not be seen as a gender-based profession. To achieve equality in social and economic development, women around the world will benefit from access to high-quality nursing care and being sensitive enough to tackle the different genders' needs and gender issues. Investing in nursing and raising its status will have the additional effects of empowering more women socially, politically and economically, and helping establish their status as important figures in their local communities.
3. **Creating stronger economies:** As most nurses are still (and likely to be for some time to come) women, developing and investing in them will, by bringing wages into the home, help empower them both economically and as community leaders. Improving health and empowering women will in turn strengthen local economies.

Based on All-Party Parliamentary Group on Global Health, 2016. Triple impact: how developing nursing will improve health, promote gender equality and support economic growth.

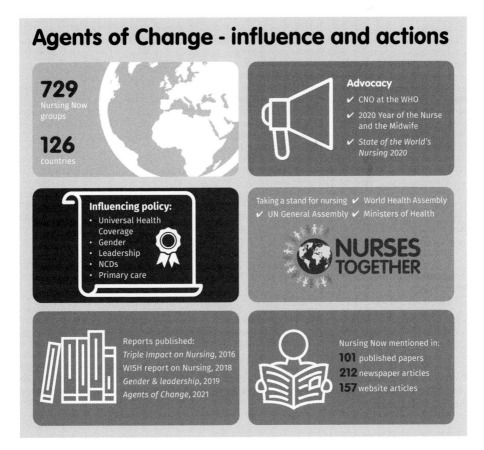

Agents of Change - influence and actions

729 Nursing Now groups

126 countries

Advocacy
✔ CNO at the WHO
✔ 2020 Year of the Nurse and the Midwife
✔ *State of the World's Nursing 2020*

Influencing policy:
• Universal Health Coverage
• Gender
• Leadership
• NCDs
• Primary care

Taking a stand for nursing ✔ World Health Assembly
✔ UN General Assembly ✔ Ministers of Health

NURSES TOGETHER

Reports published:
Triple Impact on Nursing, 2016
WISH report on Nursing, 2018
Gender & leadership, 2019
Agents of Change, 2021

Nursing Now mentioned in:
101 published papers
212 newspaper articles
157 website articles

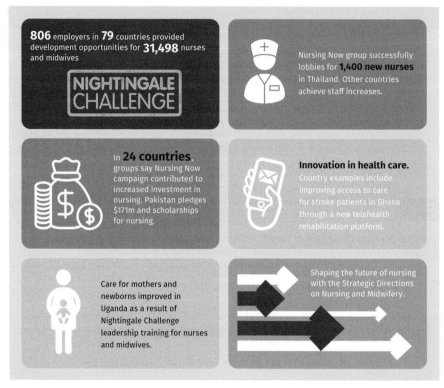

Fig. 9.2 The impact of the Nursing Now campaign globally. CNO: Chief Nursing Officer; NCDs: non-communicable diseases; WISH: World Innovation Summit for Health. (Reproduced with permission from Holloway, A., Thomson, A., Stilwell, B., Finch, H., Irwin, K., Crisp, N., 2021. Agents of Change: The Story of the Nursing Now Campaign. <https://www.nursingnow.org/wp-content/uploads/2021/05/Nursing-Now-Final-Report.pdf>.)

Nightingale Challenge worldwide. This helped to build young nurses' and midwives' skills as advocates and influential leaders in health care.

The Nursing Now campaign created a platform on which the future of nursing globally could build. The final report (2021; see Fig. 9.2) demonstrated that Nursing Now groups in 63 countries report increased investment in nursing during the campaign, with some evidence that in 24 countries investment was directly influenced by local Nursing Now groups.

The Nursing Now Challenge continues to be funded by the Burdett Trust for Nursing until 2023 and is planning for its future thereafter. This gives young leaders even more opportunity to make improvements and influence policy locally and nationally.

The recommendations in their 2021 report conclude that nursing education needs to be:

- informative (about knowledge and skills),
- formative (about professional traits and behaviours), and
- transformative (about leadership and influence).

To further promote the role of nursing, the report recommends that nursing is promoted as a science-based profession that is embedded in science, technology, engineering and mathematics (STEM) school curricula in recognition that it solves complex health issues with individuals, families and communities.

The legacy of Nursing Now urges that we as nurses view ourselves as powerful agents of change for the improvement of health and health care.

Understanding Power

In 1959 French and Raven described five bases of power: legitimate, reward, expert, referent and coercive. Six years later, Raven added an extra power base: informational (Box 9.2). To understand further how to use these, see Tips Box 9.1.

■ Time Out

Which forms of power relate to position and which relate to the personal attributes of a person?

What sorts of nursing power did the APPG on Global Health report refer to?

BOX 9.2 ■ French and Raven's Bases of Power

Legitimate—this comes from the belief that a person has the formal right to make demands, and to expect others to be compliant and obedient. A nursing example would be the power of a ward manager. However, if this role is lost the power disappears, because it is the position that holds the power, not the person.

Reward—some power positions enable them to offer rewards such as training opportunities, promotions, desirable assignments or even praise and thanks. So, reward power is often linked to legitimate power. The disadvantage of this power base is that sometimes the person in charge may not have complete control over the ability to offer the reward; for example, they may need an interview panel to offer a job. Also, if the rewards do not have enough perceived value, or are used up (such as all the job vacancies on offer have been filled), then power weakens.

Expert—this is based on a person's high levels of skill and knowledge. A nursing example may be the power of a clinical nurse specialist or advanced practitioner, or may be in roles such as digital nursing. Here the power comes from being a subject matter expert whose opinions have value and who is trusted and respected in their chosen area.

Referent—this is the result of a person being respected, liked and seen as worthy. Others may identify with them. This person also makes others feel good. In nursing this person may be a social media influencer or someone with an informal role acquired, for example, by setting up a self-help or special-interest group for fellow students, or by just being the go-to person for wise words and support.

Coercive—this comes from the belief that a person can punish others for noncompliance. This power comes from using the threat of denying privileges, firing staff or disciplining them. This type of power can be a problem because it may be abused. Using this type of power too much may mean that people leave or they may be accused of bullying.

Informational—this derives from a person's ability to control the information that others need to accomplish something. This is a particularly potent form of power and it derives not from the information itself, but from having access to it. With this type of power, a person can choose to use it as a weapon that can be withheld, concealed, manipulated, distorted or shared.

Based on French, J.R.P., Raven, B., 1959. The bases of social power. In: Cartwright, D. (Ed.), Studies in Social Power. Institute for Social Research, Ann Arbor.

Legitimate, coercive and reward power are the powers that relate to position. Expert, referent and informational power can also be found in leaders with formal roles in organisations (such as infection control nurse specialists having expert and informational power), but they can also be found throughout organisations and at any level, including student nurses.

The APPG report focused on the need to empower nurses and aspires to having more nurses in positions of legitimate power. It stressed the high level of skill and knowledge that nurses around the world possess—their expert power. It also talks about how quite often nurses are perceived as the wise women of the village or the go-to person and thus nurses can also have referent power. It mentions specifically the cultural understanding that nurses have and how that informational power can be used to find innovative solutions.

TIPS BOX 9.1

Using These Six Forms of Power

- Using positional forms of power alone can lead to unpopular and unstable leadership.
- Student nurses may sometimes have these positions of power—if they chair committees, for example.
- But at the same time it is helpful if you also develop your expertise, build your knowledge or be seen as likeable, trustworthy and helpful.
- Authentic and compassionate leadership will help you to develop expert and referent leadership.
- By understanding these different forms of power, you can learn to use the positive ones to full effect, while avoiding the negative power bases that managers can instinctively rely on.

Raising Socio-Political Awareness in Nursing

'Nurses need to make their voices heard, and use the evidence base to change the dialogue with the public, policy makers and politicians, in order to build a better future for health care.'

ACADEMIC AND FORMER RCN PRESIDENT,
ANNE MARIE RAFFERTY (2018)

In a 2019 podcast for student nurses, author and nursing academic Benny Goodman defines politics as 'the process of influencing the scarce allocation of resources'. He argues that socio-political awareness and advocacy should be included in student nurse leadership education (Tips Box 9.2). One reason that it is not, he claims, is that educators may not be equipped to deliver such education, so it may be up to you to develop your knowledge and skills around such issues as understanding the social determinants of health, human rights, how funding is allocated and used, inequality in access and outcomes, and what drives inequality.

In 1998 during a parliamentary debate, member of parliament Tony Benn described five questions to ask of those in power, which student nurses (probably via a representative group rather than directly!) could ask within the organisations in which they work and study:

1. What power do you have?
2. Where did you get it?
3. In whose interests do you exercise it?
4. To whom are you accountable?
5. How can we get rid of you?

Benn adds 'Anyone who cannot answer the last of those questions does not live in a democratic system.' Because senior leaders in health care, unlike in local authorities, are not elected, this is an interesting point!

TIPS BOX 9.2

Becoming More Politically Active

- Understand the social and political aspects that impact people's lives.
  - Read as much as you can to understand political issues.
  - Talk to the people around you, not just the people who are like you but people from all walks of life, especially those who feel disadvantaged in some way.
- Identify your issue—what is it that you feel passionate about?
- Choose your sphere of influence—the audience for your voice and whether you want your influence to be local, regional or national.
- Join relevant groups, for example, your union or professional body, a political party or an organisation such as MedAct (www.medact.org), which is a network for health workers to challenge the social, political and economic conditions that damage health and deepen health inequalities.

Based on Goodman (2019).

How to Lobby

'Oh dear! How politically naïve! Don't they realise? This is quite the wrong way to go about it. Many a time I have thought along these lines when I have met ambitious nurses.'
BARONESS JULIA CUMBERLEGE, FORMER HEALTH MINISTER AND
MEMBER OF THE HOUSE OF LORDS (2004)

Lobbying is about trying to influence the actions of those in power, usually in a national government context, although it can be used to refer to influencing anyone in authority. Baroness Cumberlege has been a staunch supporter of nurses over many years. She had to lobby for 18 years to introduce legislation so that nurses could become nonmedical prescribers. She is keen to help nurses to develop their skills of lobbying and has written and undertaken presentations on the subject (Tips Box 9.3). As well as using these tools with politicians themselves, they can also be used when you wish to lobby high-level decision-makers in universities, NHS trusts or national bodies.

TIPS BOX 9.3

Political Lobbying

- Be clear on your message: be able to describe succinctly who you are, what you are and what you do.
- Have a compelling vision: be able to describe this in as few words as possible.
- Prepare a brief synopsis of your case: What is happening? Why is it happening? How can it be changed? What are the costs involved?.
- Identify and engage your supporters: followership is an important function in understanding power and influence, and we shall examine this shortly.
- Identify your opponents: opposition, particularly political opposition, has an important function because their questions can help you to identify flaws in your arguments and plans.
- Identify your bedfellows: Cumberlege describes these as 'those you mistake for allies but when the going gets rough they evaporate and sometimes join your enemies because it is more popular and convenient for them to do so'.
- Identify your allies: people you trust to go all the way with you. These might not always be the ones who you might expect. Cumberlege cites rail and airline companies who

Continued

supported the antismoking lobby—not for health reasons but because they wanted to reduce their cleaning bills!

- Identify who you are trying to influence and put yourself in their shoes. Cumberlege
  advises that you have 30 seconds to attract their attention and 5 minutes to make your
  case! (Look up how to create an elevator pitch in Chapter 13 on leading change.)
- Explain how your idea will be a winner for them. Politicians are looking for vote-winning
  ideas and photo opportunities. Preelection, they are keen on 'save our NHS' types of
  initiatives and capitalising on the energy of pressure groups.
- Connect your issue to the objectives of the organisation and even to the chief executive's
  personal objectives. Engage nonexecutive directors of NHS trusts who may have more
  time to consider your ideas.
- When lobbying local authorities, identify the councillor who serves on the relevant
  committee—housing, highways, education etc. Finding the right councillor is easy if you
  look on the council's website, where there is usually a list of councillors and their roles.
- Avoid glossy 16-page brochures that busy people have no time to read. Instead, opt for
  an arresting single side of A4 that includes evidence on the effectiveness of your idea.
- Seeing is believing—invite those in power to visit and see for themselves.

Adapted from Cumberlege (2004).

■ Time Out

Think of an issue that you would like to lobby those in power about. Make a plan for how you
would proceed, using Cumberlege's advice.

Old Power, New Power

We are quite familiar with the concept of 'old' power: where power is spent like a currency that
is held by a few people at the top, commanding others and 'downloading' decisions from the top.
But today we have something else, called 'new power'. This is a type of peer-driven power that is
made by the many rather than the few. New power 'uploads' information and shares it openly
with colleagues. Power is not hoarded but channelled (Heimans and Timms 2018). The analogy
used is that old power is like the electronic game Tetris: a top-down game, with blocks 'falling
down on our heads' that need to be correctly stacked into lines. The new-power analogy is Mine-
craft: a game where people come together to cocreate something on those people's terms, from
the bottom up.

In their book, Heimans and Timms give several examples of the move from old power to new
power. Take what happened to Harvey Weinstein for example, who was once one of the most
powerful men in Hollywood. He could spend his 'power currency' to make or break actors and
commission or reject film projects. His mutually beneficial relationships with media and press
moguls, supported by his lawyers with their nondisclosure agreements, protected his power. But
he was toppled by widespread sexual abuse allegations that gave rise to the #MeToo movement.
This started when American actress Alyssa Milano posted on Twitter, 'If all the women who have
been sexually harassed or assaulted wrote 'Me too' as a status, we might give people a sense of the
magnitude of the problem.' This attracted responses from many high-profile women. The movement was then expanded and interpreted in subtly different ways across different nations and
languages.

Old-power and new-power mindsets and values are quite different (Table 9.1). Old power thinks about matters such as representation, being aware of the competition, confidentiality, building expertise and affiliation to the organisation. New power expects things to be done on people's terms, not that of the organisation: we see self-organisation and networked governance, transparency, a do-it-ourselves culture and affiliation that is short term. New power surges and can then disappear.

TABLE 9.1 ■ Old Power and New Power Values

Old Power Values	New Power Values
Formal, representative governance, managerialism and institutionalisation	Informal networked governance, opt-in decision-making, self-organisation
Competition, exclusivity, resource consideration	Collaboration, crowd wisdom, sharing, open-sourcing
Confidentiality, discretion, separation between private and public spheres	Radical transparency
Expertise, professionalism, specialisation	Maker culture, 'do-it-ourselves' ethic
Long-term affiliation and loyalty	Short-term, conditional affiliation
Less overall participation	More overall participation

Heimans, J., Timms, H., 2014. Understanding "New Power". Harvard Business Review, December 2014.

■ Time Out

Consider whether you have been part of a peer-driven, sharing, open, new-power initiative. How did you feel and what have you learnt from this experience?

Examples of new power that you may have been involved in:

- #RehabLegend (https://www.plymouthhospitals.nhs.uk/rehablegend)—the sharing of rehabilitation skills
- The Academy of Fab NHS Stuff (https://fabnhsstuff.net/)—a repository of fab ideas created by health commentator Roy Lilley
- #NursesActive challenge (http://wecommunities.org/)—an annual challenge to encourage nurses to take exercise
- And there are many more!

With old power you may have experienced things like safety and familiarity alongside maybe feeling too stifled to innovate. On the new-power side you may have felt freedom and excitement but maybe felt slightly out of control.

Student nurses today can engage in and use both old and new power. Let us look at a new-power example from a midwifery student in Case Study 9.2.

CASE STUDY 9.2 Alicia Burnett

'I think the whole world was experiencing this global trauma in little pockets. If we share our experiences it's a step towards healing.'

Alicia Burnett describes herself as an introvert who does not seek the limelight but is passionate about sharing the student midwife voice; circumstances caused her to step forward and help herself by helping others.

Continued

CASE STUDY 9.2   Alicia Burnett—cont'd

She was a student midwife when the COVID-19 pandemic struck. She felt that, because of the pause in her midwifery training, that part of her identity had disappeared. She also started to feel like the midwifery profession and the role and contribution of student midwives were invisible compared to that of doctors and nurses.

Alicia has always been a helper. In the autumn before the pandemic, she started helping her fellow students with their essays, ideas and professional writing and their contribution, as she put it, to the global midwifery journey. Following the publication of an article on the management of sickle cell anaemia, she was invited to become a member of the editorial board and progressed to becoming editor-in-chief of *The Student Midwife*, an online journal.

The pandemic paused her undergraduate course for a few weeks while her university worked out how to delivery her training online. She felt completely lost during this time and decided, much like Brian Webster in the Think Theory example, to start a blog called 'The Covid-19 Cohorts' to reach out to other student midwives who could share how they were managing their education, as a way for student midwives to offer support to each other. The idea developed into giving a way for student midwives to share their voices while highlighting how midwives were supporting families during the pandemic. She wanted to 'boost morale and lift up the profession'.

As International Day of the Midwife 2020 approached, Alicia used it as an opportunity to contact students all over the world. She used social media and email to write to midwifery leaders to invite student midwives to share their insights. She attracted support from Uganda, Rwanda, Iran, Greece, England, the Republic of Ireland, Jamaica and Scotland.

An online learning platform called All4Maternity (https://www.all4maternity.com) offered to host the blogs and taught her how to upload and curate the blogging site.

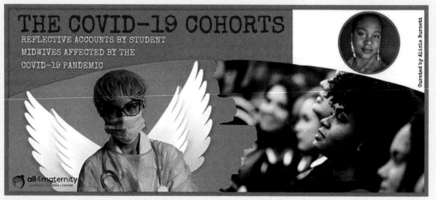

Photo courtesy: The Covid-19 Cohorts Reflective Accounts. A series of blogs edited by Alicia Burnett and published by www.All4Maternity.com. Reproduced with permission.

Alicia facilitated the writing of an article for *The Student Midwife*, one of two journals that All-4Maternity produce. This included contributions from five student midwives from around the world, who each gave an account of how the pandemic has affected student midwives in their part of the world.

As a result of Alicia's initiative, the journal has started taking more of an international midwifery focus. This culminated in their first ever international edition featuring authors from six different countries—Malta, Australia, Malawi, England, Mexico and the United States.

Alicia was acting as a servant leader, meeting the needs of others just like herself. You will recall from the beginning of this book that the servant leader sees those they lead as peers to both teach and to learn from. She leads others to reach an agreed-upon goal but does not believe that she is any better than anyone else.

In this case study we can see Alicia using new power to connect to others, to understand and share their experiences and bring healing by being together. She also helped to highlight the important work that midwives around the world do, even in a crisis. She helped a publisher to realise the benefit of considering a global perspective on midwifery, which led to the sharing of learning from other cultures and perspectives.

THE EQUAL IMPORTANCE OF OLD AND NEW POWER

■ Time Out

Think of an example of old power and then think of an example of new power. Why do they operate with that particular power dynamic?

Heimans and Timms point out that old power is not always bad and new power is not always good. There are situations when old power—with its systems, structures, empiricism and peer review—is exactly what is needed. Old power methods and values are very appropriate in research organisations, governmental bodies and NHS trusts. You really would not want new-power approaches such as self-organising and making up their own rules here!

Examples of new power include antivaccine groups that operate outside of the rules, uploading and sharing malicious and untrue data that is traded between peers. This sort of initiative calls upon nurses to understand new power and to operate in new-power ways to counteract it.

A more positive example is initiatives such as the #HelloMyNameIs campaign, which arose from the experience of a doctor, Kate Granger, who was admitted to hospital with sepsis. She observed that staff did not introduce themselves to her and felt that, as part of compassionate care, the sharing of a name helped her to make an initial connection with someone. She initiated a campaign with her husband Chris to encourage doctors and nurses to introduce themselves.

Ideas like Kate and Chris's that spread through new power are ACE:

- actionable—asking people to do something;
- connected—making people feel connected to a shared enterprise; and
- extensible—anyone can take part in your mission on their terms so they may interpret it differently and build on the initial idea. This is a significant change from old power, where people take part in an organisation's mission on that organisation's terms—the power dynamic has shifted (Heimans and Timms 2018).

The Power of Connections

Power and influence are said to be about what you know and who you know, but senior leaders are less influential than you might think. Employees who are influencers and are highly connected have twice as much power to influence change as people with hierarchical power (Herrero 2014). Just 3% of people can influence up to 90% of their colleagues (Hansgaard and Andell 2020). These 'super connectors' are trusted by their peers, make sense of things and reduce ambiguity for others (Tips Box 9.4) (North West Leadership Academy 2020).

If leaders want to get the same level of influence though top-down change as the 3% get, they need four times more people (Hansgaard and Andell 2020). Smart leaders should try to identify the 3% and engage them to understand what staff are feeling and thinking. They can then use this information to shape communications so that messaging addresses the real issues and helps to motivate people. Likewise, if those super connectors have been involved in change led by leaders, they can help by correcting any misunderstandings over a cup of tea in the staff room. Leaders should stay connected to these people for the long haul and not just use them for their own purposes.

The 3% rule also appears true for social media: these social media super connectors account for a massive 85% of retweets, but interestingly these people are not always the same people who are super connectors in their organisations (Mackenzie and Oliver 2018) (Tips Box 9.5).

■ Time Out

Who are the super connectors in your organisation?
If you use social media, who do you consider to be super connectors?
In what ways do you think that you may be able to connect with them to help with any changes or improvements that you have in mind?

TIPS BOX 9.4

Finding Super Connectors

Ask 10 people in your organisation:
- Who do you go to for information when you have concerns at work?
- Whose advice do you trust and respect?

Based on North West Leadership Academy (2020).

TIPS BOX 9.5

Becoming a Social Media Super Connector

- Pick a topic that you want to influence—this might be around education, such as curriculum development, research and student wellbeing, as well as clinical topics that you are keen on.
- Build your connections and relationships.
- Avoid 'broadcasting': sending out information without listening and without engaging others.
- Be a conversation-starter: study the work of others and add your own insights.
- Be willing to enter into debate, posting useful insights.
- Be helpful to others, bringing in people who you think will help the debate along and will share useful resources and information.
- Try to catch the mood and summarise how people are feeling.
- Be a model of trust and positive behaviours—do not gossip or bad-mouth others, and reply to messages.
- Always follow up on what you say—or people will lose trust.
- Post interesting content every day so that you build and keep your followership.
- Use pictures and colour in your social media posts to attract attention.
- Be as authentic and human on social media as you are in person.

Tipping Point Leadership: When Ideas Go Viral

The importance of new power and super connectors is not new. Malcolm Gladwell explores this in his book, *The Tipping Point* (2001). In his book he gives examples of ideas that 'tipped over' and went viral. One example that he gives is the resurgence of the shoe brand Hush Puppies, which by the early part of the 1990s saw poor sales. Then suddenly Hush Puppy bosses heard that their shoes had suddenly became fashionable in clubs and bars in downtown Manhattan. This was down to a few influential young people who started buying and wearing Hush Puppies shoes again. Annual sales increased from 30,000 pairs to 430,000 pairs in 1995. It doubled the following year and increased more the next year.

Gladwell describes what he terms the 'law of the few'. By this he refers to something you may have heard of called the Pareto principle, meaning that 80% of the effect comes from 20% of the cause. For example, health and safety officers look for 20% of the causes that give rise to 80% of the accidents. He identifies a few special people who are responsible for making ideas go viral. He categorises them into three groups (Box 9.3); as well as recognising the important role of the connector that is highlighted earlier, Gladwell also recognises two other types of people who together have huge influence—the maven and the salesperson.

BOX 9.3 ■ The Three Key Roles in Tipping Point Leadership

Mavens—human 'data banks' who have lots of information on a wide range of topics. They are also teachers and serve their own emotional needs by solving other people's problems. By wanting to help others they also gain attention, which makes them more powerful.

Connectors—people who know a huge number of people and occupy many different worlds, subcultures and niches. The more acquaintances you have, the more powerful you become. These people know who you should be connected to and can make introductions for you.

Salespeople—use not only their persuasiveness, enthusiasm, smiles on their face, their arguments etc., but they also use subtle synchronised movements. Salespeople mirror the behaviour and pattern of their 'customers', techniques that we see in neurolinguistic programming as well.

Based on Gladwell, M., 2001. The Tipping Point. Abacus, London.

Let us take a look at Case Study 9.3 to see if we can find super connectors, mavens and salespeople in action in a student nurse-led project.

■ Time Out

Which of Malcolm Gladwell's roles (maven, connector and salesperson) did the various stakeholders play to enable this project to reach a tipping point?

Is this case study an example of new power or old power in action?

CASE STUDY 9.3 **MyCOPD App**

Joy O'Gorman, a student nurse from the University of Plymouth, was undertaking a university project to promote an app to help people self-manage their chronic obstructive pulmonary disease, or COPD. She encouraged patients attending a hospital preoperative clinic to ask their GP for access to the MyCOPD app, only to find that GPs did not know about it. This made her feel like she had built up the patient's hopes for nothing.

It is notoriously difficult to influence GPs, or even to get their attention, because they are so busy and, being generalists, they have many clinical areas to cover. But luckily Joy's personal tutor was a band 8 general practice nurse and invited her to do a presentation about the app for a local general practice nursing conference. In this way Joy first got to know the general practice nurses in primary care.

In addition, when she first joined the university, Joy had already signed up to be a student digital health champion on an eco and eHealth academic programme for Cornwall and the Isles of Scilly called EPIC. Many of the local GP surgeries were part of that network, so she explained what she was doing to EPIC leaders, who were supportive, as it met their eHealth objectives. Joy harnessed the network to set up roadshows and engaged fellow student nurses as volunteers who visited GP surgeries, explained the app and got GPs signed up to using it, so now Joy had two routes into primary care.

Joy also contacted the developer of the MyCOPD app, My mHealth, to explain what she was doing and invited their support. This led to new connections between the developer and EPIC, and dedicated funding to do more with student nurses. Joy, EPIC and My mHealth presented a lecture to fellow student nurses to help make students aware of the resource and how it can support their patients. The project was also promoted as a way for students to introduce a change in practice and be able to practise their leadership skills.

The company had never had a student nurse get in touch to help before. They had been trying to persuade physiotherapists to promote the app, but explained that some physiotherapists seemed to see the app as a threat because it contained physiotherapy techniques that might challenge their role as health professionals practising face to face.

Joy also contacted the local Breathe Easy groups, which are a network of self-help groups for people with COPD, supported by the British Lung Foundation. The Breathe Easy groups started doing peer-to-peer referral, demonstrating and telling each other about the app.

When Joy spoke to senior nurses in accident and emergency, she explained that the app would help reduce emergency admission rates. When she spoke to senior nurses in outpatient departments, she argued that apps could be promoted in the waiting room TV screens.

Licensed user uptake tripled within the 6 weeks of Joy's project. It had started to reach tipping point. The board of governors for the hospital were impressed with the speed of the change, explaining that they had been working on such a change for months and months and Joy had done it in a matter of weeks. Promotion of the MyCOPD app is now under development as a quality improvement project at the local trust, so that COPD patients can access the app as part of their discharge package.

Joy demonstrates early signs of being a super connector. She already seems to have connections that she can leverage—such as her personal tutor, EPIC project leaders and even people who she has only met once, such as the employees of the company that made the app that she was promoting. She seems to have a natural affinity for extending her connections by reaching out to new people and groups such as the governors of the NHS Trust, local Breathe Easy groups and nurses in the accident and emergency department.

Joy's project is also ACE:

- actionable—she is asking each group to take some form of action that will help them;
- connected—everybody feels connected in a common enterprise; and
- extensible—notice the way that Joy changes her message to appeal to the group she is connecting to, so they can take part on their terms.

For A&E nurses, the MyCOPD project is about reducing emergency admissions, for the My mHealth company that designed the app it is about selling more licences and for Breathe Easy group members the app is a self-help tool: that idea from Carnegie about 'arousing in others an eager want' and Cumberlege's message about explaining how your idea will be a winner for the other person. These are great sales techniques!

Joy continues to be an influencer and super connector in the field of the adoption of digital technology in health care (eHealth). She argues that student nurses can enable the adoption of eHealth in the workplace and that eHealth should be a core part of the undergraduate curriculum (O'Gorman 2020).

Understanding Followership

There are many myths and preconceptions about followership, such as that leaders are active and followers are passive, or that followership is just preparation for leadership. Throughout this book, we have identified that the idea of charismatic, autocratic leadership is outdated and that distributive leadership is more effective. Followers are in fact crucial, and it is important to understand their role as active participants in making change happen (Tips Box 9.6).

'The first follower transforms the lone nut into a leader.'

DEREK SIVERS (2010)

When developing social movements, being the first follower is an underappreciated role. In his 2010 TED talk (Technology, Education and Design), Derek Sivers uses a video of a man dancing crazily at a music festival to illustrate this point. The video shows how powerful his first follower is—the person who is the first to join in and copy his crazy dancing. The leader embraces this first follower as an equal and the first follower starts to copy the leader's dance moves, which are easy to follow. Once the first follower joins in with the craziness, it makes it less risky for others to join in. He encourages them, making the leader's actions credible.

The second follower turns the individuals into a group. From there it is only a few seconds before other people start running to join in, until tipping point is reached and the group turns into a large crowd. The people who remain seated then become the ones at a social disadvantage by not joining in with a popular movement.

TIPS BOX 9.6

Followership

- Every leader of a social movement needs a first follower to give them credibility.
- If you are a leader, then you should make your actions as easy as possible to emulate.
- You can become that first follower, which is a gamble if you are seen as supporting a 'lone nut', but this pays off if the initiative grows into a movement, as you will be given credit as an early adopter.
- If you are the leader, then you should nurture and support your followers as equals.
- Make the followership as public as possible—new followers emulate the follower, not the leader.

Based on Sivers (2010).

Summary

Power is about getting things done, and influence is power in motion. Understanding power and practising influencing techniques are important for student nurses to learn, because you not only advocate for yourselves and those you care for, but may also wish to highlight the important triple impact that nurses have: better health, gender equality and stronger economies.

By understanding different forms of power, such as those described by French and Raven, you can learn to use the positive ones to full effect while avoiding the negative power bases that managers can instinctively rely on.

Students may have to rely on themselves to develop their socio-political awareness and lobbying skills, as these may not form part of the current undergraduate curriculum. A key concept here is influencing others by phrasing your arguments or requests based on what the other person wants to achieve, rather than what you do.

The old power mindset of command and control can be overthrown by a new power dynamic that is more open source and peer-driven, but both have their place and today's student nurse would be wise to understand and leverage these appropriately. Students can harness the power of influencers, mavens, connectors and salespeople if they can recognise their unique but often hidden capabilities. These people are informal leaders who may be far more trusted and effective than formal leaders.

Lastly, followers are crucial to the success of student nurse leaders. They need recognising and nurturing to give you credibility.

References

All-Party Parliamentary Group on Global Health, 2016. Triple impact: how developing nursing will improve health, promote gender equality and support economic growth.

Benn, T., 1998. Speech: European Parliamentary Elections Bill (Online). Hansard. Volume 319: debated on Monday 16 November 1998. <https://hansard.parliament.uk/commons/1998-11-16/debates/db35bbc5-17ba-4097-bcec-b18ba5057ad7/EuropeanParliamentaryElectionsBill>.

Benner, P., 2001. From Novice to Expert: Excellence and Power in Clinical Nursing Practice (commemorative edition). Prentice Hall Health, Upper Saddle River, NJ.

Chandler, G. E., 1992. The source and process of empowerment. Nursing Administration Quarterly, 16(3), 65–71.

Clayton-Hathway, K., Humbert, A.L., Griffiths, H., McIlroy, R., Schutz, S., 2020. Gender and Nursing as a Profession: Valuing Nurses and Paying Them Their Worth. Royal College of Nursing, London.

Covey, S., 1989. The Seven Habits of Highly Effective People. Simon and Schuster, New York.

Cumberlege, J., 2004. How to lobby. Nursing Management 11 (7), 29–30.

French, J.R.P., Raven, B., 1959. The bases of social power. In: Cartwright, D. (Ed.), Studies in Social Power. Institute for Social Research, Ann Arbor.

Gladwell, M., 2001. The Tipping Point. Abacus, London.

Goodman, B., 2019. Right To Health: The Social Political Role of the Student Nurse. #WeStNsPod. <https://feeds.buzzsprout.com/554065.rss> and on Spotify.

Hansgaard, J.V., Andell, B., 2020. Leaders must mobilize the company's hidden influencers to fight the strains of the corona virus. Innovisor. <https://www.innovisor.com/>.

Heimans, J., Timms, H., 2014. Understanding "New Power". Harvard Business Review, December 2014.

Herrero, H., 2014. Top influencers 2, top leadership 1 (hierarchical power in the organization is half of the 'peer-to-peer' power). Blog post. <http://t.co/Du6zCbrDBC>.

Holloway, A., Thomson, A., Stilwell, B., Finch, H., Irwin, K., Crisp, N., 2021. Agents of Change: The Story of the Nursing Now Campaign. <https://www.nursingnow.org/wp-content/uploads/2021/05/Nursing-Now-Final-Report.pdf> (accessed 17/12/2021).

Kanter, R.M., 1979. Power failure in management circuits. Harvard Business Review, July–August, 65–75.

Kanter, R.M., 1993. Men and Women of the Corporation. Basic Books, Inc., New York, NY.

Mackenzie, G., Oliver, C., 2018. The truth is out there: who makes and influences health news on social media in the UK and internationally? doi: 10.13140/RG.2.2.29928.72962.

North West Leadership Academy, 2020. Webinar: leadership masterclass: taking the power to make change happen, with Helen Bevan. <https://youtu.be/0kW09gS0J98>.

O'Gorman, J., 2020. Student nurses are the key to transforming health and care in the UK. University of Plymouth. <https://www.plymouth.ac.uk/news/pr-opinion/student-nurses-are-the-key-to-transforming-health-and-care-in-the-uk>.

Rafael, A.R., 1996. Power and caring: a dialectic in nursing. Advances in Nursing Science, 19 (1), 3–17.

Rafferty, A.M., 2018. Nurses as change agents for a better future in health care: the politics of drift and dilution. Health Economics, Policy, and Law, 13 (3–4), 475–491.

Sivers, D., 2010. How to start a movement. TED. <https://www.ted.com/talks/derek_sivers_how_to_start_a_movement#t-162286>.

Spratley, E., Johnson, A., Sochalski, J., Fritz, M., Spencer, W., 2000. The Registered Nurse Population: Findings From the National Sample Survey of Registered Nurses. Washington, DC.

The COVID-19 Cohorts: Real-Life Accounts of Being a Student Midwife During the COVID-19 Pandemic <https://www.all4maternity.com/the-covid-19-cohorts-real-life-accounts-of-being-a-student-midwife-during-the-covid-19-pandemic/> (accessed 13/01/2022).

Wolf, Z.R., 1989. Uncovering the hidden work of nursing. Nursing & Health Care, 10 (8), 463–467.

Wuest, J., 1994. Professionalism and the evolution of nursing as a discipline: A feminist perspective. Journal of Professional Nursing, 10(6), 357–367.

Communicating to Influence

OBJECTIVES

After reading this chapter and completing the activities, you should be able to:
- Explain the six steps in the communication cycle
- Use Monroe's Motivated Sequence to structure influential presentations
- Write more concisely using the inverted triangle
- Contribute effectively to meetings
- Engage a range of strategies to cope with social media feedback
- Use narrative to influence others.

Relevance to the Nursing and Midwifery Council (NMC) Code

Paragraph 7:
Communicate clearly
7.1 Use terms that people in your care, colleagues and the public can understand
7.2 Take reasonable steps to meet people's language and communication needs, providing, wherever possible, assistance to those who need help to communicate their own or other people's needs
7.3 Use a range of verbal and nonverbal communication methods, and consider cultural sensitivities, to better understand and respond to people's personal and health needs
7.4 Check people's understanding from time to time to keep misunderstanding or mistakes to a minimum

Paragraph 8:
Work cooperatively
8.1 Respect the skills, expertise and contributions of your colleagues, referring matters to them when appropriate
8.2 Maintain effective communication with colleagues

Paragraph 20:
Uphold the reputation of your profession at all times
20.10 Use all forms of spoken, written and digital communication (including social media and networking sites) responsibly, respecting the right to privacy of others at all times

Communication is a central part of delivering good nursing care, and as a student nurse you will be taught the communication skills that you will need to succeed. This chapter therefore focuses on the communication skills that you will need, not as a clinician, but as a nurse leading a team.

So far in this book we have looked at a range of relevant communication concepts such as:

- compassionate leadership: attending, understanding, empathising and helping those we lead. Chief amongst these communication skills is listening empathically and actively;
- the qualities of good communication in effective teamwork;
- having courageous conversations, including how to be assertive by communicating how you feel;
- managing conflict, including mediation and negotiation skills; and
- influencing and lobbying others by communicating succinctly.

In Section 3 of this book, where we discuss improving health and care, communications skills are needed when:

- building a shared vision when leading change;
- working creatively to solve problems, such as using the 'five whys'; and
- developing a communication strategy to assist with project management.

This chapter will build on ideas that we met in Chapter 9: how student nurses can communicate well to influence others. Leaders use a wide range of communication channels and communication styles. We shall start with some of the broad principles around communicating as a leader before exploring the different channels: written, face-to-face and digital.

The Communication Cycle

The communication cycle is a commonly known series of six steps to help leaders to tailor and refine their communications (Fig. 10.1). It can be used in any situation but is most useful when you want to communicate important or complex information to your team.

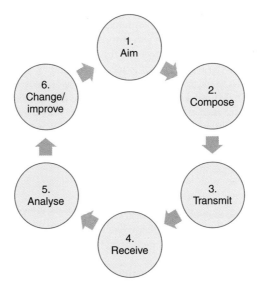

Fig. 10.1 The communication cycle. (Based on Shannon, C.E. & Weaver, W (1971). The Mathematical Theory of Communication. The University of Illinois Press; First Edition (US) First Printing edition (1971))

STEP 1: CLARIFY YOUR AIM

Answer the following questions:
- To whom am I communicating?
- What message am I trying to send? What am I trying to achieve?
- Why do I want to send this message? Do I need to send it at all?
- What do I want my audience to feel?
- What does my audience need or desire from this message?
- What do I want my audience to do with this information?

Example: I recently communicated with a branch of a national voluntary organisation that was helping me with a series of three treasure hunts in local parks to raise awareness of child asthma in our town.

The organisation had not been involved in the first event. It had gone okay and I wanted to let them know how it went, ready for next time. Having had feedback from some local people, I wanted to suggest some changes to how the next two events would be organised. The revised approach now involved recruiting more of their members to act as marshals, and it also included them using some basic asthma knowledge that I had already trained them on. I wanted them to feel happy with the revised workload and comfortable with the clinical elements.

STEP 2: COMPOSE

Now consider:
- What is the best way to communicate this message? In person, email, etc.
- What level/type of language should I use?
- Does the audience have any background information on the topic?
- Will my audience need any additional resources to understand my message?
- Am I expressing emotions in my message? If so, what emotions?
- Will the audience assume anything about me or my motives that will damage the credibility of the communication?

I asked my main contact to ring me, because I knew that this was the way she liked to communicate, so that she could ask me lots of questions. She was new to this organisation and inexperienced, so she liked to chat over the ins and outs until it was settled in her mind; otherwise I knew that she would feel anxious. I reflected that the language I should use should be straightforward and I would ask her to repeat it back to me, so that I knew that she had understood.

I thought about whether to suggest options to her, so that she could feel ownership or whether to work my revised plan out fully. I decided to do the latter because she tended to get worried if there was any uncertainty. I knew that I needed to back up my new plan in writing for her committee to agree.

I realised that the committee would want me to mitigate any risks, and I planned to review the risk assessment and the written guidance for their volunteers after I had spoken to her.

STEP 3: TRANSMIT

Ask yourself:
- Is this the right time to send this message?
- What is the state of mind of my audience likely to be, and what workload will they be experiencing when they receive this message? How should I present my message to take account of this?
- Will there be any distractions that may damage the impact of the communication? (This is especially important to consider when giving a speech or presentation.)
- Should I include anyone else in the audience?

I asked my contact to phone me when she was ready, and she told me that she was busy volunteering as an invigilator for school exams. She gave me a time and rang me as arranged, only to tell me that she was very stressed and would phone me tomorrow instead. I let her choose her time so that she would be relaxed. I knew that her husband would be in the background listening in and asking further questions, and it always helped to have his perspective too.

STEP 4: RECEIVE FEEDBACK

Feedback helps us to improve.
- Build in some type of feedback process:
  - Body language
  - Question and answer
  - Written response
  - Survey/polling
  - Phone calls
- Look for indirect feedback—that which is not communicated directly to you, such as:
  - Rumour
  - Feedback to a team member who then tells you
  - Poor take-up

My assessment of what she and her organisation needed was correct! She phoned, we chatted and she and her husband liked the new plan. What I did not expect was that her committee was meeting that evening and wanted to discuss and agree to it. I knew that there was a chance that if the new plan was communicated verbally that there might be misunderstandings. I offered to join the committee meeting in person (it was to be held virtually) to explain, but this was politely turned down. I therefore quickly revised the written guidance for volunteers and risk assessment and emailed it over.

She phoned me the following day to tell me that the committee liked the plan. I also got an email from the chairperson to answer some further questions that he had, which were answered to his satisfaction.

We agreed to visit the two local parks where we were holding our events together so that we could iron out the details.

STEP 5: ANALYSE

Reflect and learn from the feedback that you have received:
- Why did you receive this feedback?
- What does this tell you about your message?
- What could you have done differently to get the response that you wanted?
- Did the audience feel the way you expected them to feel? If not, why not?
- How should you act or behave differently to move forward?

The feedback had been good, in fact much better than I had expected. Even though the new plan was now more complex, the committee seemed to have understood it the first time.

I was glad that I had worked my ideas through in advance and just needed to put everything in writing. The park visits offered us an additional way to communicate and clarify the plans, and this face-to-face interaction served to build our relationship. The combination of written, verbal and face-to-face interaction was effective.

STEP 6: CHANGE AND IMPROVE

Use your emotional intelligence to:
- Respect the feedback that you have received. If you believe it is valid, change your message or behaviour.

- Identify resources that can help you to improve. For instance, ask colleagues for help and advice, do more testing or look up better ways to communicate.

The follow-up questions that I got were just around reassurances that were needed, so I was happy that I had communicated well. I realised that I should have asked my contact when her next committee meeting was so that I could have had my revised plan ready and not be caught off guard but, in fairness, she could have told me that earlier too.

Adapted from Mindtools.com.

■ **Time Out**

Next time that you want to communicate something to your team, try using the communication cycle.

Make a note in your diary on your reflections—did this structure help?

'Selling' Your Ideas

How might you structure your communication to motivate others and 'sell' your ideas? Imagine that you are invited to give a presentation, give a morale-boosting team talk or address the team about a health and safety issue. Monroe's Motivated Sequence (1943) is a well used and time-proven five-step method to organise presentations for maximum impact.

Let us use the example of giving a presentation to peers about the problem of people with long-term conditions having poor adherence to medication.

1. GAIN THEIR ATTENTION

Start with a shocking statistic, such as the following:

'The World Health Organisation states that the average nonadherence rate is 50% among those with chronic illnesses.'

CHISHOLM-BURNS AND SPIVEY (2012)

2. ESTABLISH THE NEED

Convince the audience that there is a problem: Use statistics to back up what you say.

'Approximately 5200 people with diabetes have a limb amputated each year, while as many as 1300 people lose their sight due to diabetic retinopathy, due to poor adherence.'

TURNBULL (2015)

Talk about the consequences of maintaining the status quo and not making changes.

'The consequences of nonadherence include a worsening of the patient's condition, increased comorbid diseases, increased health care costs, and death.'

CHISHOLM-BURNS AND SPIVEY (2012)

Show your audience how this directly affects them:

'Wasted medicines cost the NHS £800m a year' (Turnbull 2015). *'That's the equivalent of about 29,000 extra band 5 nurses a year! How much would we like to improve our staffing levels?'*

3. SATISFY THE NEED

Background:

> 'Healthcare professionals have been shown to be poor judges of adherence, identifying nonadherence no better than would be predicted by chance alone. The inability to predict adherence has been shown to be independent of seniority, professional stream (doctors versus nurses) or how long the physician has known the patient.'
>
> BURGESS ET AL. (2011)

Facts:

> 'NICE evidence reviews demonstrate that nonadherence should not be seen as the patient's problem. It often occurs because of a failure to fully agree on the prescription in the first place or to identify and provide the support that patients need later on.'
>
> (NICE 2009)

Position statement:

> 'Addressing nonadherence is not about getting patients to take more medicines per se. Rather, it starts with an exploration of patients' perspectives of medicines, their health beliefs and the reasons why they may not want or are unable to use them. Healthcare professionals have a duty to help patients make informed decisions about treatment and use appropriately prescribed medicines to best effect.'
>
> NICE (2009)

Example:

Present a case study. 'Frank is 70 and he presents with a loss of glycaemic control. He has missed his last appointment. You have the choice of scheduling another appointment in a month to check control again, revising his medications or exploring his thoughts on what is happening and how he feels he can gain control again. You decide on the latter and discover that his wife had a stroke 4 months ago and is now living in a nursing home.

You both agree that the loss of glycaemic control is down to the behaviour changes rather than a decrease in antihyperglycaemic therapy. Frank cannot cook, he has stopped going walking with friends and he admits that his wife used to remind him to take his medications. You discuss and agree that the best way forward is to simplify the medication regime and introduce a pill box. He joins a local support group and gets some help with cooking the right sort of food. He also admits that he might be feeling low and agrees to a psychological assessment.

A month later, Frank's blood glucose has improved. The agreed interventions appear to be working, although he still struggles to eat healthily, but now he has the support of peers to help him.'

Case study based on Ji and Bailey (2013).

Present counterarguments:

> 'A better word to use is concordance with treatment, rather than adherence, because that suggests debate and agreement with the patient rather than us imposing our views. Much of the evidence points towards the importance of us as nurses focusing more on person centred, understanding health beliefs and improving health literacy. People have the right to be involved in discussions and make informed decisions about their care.'

4. VISUALISE THE FUTURE

The more realistic and detailed the vision you present, the more it is likely to influence behaviour, attitudes and beliefs. Try to make the vision as believable and realistic as possible. You could start with visualising what the future would look like with no change and then go on to contrast this with how this would change if your proposals are accepted:

'Let's visualise what happens if you continue prescribing for, managing and monitoring patients without accepting that half of them aren't self-managing their medications well, for a variety of reasons. You are working in outpatients when the consultant says to Mr Shah that his foot requires amputation. You talk through the quality-of-life implications not only for him but also his wife. He may no longer be able to get out the house unaided and she may have to give up her part-time job to become his carer. They leave in tears.

Consider the opposite: you are receiving a top nursing award because you led a successful nursing programme focusing on the systematic implementation of the NICE guidance on medicines adherence (2009) in your trust for people with diabetes. This involves increasing patient involvement and understanding the patient's knowledge, beliefs and concerns about their medicines. Diabetes complications have reduced overall by 30% in a year. The estimated financial saving to the trust is £145,000. Patient satisfaction has risen by 43%.' (Important: These results are made up, not evidence, to act as an illustration).'

5. TAKE ACTION

Give your audience specific actions to help them to start solving the problem. Do not overwhelm them at this stage with too much too soon—just encourage that first step:

'I've invited a few expert patients with long-term conditions to have lunch with us now. So, let's adjourn to room 5 and chat informally with them to get their views on the issues that they see around adherence to treatment.'

■ Time Out

Some of you may naturally be more persuasive and motivational, but for others Monroe's Motivated Sequence will give you a structure.

The next time you listen to a presentation intended to persuade an audience to a desired course of action, see if you can detect Monroe's Motivated Sequence—or try it out for yourself!

Getting Your Voice Heard in Meetings

Many of those interviewed for this book, especially the ones who described themselves as introverted, spoke about how difficult they felt it was to speak up in big meetings. They talked about imposter syndrome—feeling that their ideas were not worthy—and of being overwhelmed by their more outgoing and confident colleagues. Some tips to help you speak up have been summarised in Tips Box 10.1.

TIPS BOX 10.1

- Students interviewed for this book found that **having a coach** really helped: someone who encouraged them to speak out, just once, to see how it felt. This seemed to get the ball rolling—and invited them to reflect on how that felt. Without exception, the first time was the most nerve-wracking, but the experience emboldened them to try it again.
- Not speaking up in meetings means that **your team or organisation misses out** on your valuable contribution. Make a commitment to yourself to share your experience.
- Think about where **your expert knowledge** lies before you go. Remember that student nurses are a huge asset to organisations because they often see things with fresh eyes. Your views will often offer unique insights into their team or organisation.

- **Speak up early.** This will help you to 'get it over with' and feel more relaxed, avoid others voicing your best ideas before you do or avoid the problem of trying to break into a conversation in full flow.
- Use all your **nonverbal skills**: look speakers in the eye, nod along and forward to show that you are alert and involved. Use open and confident body language rather than sitting with your arms folded while looking at the floor.
- If putting your ideas forward seems too nerve-wracking at first, jot down a few **questions to ask** either before you go (in case your mind goes blank) or during the meeting. Be careful not to ask too many questions, as it may irritate people if you delay proceedings.
- Rather than pushing yourself forward, you may want to **praise others and build on their contribution.** Alternatively, you may notice that someone was interrupted and you can encourage them to continue: 'Saeed, what were you going to say?'
- **Introverts tend to be reflective and thoughtful,** so use those skills to research and prepare. Use your listening skills and, like Barbara Stilwell in the chapter on assertiveness, summarise what is happening before offering your own considered point of view.
- If you have something important to say, speak to the meeting chairperson or secretary in advance to **get a slot on the agenda**.
- **Keep it short and convincing**: do not start with 'I'm sorry but...' or 'I may be wrong here but...', as this sounds apologetic. Instead, use 'Can I just say...' or 'I'd like to add...' This makes you sound confident, concise and efficient.

■ Time Out

What stops you from speaking up in meetings? Make a plan for how you will address this, using the tips above.

Alternatively, if you are quite confident, think about how you might use the tips to support a peer.

Write in a Way That Grabs Attention

In a health care context, time is often valuable, so it is important that your team quickly grasp the nub of what you are trying to say in your written communications (Tips Box 10.2). Student nurses can learn from journalists on how to structure their communications and write as concisely as possible, with the most important information summarised at the beginning. This is also the structure that is used when writing press releases.

TIPS BOX 10.2

The ability to write succinctly is an extremely useful skill for emails and reports, especially where the recipient is very time poor. They may scan items and only read in full those that they consider to be the most important. It is also helpful if you are working with your organisation's communications lead, as you can help them by providing the most pertinent information.

Be aware, however, that sometimes board and committee reports are structured using a template, so always ask about this first if you are writing a formal document for your organisation. Such templates often require information at the beginning of a report like the purpose, the background and an introduction, rather than just getting straight down to the facts.

■ Time Out

Read some newspaper headlines. What do you observe about the way that journalists write?

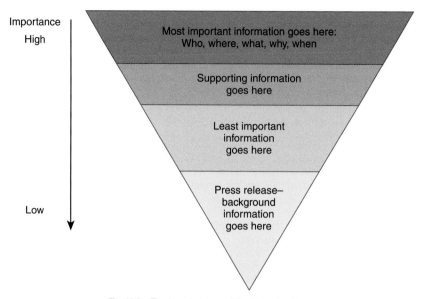

Fig. 10.2   The inverted pyramid writing structure.

The style of writing that journalists use is called the 'inverted pyramid' (Fig. 10.2).

1. **Write the most important information first:** Cover the five Ws that we discussed in the chapter on creativity: who, where, what, why and when. Aim to write this in 30 words or less. Use everyday language and avoid jargon.
2. **Add supporting information:** The bulk of the information comes next. Expand on your points or describe the issue in more detail; provide data. This information helps the reader to understand your message more clearly. Do not overload them with lots of detail so that they get lost in it.
3. **Add information of lesser importance:** You may want to include related information, such as historical detail or links to national policy or data related to the subject. Think about whether it adds to what you have already said.
4. **Add background information:** In press releases only, add your contact details and advise on how people can find out more information, such as from your organisation's website.

Refer Table 10.1 for structuring a press release.

TABLE 10.1 ■ Structuring a Press Release

Journalists are tight for time, so make their job easy by using the inverted pyramid structure so they have little or no editing to do. Include an uncluttered photograph in landscape rather than portrait mode to draw the eye. Use the following as a template for your press release:

Date:

Contact: *(Your name and contacts [phone and email])*

Immediate release/embargoed *(Think about press deadlines)*

Headline:

TABLE 10.1 ■ Structuring a Press Release—cont'd

<News release starts>

Introduction *(This should give a concise summary of the story. Who is it about? Find the strongest story angle.)*

Second paragraph *(This is the remainder of the five Ws, but with gradually less important details. Write in the third person rather than in the first person.)*

Quote *(This is your chance to say exactly what you think. A journalist may well edit the first paragraph of your press release, but they will not make major changes to your quote. Your quote should be personal and emotive; try to include a key message.)*

Fourth paragraph *(By the fourth paragraph, you are giving a bit more background. If the journalist only has a small amount of space they may well 'cut to fit', meaning this information is missed out.)*

Finish off *your press release with contact details, where people can find out more information, for example, a website or phone number.*

<News release ends>

Example of a Press Release

Date Tuesday, 26 May 2020
Contact BreathChamps@ xxxxxxxx Tel 0161 xxxxxxxx
Immediate release

News Release

Shared tips to help breathing during lockdown & Covid-19

A local community group has received Awards for All funding from the National Lottery to set up a 'Breathe Well UK' Facebook group, where citizens can share breathing tips. There is a lot of fake information on the internet and so the group will dispel myths and be a place where people can get information with confidence.

This group is about learning from each other about how to breathe better. The group is moderated by a registered nurse (Heather Henry) and a local person (C), and both have had lung problems for a long time. They will make sure that the information that is shared helps people feel better and does no harm.

C said 'Whether you've had breathing issues for a long time, are struggling at the moment, or you help others to breathe, this group is here to care, be kind and share knowledge. We know what it is like to be breathless and we can help.'

Heather runs a not-for-profit group called BreathChamps CIC. C is a patient representative on the UK Taskforce for Lung Health and also the National COPD and Asthma Audit and an active British Lung Foundation patient by experience representative.

You can join the Facebook group **here**.To get more information from the NHS on breathing tips during the pandemic, visit xxx.

Digital Leadership and Influence

Many health students interviewed for this book talked about using social media to communicate and to lead in various ways. Working with colleagues to curate social media accounts and jointly run tweet chats is a common method for starting discussions, building community, making connections and learning together.

Over the last couple of years, the range of social media accounts curated by health care students and newly registered nurses has proliferated. The topics range from developing students' leadership skills, campaigning, promoting nursing and nursing specialisms, supporting the transition from student to registered practitioner and focusing on topics of interest to students, such as the environment or student mental health.

What is clear from talking to students involved in such accounts is how they 'hand on the baton': seeking out new talent and developing their successors to take over the account, supervising and supporting each other until the new curators were ready to manage alone, before moving on.

Some students talked about creating 'Tweet cheat sheets' that decsribe how they manage social media accounts and how they mentored their successors until they were ready to manage alone.

The successor students talked about the legacy they inherited and how they sometimes felt daunted by the achievements of those who came before them. What is noticeable is how much these students successfully build on that legacy and at the same time injected their own leadership style and personality. Success seems to breed success (Case Study 10.1).

The consistency with which these accounts have been created and subsequently curated is striking. This means that the number of followers has risen because the accounts are actively curated and moderated. With a rise in followership comes influence: student leaders in this space have credibility and the ability to accurately gauge student reactions through tools such as polls and asking questions. This sort of digital leadership gives rise to the sort of expert, referent and informational power mentioned by French and Raven, discussed in the previous chapter.

CASE STUDY 10.1 **Digital Leadership: Representing Your Profession and Your Organisation on Social Media**

Alison Booker, a student dietician and former #150Leaders participant, stood for election in 2019/20 to be the student representative on the British Dietetic Association (BDA). She sees social media as a real force for positivity. She used Twitter to ask her colleagues to vote for her, and when she was elected she took over the running of the BDA student representative Twitter account:

'I felt that it was important that if I was going to be the student rep, I was going to be approachable and personable, authentic—all those things that make you a good leader. And that will enable students to engage with me. I felt that if it was a corporate account then it would be quite off-putting.'
ALISON BOOKER

Alison also made a clear distinction between her personal Twitter account and the BDA representative account. Using the BDA account she did a lot of retweeting, engaging with members and sharing BDA material. She used her personal account to tweet her personal opinion and share her work.

During the COVID-19 pandemic she noticed that morale was low among the student dieticians. She felt that continuous personal development (CPD) was very important. She engaged a former BDA student representative to help her to put on CPD webinars especially for student dieticians, with backing from a nutrition company. Afterwards, she saw a lot more student dieticians with social media accounts and greater social media engagement between student dieticians as well as more CPD opportunities.

One of the features of the #150Leaders programme is to encourage student leaders to be curious about each other's roles and consider how they might work better together. This fits with the approach being adopted in health and social care, which is about integrated care and multidisciplinary teams.

'When we first joined the @WeAHPs team (an allied health professionals peer support account on Twitter) we did a student takeover week. And in that week we explained about every single profession. And I think if we can educate students about that straight from the word go then you're on to a winner really.'
SARAH BRADDER, NEWLY QUALIFIED THERAPEUTIC
RADIOGRAPHER AND FORMER #150LEADERS PARTICIPANT

Alison Booker decided that to promote and explain her role to others she would set up personal Twitter and Instagram accounts and a write a blog called *Alison The Student Dietitian* to promote dietetics. Instagram works well for dieticians, she says, because images of food are very visually attractive. She found it quite daunting at first because there were not many dietetic accounts and blogs, and she wondered whether she should be saying certain things in her role as a student. Now she sees that many more accounts have been set up on Instagram using the hashtag #RD2B (registered dietician to be). She uses her social media accounts to try to explain the breadth of the dietician role beyond traditional weight management.

Alison also thought about how to introduce her role to others. Unlike student nurses, her profession refers to its undergraduates as 'dietetic students' and noted that people found that term confusing. Alison started to introduce herself by saying 'I'm a student dietician' which she thinks gives her profession more power because it has a clearer identity.

■ **Time Out**

Make a note of anything that strikes you about Alison and Sarah's digital leadership.

If you have more than one role and like to use social media, it is important that you are able to separate out the roles and use each account for the correct purpose.

People like to engage with people rather than accounts, so quite often, even if an account is curated by a team, the account description may be tweaked to let others know who the face is behind the tweets for a particular day or week.

Social media is a powerful way to explain your role to others and to learn about the role of other professions and disciplines. Nurses often feel that their role is poorly understood, but other disciplines also feel this way, especially amongst some of the smaller allied health professional groups, so reach out and engage across disciplines as much as you can. This will help you hugely when you become registered because teams are increasingly multidisciplinary, and you will succeed in your leadership more if you understand each other's roles.

Small changes can make a big difference. In Alison's case she not only encouraged student dieticians onto social media by putting on CPD activities but also, by tweaking how she introduced herself, it enabled others to understand her role better. Alison is clearly a trendsetter, unafraid of being the first to do something!

Blogs, Vlogs and Podcasts as Ways to Influence

As a student you may think that publishing may not be a priority and that you might be not academic enough to write, but for some it is more about getting their message across about something that they are passionate about in the most engaging way.

Blogging (an online journal or diary on the internet), vlogging (video blogging) and podcasting (a series of spoken word, audio episodes focusing on a particular topic or theme) can also be powerful and influential forms of digital leadership to communicate your thoughts to others.

'Someone said to me, you can't think about what other people think about you. It will stop you from doing so much. You just need to forget about that... Just put it out there.'
CLAIRE CARMICHAEL, NEWLY REGISTERED GENERAL PRACTICE NURSE

For Claire Carmichael, vlogging is her way of using her own experience to show that nursing is an amazing career choice. Her motivation is intrinsic—to help others and to know that she has helped people to decide on a career in nursing.

■ **Time Out**

Start a discussion with your peers on the influence of podcasts, blogs and vlogs on their nursing journey. Which ones do they follow? Do any of them create them? How have they influenced you all? What do they like about them?

Why Storytelling Influences Us

What vlogging, blogging and podcasting all have in common is that they often use the power of narrative and storytelling—and this is important and powerful.

"We dream in narrative, day-dream in narrative, remember, anticipate, hope, despair, believe, doubt, plan, revise, criticise, construct, gossip, learn, hate and love by narrative.'
BARBARA HARDY, BRITISH LITERARY SCHOLAR, AUTHOR AND POET

In the chapter on cocreation, we discussed how patient's stories are, as Brené Brown puts it, 'data with a soul', but storytelling and public narrative are also extremely powerful ways of influencing people.

Storytelling is the way that humans organise their thinking to make sense of the world. We are programmed to make patterns and associations. We assemble mutually reinforcing stories to construct common sense, stereotypes, communities, cultures and ideologies to help us to navigate our way.

Stories are in effect our mental models and are often fed by media, politics and popular culture. The other thing about stories is that they are relatable—we associate ourselves with characters and situations, and this helps the storyteller to engage their audience.

Stories are told in the form of a narrative: a description of a series of events told in a particular way to explain or understand situations. Narratives are often messy, nonlinear and contradictory, but can also cause us to viscerally respond:

> 'Narratives are powerful. They can swing juries and elections. They can fill prisons. But they can also fill the streets.'
>
> JEE KIM, LIZ HYNES AND NIMA SHIRAZI, THE NARRATIVE INITIATIVE (2007)

Storytelling has important neurobiological effects and engages the emotions, as you will perhaps have felt when watching a powerful movie such as Schindler's List. Perhaps you can still remember exactly what happened in the movie, and maybe a movie or story changed you in some way and because of it you did something differently. This is the power of story, and it is something that you can harness as a leader.

At a networking event I recently attended, I heard a nurse tell her story about her battle with long COVID, which affected me greatly and I developed a huge admiration for her. She had done her own research and was describing which medical and nonmedical interventions were helping her. I immediately contacted this nurse to tell her my story of the nonmedical respiratory interventions for long COVID that I was considering. Together we are now trying to influence system leaders to research and invest in more nonmedical interventions for long COVID.

The evidence is that giving information in the form of a story enables recall, cooperation and personal responsibility (Zak 2014; Hamilton and Weiss 2015; Mantle of the Expert online—see Fig. 10.3). Not only that, but by telling a story to people, it creates a strong connection to them that you can then go on to harness as part of your leadership, as in my example above. Zak (2014), for example, discovered that character-driven stories, especially where there is a degree of tension, stimulates the production of oxytocin in the brain. This neurochemical encourages a sense of empathy with the storyteller and a desire to cooperate. This is the power of the story told by the nurse with long COVID.

A pioneering drama teacher in the 1980s called Dorothy Heathcote worked with primary school children to develop imaginary story-based contexts to generate purposeful and engaging activities for learning. This system is now called 'mantle of the expert', and there is a website (www.mantleoftheexpert.com) dedicated to sharing that knowledge. For example, a class of children studying the Tudor period might be cast as museum experts in charge of running a Tudor mansion for the National Trust. They create all the exhibits, do their research on the Tudor period and find out the history of the mansion and its owners. The children then open the fictional museum and act as guides for guests. In doing so the children start to exhibit responsibility, which is what you as a leader are asking your team to do. There may even be some parallels here to nursing students' own simulated learning!

In terms of how stories improve recall, in my own work I use the *Three Little Pigs* story to invite children in school assembly to come up and give my puppet the Big Bad Wolf the correct inhaler using the correct technique when his asthma stops him blowing down the various

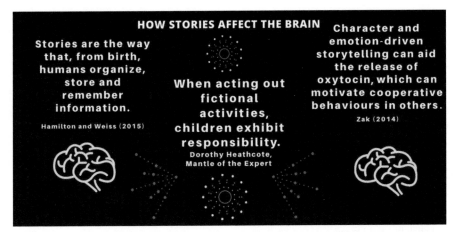

HOW STORIES AFFECT THE BRAIN

Stories are the way that, from birth, humans organize, store and remember information.

Hamilton and Weiss (2015)

When acting out fictional activities, children exhibit responsibility.

Dorothy Heathcote, Mantle of the Expert

Character and emotion-driven storytelling can aid the release of oxytocin, which can motivate cooperative behaviours in others.

Zak (2014)

Fig. 10.3 How stories affect the brain. (Based on Zak, P., 2014. Why your brain loves good storytelling. Harvard Business Review. <https://hbr.org/2014/10/why-your-brain-loves-good-storytelling>; Hamilton, M., Weiss, M., 2015. Children Telling Stories: Teaching and Using Stories in the Classroom. Richard C. Owen, New York; Mantle of the Expert. <https://www.mantleoftheexpert.com/>.)

piggies' houses. As all the children know the story already, they can more easily recall the asthma knowledge by associating it with the story. This memory technique of connecting important information to memorable stories or journeys is also often used by people in preparation for examinations.

Today's leaders are using digital storytelling to get across their message. This involves combining the art of storytelling with multimedia features such as text, audio, voiceover, photography, hypertext and video. Using accessible software such as iMovie, Microsoft Photos and WeVideo. com, student nurses can create and share their story in digital ways.

Public Storytelling

Student Nurse Gloria Sikapite takes people on her leadership journey and shows how she has developed her skills along the way, so that others will not be discouraged. She sees the sharing of her experiences as an investment in herself and in the hope that it will help others (Case Study 10.2).

CASE STUDY 10.2

Gloria Sikapite describes the culture shock of her first time at university and how she really benefitted from listening to more experienced students who helped to prepare her for what to expect. As she became more senior, she decided to offer that same help to new students. As part of a recruitment and retention project for her university, she got in touch with her student union and now presents her story at open days and fresher's weeks. She not only talks about what to expect, but also covers the opportunity offered to her by being part of the #150Leaders programme.

'I wasn't born a leader and I didn't think I was a leader. If I'm able to speak (to an audience) now, then why shouldn't you?'

Her approach is to invite her audience to get to know her before and after her experiences as a student and as a participant in the #150Leaders programme. She wants to demonstrate, using her story, that she was not always someone who was very confident.

◼ Time Out

What do you notice about Gloria's presenting style and how she goes about trying to influence new students?

One way to develop your presentation skills is to talk from your own experience and tell your story—after all, you are the expert! And it also helps with the important skill of being your authentic self (Tips Box 10.3).

TIPS BOX 10.3

Public Speaking

- I wear red lipstick because it makes me feel more put together.
- I research exactly what they want me to talk about.
- I stick to what I know.
- I present as my authentic self: I've always had good feedback. I prepare reams of notes but I don't read from a script. I'm happy to be bumbling, to be flailing my arms about. I'd rather not work myself up about coming across as uber-smart.
- I have a clear message that I want to communicate.
- I connect with my audience by looking at people and not over their heads.
- I did some drama and role-played to build my confidence.

(Based on author's interviews with health students.)

STORYTELLING TIPS

'Audiences cannot resist a well-told story even if they try.'

AKASH KARIA (ONLINE)

The best storytellers can often be seen on TED. Akash Karia is a well-known keynote speaker who has distilled from TED talks some of the main components of how to engage people using story:

- Hook your audience by beginning with a story rather than lots of introductory remarks. Here is a version of my story that I use in my respiratory work: 'What a shock I had when I suddenly found myself having major chest surgery in my second year as a student nurse, to stop my right lung from repeatedly collapsing. I had just turned 21 and was allowed home from my 21st birthday before being admitted for a planned pleurectomy. But when my chest was opened the surgeon saw emphysematous bullae and so I ended up having most of my right lung removed.'
- Introduce conflict into your story. The stronger the conflict, the greater the interest will be. For example, 'I remember the director of nursing coming to see me on the ward to give me the news that, in her opinion, I was not strong enough for a career in nursing and would probably never nurse again'.
- Engage them using lots of detail, how the characters in your story looked, what they saw, what they felt, heard, smelled, etc. For example: 'It was a hot May day, my nightie was sticking to me, so I painfully got myself out of bed to straighten myself up. I had a draw sheet wrapped around me to support my thoracotomy wound. I felt like if I coughed I might split in two.'
- Use dialogue, for example: 'Then I saw her, striding purposefully towards me. She said 'no—don't get up'. I had to laugh because she thought I was getting up from my sick bed out of respect for her!'

- Inspire your audience with positive messages. For example: 'My experience of being a patient gave me empathy as a nurse. I think about how I begged for pethidine 3 hours after the last dose and how my request was refused, making my sister cry because she saw me in acute pain and couldn't help me. I recall how my wishes were ignored and a chest drain was taken out under suction, which was excruciating; how my bare chest was examined by the consultant on a ward round, in full view of his all-male team. How my locker was never replaced in my reach after I was repositioned, so I had to bother people to ask for it to be moved. I vowed that the same standards of care would not happen on my watch.'
- Leave your audience on an emotional high. For example, did I finish my training? Well, I guess you know the answer: 'It took me precisely 3 months longer to get to my finals. I got out of doing lots of night duty, because staff were short on the ground at night and I was not allowed to lift (yes we still did manual lifting back then). I didn't have to do my planned allocation in gynae theatre with the 'Dragon Sister' either. So, I think that was a bargain! And to that director of nursing I say—I hope that I have made a difference in my career. Now here I am writing about leadership for student nurses. Who would have thought it?'
- Have a final takeaway message, for example my message is: 'You can overcome adversity, learn from it and come away stronger.'

AUTHOR'S STORY BASED ON KARIA'S (ONLINE) MAIN TENETS OF STORYTELLING

STORY OF SELF, STORY OF US, STORY OF NOW

In a later chapter on leading change we shall expand on this idea of storytelling to include how communicating your values in your story can engage people's emotions and encourage them to act. We shall also discuss how to structure your story into three parts: starting with your personal story (story of self), before relating this to something that your audience shares (story of us), before guiding them towards a call to action (story of now).

In my story I take you from telling you about my operation, through to sharing my values around standards of care that I hope you can relate to. This might all lead up to the third part of my story where I might want to galvanise you into action around a theme of personalised care! Fortunately, I am sparing you that.

▨ Time Out

- Try using storytelling to influence others: your own story, or maybe the story of a patient you have worked alongside.
- Then ask trusted colleagues for feedback: did storytelling make a difference to the way the presentation was received?
- Take care to only disclose what you would be comfortable sharing in the public domain. (I have shared my operation story lots of times, and the director of nursing and the Dragon Sister are no longer with us!)

Coping With Feedback on Social Media

All student nurses and registered nurses are obliged to follow the NMC's guidance on social media, which was first published in 2015. However, the NMC does not offer guidance on how to cope with the consequences of being 'out there' on social media (Tips Box 10.4, 10.5 and 10.6).

As a vlogger and blogger, Claire Carmichael's aim is to inspire people to come into nursing and be the best nurses that they can be. In doing this she shares some of her personal journey. And this may be why she is seen as an inspirational, authentic leader and maybe even an 'influencer'—someone who influences in this case not brands or goods, but promotes the nursing 'brand'.

Her vlogging means that to some she is instantly recognisable. Through answering questions on her social media pages, she was viewed by one student as her 'social media mentor', even though they had never met. This student ran up to talk to her, embracing her as a friend. This experience, which has happened at other times too, was not anticipated by Claire and at first she had difficulty understanding what was happening and accepting that she is seen as a leader by those aspirant nurses or fellow students.

TIPS BOX 10.4

Dealing With Social Media Supporters

- Accept that by being on social media you will influence people, so use that influence responsibly.
- You may not know your supporters, but they may feel that they know you. Manage their reaction with calm kindness.
- You may have no real idea of the positive impact that you have on others until you meet them.
- You may have to do a reality check to understand, like Claire, the positive effect that you are having on others.
- Alternatively, you must keep your ego in check and avoid pushing personal agendas, such as seeking money or free goods (see the NMC code!).
- You can of course use your platform to give voice to professional causes.
- As an influential person, you may get invited to involve yourself in many things. Think about your circles of concern, control and influence, and do not overload yourself, especially regarding issues that you probably cannot control.
- Set boundaries for yourself and be able to say no, with kindness.
- Look out for opportunists: these are people who are keen to work in partnership with you because of your influence alone. If they are not interested in your work, then politely back away!
- At all times, abide by the NMC code and their guidance on using social media responsibly.

Adapted from Griffin (2021).

Reaction of Others and Managing Envy

'Being a leader is not very easy, especially when you have friends in the same area that you're being a leader. You can distinguish friendship role and leadership role.'

GLORIA SIKAPITE, ADULT STUDENT NURSE

'I've gone past pinching myself and feeling lucky and realised... how can I use this opportunity to do something that I'm passionate about? I've just got to go with it and not be fearful of back-lashes and people hating you because you're linked with a particular organisation. Or you're in a leadership role and people accuse you of not caring about the masses.'

ANONYMOUS THIRD YEAR ADULT STUDENT NURSE,
TALKING ABOUT HER DECISION TO TAKE UP A NATIONAL ROLE WITH A UNION

Let us continue with Claire Carmichael's story. She was recognised by her university for her leadership work, winning various awards, but then she noticed that two of her friends had blocked her on social media and so she contacted them to find out why. They told her that they could not cope with how positive she was about nursing. Later at an awards ceremony she noticed that a friend was making negative comments, so she asked to speak to her privately about it. Her friend admitted her envy at Claire winning lots of awards and, despite Claire's efforts, the friend could not accept it. See Tips Box 10.5 for ways to deal with envy in others.

TIPS BOX 10.5

Dealing With Envy

- Lead with what you believe in—your values—rather than ego or desire for promotion and people will have less to fight against.
- Use your emotional intelligence to tune into how people may be responding.
- Ask to speak to the person whose envy may be negatively affecting you—do not let it slide.
- Listen to what they say and invite them to listen to you (look back at the chapter on being assertive).
- Try to resolve it, but recognise that sometimes this cannot be done and you may have to walk away from negative people and be around people who are positive and supportive.

Based on the author's interviews with student nurse leaders.

Dealing With Internet Trolls

An internet troll is someone who makes inflammatory or upsetting comments on social media, sometimes for their own amusement and sometimes to pursue their own specific agenda. If you have had a presence on social media, you may have come into contact with them. See Tips Box 10.6 for ideas on how to handle this.

TIPS BOX 10.6

Dealing With Trolls

Teresa Chinn is a registered nurse and highly regarded professional social media community development specialist. She is the founder of a network of social media nursing accounts called WeCommunities. In a 2019 podcast Teresa offers advice to others on managing disagreements on social media. She reminds us that although we have an NMC code to follow, the public generally does not! Her first point is that we are in control of our social media use and that it should not control us.

You need to be clear about the purpose of your social media messages and should never react out of anger, when tired or after drinking alcohol. If someone is upsetting you, reflect on whether this is a disagreement or a troll. Think why something upsets you—you may be tired, the comment may have triggered personal experiences, you may be just having a bad day or you may have interpreted the message in a way not intended by the sender. Take a break and come back to it.

Disagreements based on reasoned argument and evidence should of course be welcomed. We can always learn from others, broaden our horizons or disagree respectfully. But if you receive abuse, especially if it diverges from the topic being discussed, then consider whether this is 'trolling'. Teresa suggests that you offer three chances: invite them first to expand and clarify, then invite them to offer research or evidence to back up their point, followed by an invitation to agree to disagree. The last resort is to unfollow or block accounts.

Teresa advises that it is unwise to 'feed the trolls'—this means ignoring them rather than giving them the satisfaction of seeing you upset or angry. It is helpful, she says, to look at the person's social media history and judge whether a person has abused and upset others.

Racist, sexist, discriminatory, abusive, offensive language, including inciting hatred, is unlawful. If you feel unsafe or threatened take screen shots as proof, block the person and report the account to the provider and to the police. Most social media sites will have advice on what to do.

Based on Chinn (2019).

Summary

There are many well-practised ways to communicate to influence others and a body of scientific knowledge to enable us to deliver an effective story or narrative. Student leaders can use the communication cycle to plan and reflect on the way they communicate, based on their intended audience. They can use the inverted pyramid to get their message across concisely and effectively. Students can become more persuasive by using Monroe's Motivated Sequence to get attention, establish the need, satisfy the need, visualise the future and start to take action. In meetings, there are various techniques that can be used to get over the fear of speaking out, plus finding a coach to guide and encourage you can be helpful.

In the digital world, many students are leading the way to influence others using digital storytelling, social media accounts, podcasts, blogs and vlogs. They need to be prepared for the reaction, both positive and negative, and of course abide by the NMC's social media guidance and code.

Storytelling is one of the most powerful ways of influencing others, engendering feelings of empathy, cooperation and a sense of responsibility. Stories help people to remember the information that is given. Effective storytelling needs to attract and maintain attention by including conflict, detail and dialogue, and positive messages that leave your audience on an emotional high.

References

Burgess, S., Sly, P., Devadason, S., 2011. Adherence with preventive medication in childhood asthma. Pulmonary Medicine, 973849.

Chinn, T., 2019. Disagreeing or Trolling? #WeNursesPod. Available on Spotify.

Chisholm-Burns, M.A., Spivey, C.A., 2012. The 'cost' of medication nonadherence: consequences we cannot afford to accept. Journal of the American Pharmacists Association, 52 (6), 823–826.

Griffin, T., 2021. How to Handle Fame. wikiHow. <https://www.wikihow.com/Handle-Fame>.

Hamilton, M., Weiss, M., 2015. Children Telling Stories: Teaching and Using Stories in the Classroom. Richard C. Owen, New York.

Ji, L., Bailey, C., 2013. Case study: patient with poor glycaemic control due to poor adherence to medication. The Global Partnership for Effective Diabetes Management. <http://www.effectivediabetesmanagement. com/download/Poor_adherence_1_20May2013.pdf#.~:text=Case%20study%3A%20Individual%20 with%20inadequate%20glycaemic%20control%20due,Effective%20Diabetes%20Management%20is%20 supported%20by%20an%20unrestricted>.

Karia, A., TEDTalks: Storytelling. 23 Storytelling Techniques From the Best TED talks. <www.Akash-Karia.com>.

Kim, J., Hynes, L., Shirazi, N., 2007. The Narrative Initiative. <https://narrativeinitiative.org/wp-content/ uploads/2019/08/TowardNewGravity-June2017.pdf>. (accessed 17/12/2021).

Mantle of the Expert. <https://www.mantleoftheexpert.com/>. Based on the work of educationalist Dorothy Heathcote, this website describes how children learn through story.

Monroe, A.H., 1943. Monroe's Principles of Speech (military edition). Scott, Foresman, Chicago.

National Institute for Health and Clinical Excellence, 2009. Medicines adherence: involving patients in decisions about prescribed medicines and supporting adherence. Clinical guideline [CG76].

Nursing and Midwifery Council, 2015. Guidance on using social media responsibly. <https://www.nmc.org. uk/standards/guidance/social-media-guidance/>. (accessed 17/12/2021).

Shannon, C.E., Weaver, W., 1971. The Mathematical Theory of Communication, first ed. (US). The University of Illinois Press, Urbana.

Turnbull, A., 2015. Wasted medicine 'costs the NHS £800 million'. Independent Nurse, 8 October. <https:// www.independentnurse.co.uk/news/wasted-medicine-costs-the-nhs-800-million/108229/>.

Zak, P., 2014. Why your brain loves good storytelling. Harvard Business Review. <https://hbr.org/2014/10/ why-your-brain-loves-good-storytelling>.

Improve Health Care

CHAPTER 11

Navigating Organisations and Systems to Improve Health Care

OBJECTIVES

After reading this chapter and completing the activities, you should be able to:
- Describe what is meant by a complex adaptive system
- Identify the difference in skills needed to lead across a system compared to leading in one organisation
- Define place-based care and integrated care
- Explain the difference between simple, complicated and complex problems
- Explain the link between the culture of an organisation, the climate and the quality of patient care.

Relevance to the Nursing and Midwifery Council (NMC) Code

Prioritise People
  1 Treat people as individuals and uphold their dignity
  1.1 Treat people with kindness, respect and compassion
Listen to People and Respond to their Preferences and Concerns
  2.1 Work in partnership with people to make sure you deliver care effectively
Practise Effectively
  8 Work cooperatively
  8.1 Respect the skills, expertise and contributions of your colleagues, referring matters to them when appropriate
  8.2 Maintain effective communication with colleagues
Promote Professionalism and Trust
  20 Uphold the reputation of your profession at all times
  20.1 Keep to and uphold the standards and values set out in the code

Continued

20.2 Act with honesty and integrity at all times, treating people fairly and without discrimination, bullying or harassment

20.3 Be aware at all times of how your behaviour can affect and influence the behaviour of other people

20.8 Act as a role model of professional behaviour for students and newly qualified nurses, midwives and nursing associates to aspire to

For you as a student nurse to make improvements in health and care, you need to have an understanding of how organisations and cultures work. You may have worked in large organisations before coming into nursing and will therefore have an appreciation of how complex organisations like universities, NHS organisations and independent, voluntary, community and social enterprise (VCSE or third sector) operate.

You will know that such organisations work within a system. For example, if you are working in accident and emergency (A&E) you may see homeless people who may have physical, mental health or learning problems, perhaps with associated substance misuse or criminal convictions. This means that the health system must work seamlessly with housing, social care, criminal justice and relevant voluntary and community organisations such as hostels if it is to make a positive difference.

'Understanding systems is of even more importance from a student view when we represent two organisations, the university and the NHS, as well as move around different wards/hospitals and placements on a regular basis.'

ADAM ACOTT, NEWLY REGISTERED NURSE

As students you straddle both university and various placement settings. Universities likewise work with partners such as schools and colleges, scientists, business organisations and professional bodies, as well as the public sector and VCSE organisations.

This chapter will help you to differentiate between the skills needed for 'system leadership', where you are not 'in charge', and leadership within your own organisation. This will help you to understand what you see when you first look at large organisations and systems. You will also be able to identify leaders who role model the right behaviours in the right context.

The model of leadership that you adopt when working within a system is different from the one you use within your organisation and your team, because you are relying more on 'relational' working (building your relationships by sharing common values and goals) and less on organisational accountability. It is also important to develop a 'balcony view' of what is happening across the system and about setting the right conditions for change to happen, rather than trying to make things happen.

We shall start this chapter by understanding how systems operate and then move on to understanding organisational culture and climate. Both are important if you are to lead improvements.

Machine Thinking and Complex Adaptive Systems

Planned changes and improvements are typified by linear thinking—'we are doing X to deliver Y change and to do this we will do ABC'. It is logical and it is undertaken by a series of organised steps. It is led through the art of crafting the change story, and the knowledge is explicit: we know what we are doing, why we are doing it and how best to do it.

It is the sort of thinking that is used in manufacturing, where processes are streamlined and the phrase 'one best way' comes to mind. This emerged from a theorist in the early 1900s called Frederick Taylor, who worked to optimise and simplify manufacturing jobs.

However, people do not behave like the machines used in Taylor's scientific management principles (1911). They are not always rational, linear thinkers, so it is not surprising that change often goes awry. Change is threatening, and we shall discuss in Chapter 13 how people react to change and how you might respond empathically to that, but we also need to examine something called complexity theory. This is about understanding how organisations in complex environments adapt to and cope with conditions of uncertainty.

Health and care organisations are not aggregations of individual entities but are characterised by complex, dynamic networks of interactions that adapt to conditions and self-organise in response to events. The phrase often used in health and care is that organisations operate in 'complex adaptive systems'. In these circumstances, the capabilities of leaders need to change from trying to control events to setting up the enabling conditions for positive change to occur.

A common way to describe the difference between mechanistic thinking and a complex adaptive system is the analogy of inviting a group of businesspeople to organise children's play time at a school. The managers might spend some time organising activities and time slots, but the result might be that the children completely ignore this and dash excitedly around. If the managers then watch how the teachers manage play time, their approach is completely different. They set the enabling conditions by creating a few boundaries and rules for play time, within which the children organise themselves.

Nursing practice itself, often described as both an art and a science, is now being described as a complex adaptive system (Kiviliene and Blazeviciene 2019) as nurses observe, guide and adapt their care to what is happening. It is just like planning a party—organise the right venue; invite the people you know based on who you think will work together to make the party swing; encourage the building of relationships between the guests; put on the right entertainment, music, food and such at the right time; watch over your guests and adapt—and you are all more likely to have a good time.

Changes are categorised by:

- A high degree of connectivity between the parts of the system
- Self-organisation
- Emergent rather than planned solutions
- Observing and responding to patterns
- Systems being governed through just a few simple rules

(Health Foundation 2010; Henry 2014).

Part of your thinking, therefore, as you consider the change or improvement that you have in mind is how much certainty and agreement there is about what is proposed (see Fig. 11.1). Where there is high certainty and agreement, then planned change, with mechanistic thinking,

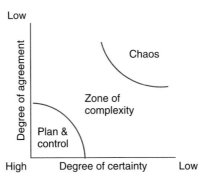

Fig. 11.1 Certainty–agreement diagram. (Stacey, R.D., 1996. Complexity and Creativity in Organizations. Berrett-Koehler Series. Berrett-Koehler, San Francisco, CA.)

is more likely to work. Where there is less certainty and agreement, the more likely you are to enter the 'zone of complexity' and become an enabler rather than a leader.

Place-Based Care and Integrated Care

Over the last decade or more, health and care leaders have increasingly realised that the parts of the system such as the NHS, voluntary sector, social care, business, housing, education and so on have often operated in isolation from each other. Yet you only need to step into a GP waiting room, a ward or an A&E department to know that the reasons that many people are there relate to problems such as poor housing, lack of social care and unemployment. There remain unacceptable variations in healthy life expectancy from 7 years in Northern Ireland to up to 19 years for example in England (Department of Health Northern Ireland, 2021; NHS England, Place Based Care, online). Today there is a move towards 'place-based' care, which is about recognising that to make a significant change to health outcomes at a population level, it is necessary to not just treat disease or the causes of disease but to address the wider determinants of health and to consider the impact of psychosocial and protective factors for the place that you are in.

> *'Integrated care is about giving people the support they need, joined up across local councils, the NHS, and other partners. It removes traditional divisions between hospitals and family doctors, between physical and mental health, and between NHS and council services. In the past, these divisions have meant that too many people experienced disjointed care.'*
> NHS ENGLAND, WHAT ARE INTEGRATED CARE SYSTEM (ONLINE)

Integrated care systems (ICSs) have existed for a few years now across various parts of the UK. They are partnerships between NHS, local councils and other important strategic partners such as the VSCE sector to meet the health and care needs across a defined geography. They coordinate services and plan in a way that improves population health and reduces inequalities between different groups.

Understanding Health and Care Systems

A system can be defined as an interdependent group of items, people, or processes working together toward a common purpose. Take for example the various teams, functions, processes and pieces of equipment that work together to achieve the common purpose of operating successfully on somebody. Immediately you can bring to mind the theatre itself, clinical and theatre staff, all the equipment and all the imaging and pathology testing that happens. But what about the porters, the maintenance teams, the teams who clean and return the instruments and the people who procure gloves, masks and gowns and so on? They are part of the system too.

Then stretch that same idea out to consider how, for example, the wider system operates to support people with alcohol dependency. The system might then include police, local authority licencing, publicans, off-licence owners, hostels, domestic abuse charities and recovery organisations as well as the NHS.

Think also about the boundaries of the system—where it starts and where it ends and the interface with wider systems. For example, after someone has had major surgery, they may need to enter the rehabilitation system.

To make improvements to a system you need to be able to understand it first rather than try to implement a project based on your personal perception of the part of the system in which you are involved. This is sometimes called 'silo working' or 'silo thinking'.

Simple, Complicated and Complex Systems

Systems can also be simple, complicated and complex. A simple system might be a preoperative assessment. A complicated system might be an organ transplant system involving transplant coordinators, the harvesting and transporting of donor organs, consents from donors or their families as well as recipients and their families, all the ethical considerations as well as the procedure itself and follow-ups needed to prevent rejection. In complicated systems you can disassemble the parts and understand how they all work together.

By contrast, in a complex system it is not enough to know the parts. The way they interact may result in unexpected or emergent ways, so it is important to investigate the dynamics between the various parts of the system. The human body, a city traffic system or a national public health system are examples of complex systems. In complex systems, we cannot assume that a solution will have the desired outcome.

■ Time Out

Think of a system that you are part of, at work or at home, that is set up to achieve a shared purpose. Would you define it as simple, complicated or complex? Examples might include your child's school system, a slimming group or a study group.

Understanding People's Experience of the System

It is important here to distinguish between a person's experience and their satisfaction with it. Their experience of care focuses on what actually happens during interactions between the person/people giving care and the person receiving it. Their satisfaction focuses on whether interactions between the caregivers and the person live up to expectations. To achieve truly person- or community-centred improvement, it is important to first understand and value the experience of the person's family and community who are involved and what matters most to them. Look back to the chapter on codesign where we discussed the ways to understand patient experience.

Understanding System Flow

System flow is about understanding how people move through the system, and this will give you insight on where you might want to make improvements. This means mapping out the entire process and understanding all of the steps, quality issues, bottlenecks and data. We shall explore this more in Chapter 14 on leading improvement.

Understanding Perverse Incentives

Another thing to watch out for when working in a system are incentives that can produce unintended and undesirable results. The most direct kind of unintended consequence is known as the 'cobra effect', which unintentionally rewards people for making issues worse. This term arose from an anecdote about the time of British rule in India when there was concern about the number of venomous snakes. The British offered a bounty reward for each snake killed. This led people to breed cobras to cash in. When the British discovered this, they removed the reward, leaving the breeders to let their cobras return to the wild. The population of cobras became a greater problem than it was before.

■ **Time Out**

Can you identify any unintended consequences in the health and care system—past or present?

Some would argue that Payment by Results (PbR), which was a system of paying NHS health care providers a standard national price or tariff for each patient seen or treated, led to gaming of the system. Perverse behaviours have been found, including 'upcoding', where hospitals systematically categorise patients into coding groups that have a higher level of reimbursement procedures. Another is so-called 'cream-skimming', or adverse selection, meaning the selection by providers of services for patients which are expected to be (more) profitable (Mays et al. 2011). The PbR system was anecdotally seen as making providers compete with each other, which inhibited integrated working. PbR was suspended in 2020, and providers returned to 'block contracts' (a block payment made to a provider to deliver a specific, usually broadly defined, service).

The Principles of Systems Leadership

Because as a student you straddle the university, research bodies, the NHS, social care and beyond, it is helpful to understand how leaders work across boundaries. Likewise, if you have a leadership role in a professional body or trade union around issues such as safe staffing, health and safety or the development of undergraduate education, you may be involved in big changes where people are leading, but are not 'in charge'. This is called systems leadership, and it is about influencing others rather than pulling management levers (Tips Box 11.1).

Systems leadership is particularly useful when faced with large, complex, intractable problems where you cannot solve the problem on your own and need to work with other departments or organisations. These are sometimes called 'wicked problems' and we shall discuss these more in the chapter on problem solving. There may be lots of uncertainties and maybe not enough resources to meet the challenge, and so you need the energy, ideas and expertise of others, including citizens.

Examples of issues that may demand systems leadership include less time for care, delayed transfers of care, rising waiting lists for elective treatment and unsafe staffing levels.

COMMON PURPOSE

When things go wrong and there is a blame culture, it seems easier for organisations to retreat behind organisational boundaries or wait until the organisation is instructed on what to do by a higher authority. These actions can make matters worse, and in systems leadership we need to do the reverse and come together to find new and joined-up solutions. It draws on some of the ideas that we have met earlier in this book, that leadership does not depend on job title—that idea of distributed leadership—and the need for a common or shared purpose. These concepts are a central part of the NHS Change Model that shall be explored further in this section on managing change, making improvements and project management. Common purpose is about bringing partners in the system together by asking questions such as 'what do we want life to be like for people in this place?' and 'who else needs to be in the room that isn't?' such as citizens or subject experts. It is also about building trusting relationships. The mantra here is that 'systems move at the speed of trust'.

Systems leadership has been promoted since 2013 by a national systems leadership programme. In the resources section you will find links to resources across the United Kingdom on system leadership and integrated care.

TIPS BOX 11.1

How to Lead When You Are Not in Charge: Top Tips on Systems Leadership from the Leadership Centre

One of the most influential organisations that has been training systems leaders at all levels is the Leadership Centre (www.leadershipcentre.org.uk). Here are their top tips:

- Service users/citizens must be the centre of the work.
- It is about relationships and trust, not structures and hierarchies.
- You can start small, and from where you are.
- Use narratives and framing to change the way people perceive issues.
- Work with coalitions of the willing.
- Make connections, form networks and use offline conversations to build support.
- Look to make progress rather than solving an issue in one fell swoop.
- See yourselves as systems leaders, not as passive recipients.
- There will always be setbacks, and you will more often than not have to take the scenic route.

Based on Sorkin (2016).

■ Time Out

At this stage in your career, you are unlikely to be involved in the sort of large-scale change that requires systems leadership, so this section is about building your awareness of the principles and noticing what you are seeing, so you are not blindsided later on. There may, however, be smaller-scale changes that might benefit from you using some of the principles.

There is a link to an excellent webinar in the resources section from NHS England featuring Debbie Sorkin explaining systems leadership, plus a link to a report on system leadership called 'The Revolution Will Be Improvised Part II'.

Watch the webinar and then try to observe systems leaders in action in your area. One way to do this is to attend a board meeting (virtually or in person) of an NHS Trust or ICS partnership that is open to the public. You can find this out by searching for '[name of organisation or partnership] public board meeting' on the internet. You could also ask to shadow a director or chief executive who will be attending such a meeting, so you can debrief afterwards.

Write some reflections on what you observe and whether they are using Sorkin's top tips.

Adaptive Leadership

Another leadership approach that deals with complex change is called adaptive leadership. This is not a leadership style like the ones we discussed in Chapter 1, but a framework that incorporates various leadership styles. Adaptive leadership was developed by Ron Heifetz and Marty Linsky in their book *The Practice of Adaptive Leadership*, and it refers to the idea of being able to adapt quickly in a rapidly changing environment.

Adaptive leadership separates out those problems that have technical solutions (much like we see when we separate complicated from complex problems) and those where there is no road map to a solution and people have to adapt what they do.

Change is primarily about facing the discomfort of loss. This may be in terms of people feeling that their competence is challenged, feeling outside of their comfort zones and unable to operate, or being concerned about losing their job or status. Response to change will be examined further in Chapter 13 on leading change.

DANCING ON THE EDGE

Sometimes what people need in situations of change is not formal authority and stability. Instead, they may need to challenge the systems whilst at the same time keeping people on side. Adaptive leaders 'dance on the edge' which means operating on the edge of their authority. A clinical example might be that an authority figure such as a surgeon needs to explain that they could operate to fix a person's problem but instead has to deliver a hard lesson about that person's lifestyle—maybe to lose weight—whilst at the same time maintaining trust and supporting them to make a painful change.

DANCE FLOOR AND BALCONY

In complex change it is often difficult to see what is going on because you are too close to the action. In adaptive leadership, leaders alternate between being on the 'dance floor', where they can see the everyday activities, and then getting on the 'balcony', where they can gain an overview of the whole system. The metaphor suggests that if you are on the balcony at a party then you can see who is dancing, who is not enjoying themselves and who is leaving. The leader alternates between being in the fray and enacting change and being on the balcony and viewing the response of the whole system. An actual example of this in action is when, during a council meeting, a leader made a major announcement (dance floor) and then resisted his normal urge to talk more, maybe to apologise or explain further, and just let the information sit whilst he listened and observed the reactions of others (balcony). As a result, he built up levels of trust by allowing others to express their feelings without interruption (Patterson 2020).

EXPERIMENTAL MINDSET

Because of the uncertainty of even being able to determine what the problem is, another component of adaptive leadership is about adopting an experimental mindset. By making small changes and adopting a mindset of experiment where you are observing, learning and making small corrections, your ego will be less bound up with the success of the experiment and ideas can be let go of. This means being open to making mistakes and being courageous enough to admit it.

Dancing on the edge, alternating between the dance floor and balcony, and adopting experimental mindsets are just a small snapshot of the many components of adaptive leadership. You will be able to find many videos and articles on the internet to explain more and help you expand your ability to adapt. Note that adaptive leaders often take risks and see rules more as guidelines, so be prepared to expect some ripples or waves if you decide to adopt some of these principles!

■ **Time Out**

Think of a situation where you may benefit from getting off the dance floor and onto the balcony. How might you do that?

Like the council leader, you may want to spend less time talking and explaining, and more time observing the effect of a change or improvement that you might be leading and making small changes to your experiments. Try it out and make some notes on what happened.

Leadership, Culture and Climate

Having looked at how systems operate and how leaderships skills change when you are working across a system where you are not in charge, let us now turn to leading organisations and how leaders might create the best culture within which staff and patients can flourish.

TABLE 11.1 ■ Types of Culture and Climate

Culture: 'The Way Things Are Done'	Climate 'The Atmosphere and Personality'
Clan culture—an extended family; mentoring, nurturing and participation can be seen; e.g., a small family business	People-oriented climate—a focus on perceptions of individuals who are working in the organisation
Adhocracy culture—dynamic, risk-taking and innovative; e.g., Silicon Valley innovators	Innovation-oriented climate—encourages creative or new ways of doing tasks
Market-oriented culture—result oriented and focused on the job, competition and achievements; e.g., banking	Goal-oriented climate—a climate that focuses on achieving organisational goals
Hierarchically oriented culture—rigid structures, controls, formal rules and policies; maintenance of stability, consistency and uniformity; e.g., armed services	Rule-oriented climate—based on established rules, policies and procedures in an organisation

Based on Longo (2012).

Organisational culture is a complex concept that reflects the values and beliefs that underpin how well that organisation might perform. It is often referred to colloquially as 'the way things are done around here' (Watkins 2013). The term culture is sometimes confused with organisational climate. Culture is about the norms, values and behaviour adopted by the employees within the organisation, whereas climate is about the atmosphere of the organisation that is created based on the culture. Climate can be thought of as the 'personality' of a place. It determines the work environment in which the employee feels satisfied or dissatisfied. Because satisfaction determines or influences the efficiency of the employees (Gunter and Furman 1996), we can say that the organisational climate is directly related to the efficiency and performance of the employees. Table 11.1 shows the different types of culture and climate.

The proverb 'do as you would be done by' is a useful maxim to bear in mind as you develop your leadership style as a student. The evidence shows that leadership is the most influential factor in shaping organisational culture (West et al. 2015) and likewise culture influences the way that staff feel and behave (climate), which in turn affects the care that they give. In essence, what leaders focus on, talk about, pay attention to, reward and seek to influence tells staff what the leadership values and therefore what they, as organisation members, should value. We talked about high-profile failures in the chapter 8 on assertiveness and courageous. For example, how at Mid Staffordshire NHS Foundation Trust the leaders focused on targets and not people, eventually leading to poor morale and motivation, which eventually affected the attitude of staff, leading to poor standards of care.

By observing how leaders in the organisations that you work or study in go about influencing culture, you will be able to identify positive leadership characteristics and start to model them. We shall start with understanding the components that are necessary for creating a positive culture and how these are built into the inspection framework of provider organisations such as NHS trusts, before we explore some of the components in more depth.

The Care Quality Commission's 'Well-Led' Framework

Following the Francis Report into the failures of care at Mid Staffordshire NHS Foundation Trust, and the government's response to the report, in 2014 the Care Quality Commission

(CQC), which is the organisation that regulates NHS trusts, introduced five key lines of enquiry as part of its 'well-led' domain. These lines of enquiry derive from research undertaken by The King's Fund and the Center for Creative Leadership into leadership and culture and the factors that help build a positive culture (Steward 2014).

The five areas that boards should focus on to ensure their organisation is well led are:

1. Inspiring vision—developing a compelling vision and narrative
2. Governance—ensuring clear accountabilities and effective processes to measure performance and address concerns
3. Leadership, culture and values—developing open and transparent cultures focused on improving quality
4. Staff and patient engagement—focusing on engaging all staff and valuing patients' views and experience
5. Learning and innovation—focusing on continuous learning, innovation and improvement

STAFF ENGAGEMENT—HARNESSING STAFF ENTHUSIASM

■ Time Out

Search the internet for the papers for your local NHS Trust board meetings. Find a recent paper that reports on how well the trust is doing on its five 'well-led' key lines of enquiry.

'One of the problems of leadership in large organisations is the institutional bureaucracy... how to really operate as a leader within the complex hierarchy.'

FAYE DENNIS, POSTGRADUATE STUDENT

One of the most important influences on organisational culture that is included in the CQC's inspection framework is whether and how staff and patients are engaged.

Two Scenarios Illustrating Staff Engagement

Imagine that you are looking for your first job as a registered nurse. You have read this book and you are aware that you need to look out for a well-led organisation and not just a good job in the specialism that you desire.

You have your eyes on a couple of organisations, and you decide that it would be a good idea to arrange a lunch to meet friends who work in these organisations and find out about the culture of their organisations and whether you will be happy there.

Your first friend arrives and looks harassed. She has not stopped all week. 'Every day the same old thing,' she says, '...and every week we are told how we are doing on our targets. We all know our place in the hierarchy, and decisions are made by the big bosses. I've no idea where we are going as an organisation and what our priorities are and why. I have some ideas about how we might improve our wound-healing rates but every time I mention something I get ignored or worse belittled because I am still very junior. I don't feel trusted to use some of the improvement tools that I have been learning about. We are told we are valued but I don't feel that.'

Your other friend has a different story to tell: 'I love working at this trust,' she says. 'We have this target for quality improvement that is about a new zero-tolerance strategy towards hospital- and community-acquired pressure ulcers and falls in hospital. We've got a new-fangled performance improvement directorate, and last week I went on a course there to learn about clinical audit. Now my ward manager has OK'd my proposal to do an audit on our falls and he's helped me to establish a team to do it. We've got this new policy on bullying and harassment, and to be honest I thought it was a bit of window dressing. But there's this health care assistant that I know and she didn't really speak to student nurses or us newly registered nurses with respect. She's been pulled up on it, and honestly the atmosphere on the ward has changed as a result. I feel much happier now and the students are more engaged.'

■ Time Out

> The culture in these two organisations is vastly different. It is fairly obvious here who is the happiest with their organisation's culture. From your reading of these two accounts, what leadership features are encouraging your second friend's enthusiasm for her work? Let us reflect on these six factors in the earlier scenarios. These are shown in Box 11.1.

Health care is about people helping people, and more engaged staff are more likely to bring their heart and soul to work, going the extra mile for their patients. A well-known example is staff at Wrightington Wigan and Leigh NHS Foundation Trust wheeling the bed of a lady on an end-of-life care pathway into the hospital car park so that she could say goodbye to a horse she had cared for over many years. But more often the NHS favours hierarchical and heroic leadership, with more 'pace-setting' styles that focus on the delivery of targets rather than on engaging staff and listening to patients.

Engaged staff deliver better health care: organisations with engaged staff deliver better patient experience, fewer errors, lower infection and mortality rates, stronger financial management, higher staff morale and motivation, and less absenteeism and stress (West et al. 2012). Collins (2015) presented six factors that, according to the evidence, encourage staff engagement and enthusiasm.

Compassion

COMPASSION AND CULTURE

'We know that there is sometimes a toxic culture on wards. But we'll never fix that unless we start teaching students about kindness, about compassion, about knowing yourself. To give them the courage to be the change that they're expected to be. Give us the toolkit.'

NATALIE ELLIOTT, STUDENT NURSE

In December 2012, the Department of Health (DH) published *Compassion in Practice: Nursing, Midwifery and Care Staff: Our Vision and Strategy*. The strategy set out '6Cs'—care, compassion, competence, communication, courage and commitment—that are fundamental to the philosophy of nursing. The document stated that each nurse should regard themselves as 'leaders in our care setting and role model the 6Cs in our everyday care of patients' (DH 2012).

Compassionate leadership encompasses a sensitivity to the challenges that colleagues in health and care face and a commitment to help them respond effectively to those challenges and to thrive at work.

As we saw in the chapter 3 on leadership behaviours, compassion has four components: attending, understanding, empathising and helping. This means that it is important for leaders at all levels to be truly present to practise listening with fascination, to hear what the obstacles are and what resources are needed, and to enable staff to find a way to overcome them.

BOX 11.1 ■ Six Building Blocks to Harness Staff Enthusiasm and Engagement

A compelling, shared strategic direction: The second friend in the scenarios knew about and approved of the direction of her trust in terms of addressing pressure ulcers and falls. Moreover, the organisation backs up the vision with resources. Successful organisations embed their visions in how they measure success and how these are embedded in staff objectives and become part of the norms, stories, rites and rituals: 'how we do things around here'.

Collective and distributed leadership: We met this in the first section of this book where we discussed how the NHS is encouraging a movement towards people at every level being leaders rather than relying on top-down leadership. In our scenarios, one friend was blocked from making improvements whereas the other was empowered by her line manager who had the authority to do so. It takes time and effort to shift cultures in this way and invest in staff skills.

Supportive and inclusive leadership: This includes involving staff and patients in decisions and encouraging staff to collaborate to solve organisational challenges, such as reducing falls, for example.

Staff have tools to lead service transformation: One friend had been supported by a new performance improvement directorate to learn about clinical audit (we shall discuss improvement tools later in Chapter 14) but the other was thwarted and unsupported. Salford Royal NHS Foundation Trust, for example, has set up such a directorate to empower their staff to make and measure improvements. On every ward at Salford Royal is a whiteboard to publicly report on things like how many days since the last infection or fall and what the staffing levels are (King's Fund, 2014).

A culture of integrity and trust: The first friend in our scenario was belittled when she voiced her ideas, and she noticed that this was at odds with the espoused statement of valuing staff. But the second friend was taken seriously and supported, and she also noticed that leaders were true to their values of tackling bullying and harassment in addressing the actions of a health care assistant. Chief executive Sir David Dalton's efforts to make Salford Royal NHS Foundation Trust the safest trust in the country included him working alongside staff for 1 day per month to see first-hand what the issues were (King's Fund, 2014). He feels this is important if he is to be a credible and authentic leader.

Staff engagement is on the agenda of the board: Clinical effectiveness, patient safety and patient experience are the three essential components of quality that an NHS organisation must focus on, but all of these require engaged staff to deliver them. Well-performing organisations take this seriously; for example, Wrightington, Wigan and Leigh NHS Foundation Trust's Chief Executive has monthly meetings with staff side representatives.

It takes courage to be truly present for those we lead. It is hard to hear the truth and to show vulnerability. Sometimes this means a leader admitting that they do not know what to do, but being open and honest helps to build trust and confidence.

Compassion is important to most health and care staff, and the better the fit between staff values and organisation values the greater the commitment, engagement and satisfaction (Greguras and Diefendorff 2009). The leadership required to foster compassion is more about support rather than direction, and enabling rather than controlling interventions (West et al. 2014).

If someone at work shows compassion towards you, you start to feel differently about yourself; for example, you might see yourself as being capable or being worthy. You also feel differently about the other person, viewing them and their organisation as kinder (Dutton et al. 2014). When this happens, you start to feel that the organisation supports you and you may feel more satisfied with your job and more committed to it (Lilius et al. 2011). There is considerable evidence that this is also true in patient care. Compassion is associated with high levels of patient satisfaction, care quality and even organisational financial performance (West and Chowla 2017).

COMPASSION DURING A PANDEMIC

Michael West, speaking in 2020 on a webinar hosted by Quality Improvement Connect (QI Connect), talked about the shift in compassion that people experienced during the COVID-19 pandemic, with an 'outpouring of compassion from person to person, staff to staff and staff to communities.' In terms of inclusion, people also came to realise the disproportionate impact on Black and minority communities, and this drew attention to discrimination and racism and its effect on health and lives (NHS England, Online).

■ Time Out

Watch Michael West's webinar, hosted by Health Improvement Scotland's QI Connect, where he reflects on compassion during the COVID-19 pandemic.
The webinar is available on YouTube (https://youtu.be/YIkXOR0fRGQ) or just search for 'QI Connect with Michael West, Thursday 17th September 2020'.
Which of his messages particularly resonate with you?
What can you, as a student nurse, do to create a better culture of compassion?

ROLE MODELLING COMPASSION

You may have taken away many points from what Michael said, but one of the first things might be about yourself as a role model. The NMC code (NMC 2018) states that nurses must 'act as a role model of professional behaviour' and 'be aware at all times of how your behaviour can affect and influence the behaviour of other people'. To support this, the NMC published *Future Nurse: Standards of Proficiency for Registered Nurses* (NMC 2018), which comprised of seven standards, or platforms. One of these platforms is 'leading and managing nursing care and working in teams', which involves nurses providing leadership by 'acting as a role model for best practice in the delivery of nursing care' (NMC 2018).

Trzeciak and Mazzarelli (2019) describe research that concluded that trainee doctors experience a hidden curriculum whereby they learn—or do not learn—compassion from their mentors. So being a role model as a student leader is vital, as is challenging how your role models might use language that depersonalises patients, such as 'the hernia in room 4' or 'bed blocker' or worse. Leaders' affective states also influence the mood of those around them—a concept known as 'emotional contagion' (Hatfield et al. 1992). In summary, the mood, behaviour and language of leaders can ripple through an organisation to strongly influence culture.

SELF-COMPASSION

You might also have picked up on Michael West's point about self-compassion: I see many posts on social media from students who are harsh self-critics. It may be helpful to review your self-talk and think about moving towards attending to oneself, understanding the challenges that we face, empathising and caring for ourselves and taking intelligent action to help ourselves.

■ Time Out

Think about how you would respond to a friend who is going through hard times. Write down what you would typically do, including the tone that you would speak in.
Now think about how you respond to yourself when you are struggling, what you would typically do and the tone in which you talk to yourself.

Continued

Notice if you spoke to yourself differently compared to how you would speak to a friend. If so, ask yourself why. Consider what factors come into play that lead you to treat yourself differently than you do your friend.

Write down how you think things would change if you responded to your struggling self in the same way you typically respond to a struggling friend.

Based on Kristin Neff, https://self-compassion.org/.

West also talked about creating the conditions for psychological safety for health and care staff by combining compassionate leadership with compassionate teamworking so we can create trust, avoid blame, value diversity and show mutual support and compassion.

OVERWORKING AND COMPASSION

Staff are the NHS's greatest asset, but a number of challenges are taking a significant toll on the workforce. These include coping with rising demand amid workforce shortages, exacerbated by vacancies and staff sickness. The 2018 NHS staff survey, for example, reported that 40% of NHS staff had felt unwell as a result of work-related stress in the previous 12 months, 13% said they had experienced bullying or harassment from managers and 19% experienced it from other colleagues. This affects workplace culture.

Over the last few years there has been an increasing realisation that supportive and compassionate leadership helps teams to cope with the demands of their jobs and improve the quality of care (Shipton et al. 2008, NHS England, 2019). Leaders, especially clinical leaders, can have a key role in influencing this. However, the attractiveness of leadership roles to clinicians is affected by financial and operational pressures and blame cultures (Anandaciva et al. 2018). This has led to a concerted effort to identify and develop the leadership capabilities of future clinical leaders and a shift in national strategy towards an ambition for 'collective, compassionate and inclusive' leadership. (See NHS 2020 'People Plan' and 'People Promise'.)

COMPASSION AND INNOVATION

Compassionate leadership creates the necessary conditions for innovation to thrive (West et al. 2017). We may remember from the chapter on problem solving that there are four basic stages: problem identification and exploration, idea generation, evaluation and implementation. West and colleagues (2017) suggest that a compassionate approach can facilitate the completion of these four stages in a more creative and innovative way, by practising the four activities of compassion: attending, understanding, empathising and helping. This makes sense; if you are really listening, understanding and bringing to the table thoughtful and intelligent action, then that could facilitate new and useful solutions.

THE CHALLENGES OF COMPASSIONATE LEADERSHIP

The criticism of compassionate leadership is that it can be perceived as 'too soft'; performance management can be perceived as bullying, the individual may be seen to take precedence over the organisation, or that compassion itself is seen as time consuming (West 2020). Leadership development experts Hougaard and colleagues (2020) claim that what is actually needed is 'wise compassionate leadership' (Fig. 11.2).

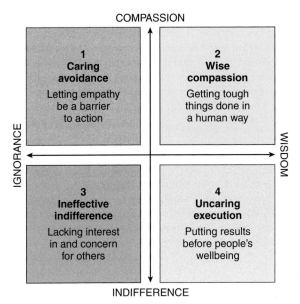

Fig. 11.2 The wise compassion leadership matrix. (Source: Hougaard, R.J., Carter, J., Hobson, H., 2020. Compassionate Leadership Is Necessary — but Not Sufficient. Harvard Business Review.)

Hougaard and colleagues identify four types of leaders based on the two criteria of compassion and wisdom. He describes those with high levels of compassion and wisdom as leaders who get things done in a human way. He contrasts these with those who are not wise but are compassionate and let empathy be a barrier to action. Those low on compassion but wise may put results before people, and lastly those who show neither wisdom nor compassion may lack interest and concern for others.

Summary

Health and care systems—groups of organisations working together—are essential to improve person- and community-centred health and care. Likewise, universities work within a wide range of partnerships to further education and research. Both student nurses and registered nurses now need to understand how systems work and the skills required to lead within systems. These are much more about developing relationships, because 'systems move at the speed of trust' and about developing a common purpose based on shared values. At this stage, your task as a student nurse is to start to understand and interpret what you are seeing and identify role models who typify the right sort of leadership characteristics.

In situations where there is little certainty and agreement about how to tackle a complex problem, the role of the systems leader becomes about enabling rather than leading and setting the right conditions so that solutions start to emerge. Leaders need to take risks, adapt, 'dance on the edge', experiment and take a 'balcony' view of what is happening. This requires nurses to embody each of the 6Cs of *Compassion in Practice* (2012): care, compassion, competence, communication, courage and commitment.

Organisational culture (the way things are done around here), climate (the atmosphere of a place) and the attitude and behaviour of role models have an impact on staff wellbeing and motivation and thus their ability to make improvements. This, plus the potential for burnout, impacts the quality of patient care, safety and even an organisation's finances.

Compassionate leadership is an evidence-based way to create a supportive culture and climate in which improvement can take place. Compassionate leaders cultivate a shared vision, engage staff, are supportive and inclusive and encourage leaders at all levels to make improvements based on what staff on the ground see. By attending, understanding, empathising and helping they encourage more innovative solutions. They show integrity and authenticity and avoid a top-down bureaucratic leadership culture. This does not mean being soft on tough decisions but is about getting things done in a more human way.

Resources

Health and Social Care Board Northern Ireland. Integrated Care Partnerships (ICPs). <http://www.hscboard.hscni.net/icps/>.

King's Fund report, 2021. Developing place-based partnerships: The foundation of effective integrated care systems. <https://www.kingsfund.org.uk/publications/place-based-partnerships-integrated-care-systems>.

Leadership Centre. Leadership for place-based working. <https://www.leadershipcentre.org.uk/>.

Leadership Centre, 2016. The revolution will be improvised - Part II. <https://www.leadershipcentre.org.uk/publications/>. (accessed 24/04/2021).

Let's Talk Leadership. <https://www.letstalkleadership.org/>.

NHS England. Integrated Care. <https://www.england.nhs.uk/integratedcare/>.

NHS England, 2018. Webinar: 'Systems Leadership', featuring Debbie Sorkin. <https://youtu.be/-B5U-Kie4Yc>.

NHS Wales, 2019. Planning Framework 2020/23. <https://gov.wales/sites/default/files/publications/2019-09/nhs-wales-planning-framework-2020-to-2023.pdf>.

NHS Wales. Health Education and Improvement Wales: Online resource on Compassionate Culture - the role of compassionate leadership. <https://nhswalesleadershipportal.heiw.wales/repository/tree?sort5recommendation&language5en>.

Scottish Government, 2019. Ministerial Strategic Group for Health and Community Care. Health and Social Care Integration: progress review. <https://www.gov.scot/publications/ministerial-strategic-group-health-community-care-review-progress-integration-health-social-care-final-report/>.

References

Anandaciva, S., Ward, D., Randhawa, M., Rhiannon Edge, R., 2018. Leadership in today's NHS: Delivering the impossible. The King's Fund and NHS Providers, London. <https://www.kingsfund.org.uk/publications/leadership-todays-nhs>.

Collins, B., 2015. Staff engagement: Six building blocks for harnessing the creativity and enthusiasm of NHS staff. The King's Fund, London.

Department of Health, 2012b. Compassion in Practice. Nursing, Midwifery and Care Staff: Our Vision and Strategy.

Department of Health Northern Ireland, 2021. Health Inequalities Annual Report 2021.

Dutton, J., Workman, K., Hardin, A., 2014. Compassion at Work. Annual Review of Organizational Psychology and Organizational Behavior. 1, 277–304.

Gunter, B., Furman, A., 1996. Biographical and Climate Predictors of Job Satisfaction and Pride in Organization. The Journal of Psychology, 130 (2), 193–208.

Greguras, G.J., Diefendorff, J.M., 2009. Different fits satisfy different needs: Linking person environment fit to employee commitment and performance using self-determination theory. Journal of Applied Psychology, 94 (2), 465–477.

Hatfield, E., Cacioppo, J.T., Rapson, R.L., 1992. Emotional Contagion. Current Directions in Psychological Science, 2 (3), 96–100.

Health Foundation, 2010. Complex Adaptive Systems. <https://www.health.org.uk/sites/default/files/ComplexAdaptiveSystems.pdf>. (accessed 23/12/2021).

Heifetz, R., Linsky, M., 2009. The Practice of Adaptive Leadership. Boston. Harvard Business Press.

Henry, H., 2014. Complexity Theory in Nursing. Independent Nurse, 3rd November.

Hougaard, R.J., Carter, J., Hobson, H., 2020. Compassionate Leadership Is Necessary — but Not Sufficient. Harvard Business Review. December 4th.

King's Fund, 2014. Video: Chris Ham in conversation with Sir David Dalton. <https://www.kingsfund.org.uk/audio-video/chris-ham-conversation-sir-david-dalton>. (accessed 25/04/2021).

Kiviliene, J., Blazeviciene, A., 2019. Review of complex adaptive systems in nursing practice. Journal of Complexity in Health Sciences, 2(2), 46–50.

Mays, N., Dixon, A., Jones, L., ed., 2011. Understanding New Labour's market reforms of the English. NHS. King's Fund, London.

NHS England, 2018. National NHS Staff Survey. <https://www.gov.uk/government/statistics/national-nhs-staff-survey-2018>. (accessed 25/04/2021).

NHS England, 2019. NHS Long-term Plan. <https://www.england.nhs.uk/long-term-plan/>.

NHS England, 2020. NHS People Promise. <https://www.england.nhs.uk/ournhspeople/online-version/lfaop/our-nhs-people-promise/>.

NHS England, 2020. We are the NHS: People Plan for 2020/2021—action for us all. <https://www.england.nhs.uk/publication/we-are-the-nhs-people-plan-for-2020-21-action-for-us-all/>.

NHS England. Place-based Approaches for Reducing Health Inequalities. <https://www.england.nhs.uk/ltphimenu/placed-based-approaches-to-reducing-health-inequalities/place-based-approaches-forreducing-health-inequalities/>.

NHS England. What are integrated care systems. <https://www.england.nhs.uk/integratedcare/what-is-integrated-care/>. (accessed 22/04/2021).

NHS England. Workforce Race Equality Standard. <https://www.england.nhs.uk/about/equality/equality-hub/equality-standard/>.

Nursing and Midwifery Council, 2018. The Code. <https://www.nmc.org.uk/standards/code/>.

Nursing and Midwifery Council, 2018. Future Nurse: Standards of Proficiency for Registered Nurses. <https://www.nmc.org.uk/standards/standards-for-nurses/standards-of-proficiency-for-registered-nurses/>.

Lilius, J., Worline, M., Dutton, J., 2011. Understanding Compassion Capability. Human Relations 64. 10.1177/0018726710396250.

Longo, R., 2012. Main differences between organisational culture and organisational climate; Milan: HR Professionals. <https://rosariolongo.blogspot.com/2012/01/main-differencesbetween-organisational.html>.

Patterson, J., 2020. Adaptive Leadership: The Dance Floor & The Balcony. Let's Talk Leadership. <https://www.letstalkleadership.org/blog/adaptive-leadership-the-dance-floor-amp-thebalcony>. (accessed 13/06/2021).

Sorkin, D., 2016. Systems Leadership for Beginners: what it is, how it works, and why it helps. <https://www.nationalvoices.org.uk/blogs/systems-leadership-beginners-what-it-how-itworks-and-why-it-helps>. (accessed 22/04/2021).

Shipton, H., Armstrong, C., West, M., Dawson, J., 2008. The impact of leadership and quality climate on hospital performance. International Journal for Quality in Health Care, 20 (6), 439–45.

Stacey, RD., 1996. Complexity and Creativity in Organizations. Berrett-Koehler Series. Berrett-Koehler, San Francisco, CA.

Steward, K., 2014. Exploring CQC's well-led domain: How can boards ensure a positive organisational culture? King's Fund. <https://www.kingsfund.org.uk/publications/exploring-cqcs-well-led-domain>. (accessed 23/12/2021).

Taylor, F., 1911. The Principles of Scientific Management. Harper & Brothers, New York and London.

Trzeciak, S., Mazzarelli, A., 2019. Compassionomics: The Revolutionary Scientific Evidence That Caring Makes a Difference. Studer Group. Pensacola.

Watkins, M.D., 2013. What is organisational culture and why do we need it? <https://hbr.org/2013/05/what-isorganizational-culture>. (accessed 18/09/17).

West, M., Eckert, R., Armit, L.L., Lee, A., 2015. Leadership in Health Care: A Summary of the Evidence Base. Faculty of Medical Leadership and Management.

West, M., Dawson, J., 2012. Leadership and engagement for improvement in the NHS: Together we can. King's Fund, London.

West, M., Topakas, A., Dawson, J.F., 2014. Climate and Culture for Health Care Performance. In: The Oxford Handbook of Organizational Climate and Culture, Oxford University Press, Oxford, 335–359.

West, M., Eckert, R., Collins, B., et al., 2017. Caring to change: How compassionate leadership can stimulate innovation in health care. King's Fund, London.

West, M.A., Chowla, R., 2017. Compassionate leadership for compassionate health care. In: Gilbert, P., ed., Compassion: Concepts, Research and Applications. Routledge, London, pp. 237–257.

West, M., 2020. QI Connect with Michael West. Thursday 17th September. QI Connect (online). <https://youtu.be/YIkXOR0fRGQ>. (accessed 26/04/2021).

CHAPTER 12

Becoming a Critical Thinker, Problem Solver and Decision Maker

OBJECTIVES

After reading this chapter and completing the activities, you should be able to:
- Apply the stages of critical thinking to a problem
- Describe the stages of a creative problem-solving process
- Apply a range of creative techniques to each stage of the process
- List the factors that can enhance or kill creativity
- Explain the role of intuition in judgement
- List common biases that affect sound judgement.

Relevance to the Nursing and Midwifery Council (NMC) Code

Practise Effectively
Paragraph 9: Share Your Skills, Knowledge and Experience for the Benefit of People Receiving Care and Your Colleagues
- 9.2 gather and reflect on feedback from a variety of sources, using it to improve your practice and performance
- 9.3 deal with differences of professional opinion with colleagues by discussion and informed debate, respecting their views and opinions and behaving in a professional way at all times

Student nurse leaders need to be able to solve problems and then make decisions effectively. For both activities critical thinking is required. Creative skills and techniques enable nurses to conceptualise new and innovative approaches, and so they are essential for the generation of options or solutions required by leaders. In clinical leadership contexts, students will also need to ensure that decisions are evidence based.

The skills of critical thinking and reflection in and on practice are taught as part of your undergraduate course, usually in an academic context. Here we will be focusing on critical thinking

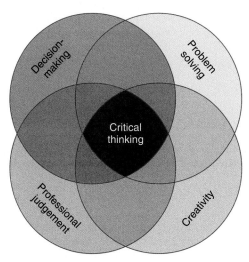

Fig. 12.1 Problem-solving and decision-making model. (Welch, R. Making Decisions and Solving Problems. <https://nursekey.com/making-decisions-and-solving-problems/>.)

in a leadership context, using a worked example. Then we shall go on to focus on some creative tools and techniques that managers and leaders commonly use in problem solving and decision-making, and provide resource links for the exploration of more ideas.

Part of making decisions is to use sound judgement, and we shall explore ways to make more robust judgements by being aware of our emotions and biases.

Fig. 12.1 demonstrates the relationship between these concepts of problem solving, creativity, decision-making and professional judgement. Each of these requires critical thinking and reflection, and so is central in the Venn diagram. Critical thinking is the concept that interweaves and links the others.

Critical Thinking

Critical thinking is more often associated with clinical practice rather than leadership practice but is important for both (Porter-O'Grady et al. 2005). As we have discovered, health and care systems are characterised by increasing complexity, and so critical thinking is an essential skill to be acquired and honed during your leadership journey.

Price and Harrington (2013) define critical thinking as: a process where different information is gathered, sifted, synthesised and evaluated, in order to understand a subject or issue. Critical thinking engages our intellect (the ability to discriminate, challenge and argue), but it might engage our emotions too. To think critically we need to take account of values, beliefs and attitudes that shape our perceptions. Critical thinking, then, is that which enables the nurse to function as a knowledgeable doer—someone who selects, combines, judges and uses information in order to proceed in a professional manner.'

Critical thinking processes can be used with individuals (patients, carers, team members, etc.), and also in teams and organisations, where collective wisdom can be applied. The role of the leader is to explore all sides of an issue by mediating and moderating, balancing the information from a number of sources, assessing it and making judgements.

Critical thinking has a powerful influence on the decision-making and problem solving that nurse leaders are faced with daily. Many academics have sought to define the elements of critical thinking. The skills that typify it include analysis, inference, deductive and inductive reasoning, evaluation, explanation and self-regulation (Zori and Morrison 2009, Porter-O'Grady et al. 2005).

Let us examine these skills in more detail by examining a common nurse leadership issue: why are your patients not adhering to their asthma treatments? As you think through these stages, using a worked example, try to work through a problem that you are also battling with, using critical thinking.

CRITICAL THINKING: ANALYSIS

This stage is about examining notions and ideas, looking at the central arguments and issues and separating out concepts, themes and key points.

■ Time Out

For our worked example, we are looking at the critical-thinking process of a student nurse called Nusrat on placement in general practice. She is in her final year of training and keen to work in primary care. Nusrat has been asked by the team to investigate the problem of poor adherence to asthma treatment in adult patients. She is happy to do this, not least because she has had asthma all her life.

What steps might she take in the analysis stage?

Nusrat may:
- Talk to GPs, receptionists, pharmacists dispensing inhalers, specialist nurses and general practice nurses (GPNs) for their thoughts.
- Work with the practice manager to run reports on the clinical system to discover the extent of nonadherence. Search on the clinical codes to look at rates of repeat prescribing of preventer and reliever inhalers and see whether there is any link to exacerbation rates.
- Sit in with the GPNs when they undertake asthma reviews with their patients and listen to patients talk about how they self-care.
- Talk to people in the community about the issue, such as by visiting a local Breathe Easy group (a self-help group for people with lung conditions).
- Undertake a literature search on reasons for nonadherence and guidance on improving adherence.

CRITICAL THINKING: INFERENCE

At this stage of critical thinking, Nusrat tries to establish a framework or hypothesis by drawing some conclusions from what she has found out. She discovers some conflicting findings:
- The data from the clinical system indicates that some patients are having regular prescriptions for their preventer inhalers and some are not.
- Likewise, some patients are ordering very few reliever inhalers and some are requesting 12 or more reliever inhalers a year, indicating significant variance in overuse and poor control.
- As might be expected, those who are ordering fewer preventers are ordering more reliever inhalers.
- Some patients have not ordered any new inhalers at all in the last 12 months.
- During asthma reviews some patients admit that they often forget to take their preventer inhalers, but the majority say that they remember most of the time. Nusrat notices that

inhaler technique is not always checked at every appointment and when it is, the majority of patients demonstrate poor technique.

- The clinicians in the practice and in the local pharmacy complain that patients generally say they adhere to treatment, but that symptom control is poor and they suspect poor adherence. The pharmacist talks about patients 'abusing reliever medications'.
- The Breathe Easy group members say that it is often hard to get an appointment for an asthma review and that sometimes people who must pay prescription charges cannot afford them. Some resort to using their children's inhalers. Nusrat notices that members have a good level of understanding of asthma self-care.
- Nusrat finds the evidence on reasons for poor adherence is extensive. National guidance refers to the importance of structured review, patient education and good consultation techniques. She discovers from research that:
  - Between 30% and 50% of prescribed medication for long-term conditions is not taken as recommended.
  - Clinicians are poor judges of adherence.
  - Psychosocial factors are as important as biomedical factors.
  - Inhalers with dose counters and electronic monitoring devices are gold-standard ways of monitoring adherence.

▓ Time Out

What can Nusrat infer from the information so far?

Nusrat infers that:
- Poor inhaler technique may be a cause of poor control rather than not taking preventer inhalers per se.
- There are some really worrying signs of poor adherence to preventers.
- Cost of treatment may be an issue for those paying for prescriptions.
- If clinicians are poor judges of adherence, then what they think should not be relied on.
- Dose counting might help with monitoring of adherence with some patients.
- Some patients who have not ordered any medication in 12 months might no longer have any symptoms of asthma (be in remission) and could be removed from the asthma register.

CRITICAL THINKING: DEDUCTIVE AND INDUCTIVE REASONING

In deductive reasoning, if something is true of a class of things in general, it is also true for all members of that class. Deductive reasoning predicts what the observations should be if the theory were correct. We go from the general—the theory—to the specific—the observations. A hypothesis is tested, such as 'All men are mortal. Harold is a man. Therefore, Harold is mortal.' The conclusion here is logical and true.

But sometimes it is not, such as the example 'All bald men are grandfathers. Harold is bald. Therefore, Harold is a grandfather.' The conclusion doesn't match the hypothesis.

▓ Time Out

Are there any examples of deductive reasoning in what the student nurse had found so far? Are there any findings that they should be wary of, that is, the hypothesis might not hold water?

Let us take the hypothesis 'all people who order no medication for 12 months no longer have asthma. Mr Shah hasn't ordered any medication; therefore, he no longer has asthma.' But this might not be true. Maybe he has been visiting his family in Pakistan or maybe he is using his wife's inhalers, because she does not pay for her prescriptions because she has diabetes, whereas he does.

Looking at the findings so far, Nusrat could be forgiven for thinking that any hypothesis at this stage could be wrong.

Inductive reasoning is the opposite of deductive reasoning. Here it is about making many observations, discerning a pattern, making a generalisation and inferring an explanation or a theory.

■ Time Out

Are there any patterns or generalisations in the data so far that Nusrat could test out?

A likely pattern to test out further is around whether the patients know what they should be doing to adhere to treatment, but their health beliefs influence their levels of adherence. For example, they may worry that taking inhaled steroids every day might lead to side effects or not believe that any real harm will come to them by missing doses (see for example Hochbaum's 1958 Health Belief Model).

CRITICAL THINKING: EVALUATION

Evaluation involves testing the viability, reliability and credibility of the data gathered so far and whether that leads to a logical conclusion in which the leader has a high degree of certainty.

■ Time Out

How certain should Nusrat feel at this stage? What further information might she want to include in their evaluation?

If Nusrat is hypothesising that health beliefs are a major factor in adherence to asthma treatment, then she might want to go back to the Breathe Easy groups and ask them questions about what they believe about their asthma treatment. Nusrat reflects that a self-help group may be more highly motivated and decides to compare what they say to what people with asthma talk about on social media or in the local community. From this comparison she can make some inferences about health beliefs locally.

Nusrat discovers that the attitude of local people who she has spoken to is that they do not take their asthma symptoms very seriously and tolerate poor control. She discounts what she finds being discussed on social media in other countries, where clinical guidelines and health systems are different. But locally she finds that people with asthma like to share self-help tips, some of which are clinically inaccurate, such as 'milk causes phlegm'. She also hears many times how difficult it is, if someone's asthma is getting worse, to get an urgent appointment.

She investigates consultation techniques that might help the clinicians at the practice to uncover health beliefs and barriers to self-care, and she finds that motivational interviewing would be of benefit.

'Motivational interviewing is about arranging conversations so that people talk themselves into change based on their own values and interests.'

MILLER AND ROLLNICK (2012)

She begins to understand that just providing people with self-care information will not necessarily change their behaviour. By listening to the patients talk about what they believe about asthma, such as how susceptible they believe they are, or what barriers there may be to them self-caring, then the clinician and patient can reach a negotiated agreement, where the patient takes responsibility for their own condition and decides what they will or will not do. This approach is very much person-focused, and the term used is concordance with treatment rather than adherence (where the patient agrees to the clinician's terms).

CRITICAL THINKING: EXPLANATION

Nusrat now needs to draw together a conclusion and explain her reasoning. To do this she must state her methods, concepts, evidence, circumstances and criteria—everything that she has undertaken in the previous stages. At this stage her main conclusion is that people's health beliefs have a bearing on whether they adhere to asthma treatment and that there may be barriers, such as difficulties getting appointments or cost of treatment. There may also be gaps in clinical care, such as checking inhaler technique, choosing an appropriate inhaler device and not using dose-counting devices when closer monitoring might be helpful, such as when someone has been hospitalised for asthma recently.

CRITICAL THINKING: SELF-REGULATION

But before she draws her conclusions and explains her thinking back to the practice staff, Nusrat needs to look back at her cognitive processes and double check for validity, veracity and accuracy. This is called self-regulation. She is looking for personal bias, inaccurate and incomplete information and any missing contextual clues.

▓ Time Out

If you were Nusrat, what might you question about your critical-thinking processes so far?

Nusrat herself has asthma, so she might ask herself if her own experience has influenced her thinking. Also, she has not checked her thinking so far with any of the practice staff since she started. It may be that the clinical staff are using motivational interviewing techniques or have done so in the past and can advise on whether it was successful or not and why. Also, she might reflect on whether low income, ethnic and/or cultural diversity in the community might have a bearing on adherence to asthma treatment.

CRITICAL THINKING: JUDGEMENT BIASES

The process of judgement involves integrating different aspects of information about people, objects or situations to arrive at an overall evaluation. Judgements feed into decision-making as we evaluate or assess situations and then use this information to make choices. For example, we may assess someone with a learning disability to be at risk of injuring themselves (a judgement) and then choose what intervention to make (a decision).

During the self-regulation process, Nusrat needs to watch out for well-known judgement biases.

Availability bias—We assume that recent, familiar and vivid events are more frequent when they come to mind more easily. Older people, for example, are often fearful of crime when the police data suggests that the crime figures are much lower than they suppose. If Nusrat has witnessed several people in clinic with poor inhaler technique recently, then she might think this is the norm.

Confirmation bias—We stick to our original judgements and fail to notice evidence that does not confirm our beliefs. This might happen, for example, when you are building an argument for a written assignment and you look for evidence that supports it and ignore contradictory evidence.

Overconfidence—We may become more confident about our own ideas and actions than may be justified. For example, many of us will have come across patients who believe that they will not get lung cancer from smoking.

Hindsight bias—Looking back, we believe that we were more certain about a judgement initially that we in fact were. This can lead to overconfidence in future judgements.

Nusrat has witnessed several people in clinic recently with poor inhaler technique, and so she cautions herself that availability bias may come into play and that she might think this is the norm.

PROFESSIONAL JUDGEMENT AND INTUITION

'Intuition is no mysterious talent. It is the direct by-product of training and experience that is stored as knowledge.'

HERBERT SIMON, COGNITIVE PSYCHOLOGIST

Despite following a critical-thinking process, sometimes there is doubt about the right course of action, and this means that we may have to use our professional judgement, which may in part rely on our intuition. This section on critical thinking ends with what the evidence is for using our nursing judgement.

Expert judgement in many professions is often wholly or largely intuitive (Claxon 2006). Perhaps the most well-known nursing theories around intuitive judgement in nursing are by Benner (1984), who suggests that expert nurses mainly use intuition, which is defined as 'knowing without necessarily having a specific rationale or making explicit all that goes into one's sense of a situation'. The unconscious mind processes information more quickly than the conscious mind, and it learns through being exposed to patterns and thought experience (Berry and Deines 1993). Intuitive decision-making often incorporates complex information that cannot even be verbalised (Claxon 1997).

Sometimes you may have had a problem-solving experience where your mind feels blocked. A period of incubation, where you are not thinking about the problem often helps. Maybe you have a cup of tea or you sleep on it and when you come back the solution becomes clearer. Using intuition in creative problem solving is described as having four stages (Wallis 1926):

1. Preparation—where data is gathered and the stages of problem solving are worked through
2. Incubation—where the problem is not worked on or attended to
3. Illumination—where an intuitive solution emerges into consciousness
4. Verification—where a purposeful analysis is applied to check the intuition out

Intuition is, however, fallible—it can be hard to differentiate between intuition and hunches, wishful thinking or plain prejudice.

In situations where there is a correct answer to a problem, then the conscious mind performs better. Take, for example, a problem where there are two ropes hanging from the ceiling and the task is to tie them together. Several other props such as a stapler or scissors are made available. However, the ropes are too far apart to grasp one and then the other. What an experimenter then does is ask the subject of the experiment to 'think'. This allows the conscious mind to work out what the subject needs to do. Eventually they realise that they need to tie the stapler to one rope to create a pendulum that will allow the subject to grab both ropes.

SUMMARY: CRITICAL THINKING

There are several stages that take us through the critical-thinking process (Fig. 12.2). Each stage builds on the last, with a series of checks and balances to help leaders to make sound judgements. To help avoid bias, not only must leaders be aware of it through self-reflection, but also put together diverse teams who can constructively challenge each other. Sometimes, where there is insufficient information, professional judgement is needed, but this can be subject to bias. There is evidence that intuition, based on experience, can be helpful here.

The Creative Problem-Solving Process

By bringing creativity into your problem-solving approach, you can get an even better variety of potential solutions and ideas. This section is designed to offer student nurses a well-known problem-solving process based on Osborne (1953), starting with exploring the problem right through to action planning. We shall go through one or more examples of problem-solving techniques per stage, to get you started. The Reference list guides you towards classic texts on creativity, and the Resources section directs you to an archive library where these texts can be borrowed for free. Fig. 12.3 outlines the process and the methods that we shall go through.

DIVERGENT AND CONVERGENT THINKING

As we go through the problem-solving stages, we need to generate many ideas and then choose the best ones to take us through to the next stage. The process of exploring differing options is called divergent thinking or 'lateral thinking', and the commonest example that you may recognise is 'brainstorming'. This type of thinking requires you to free your mind and find multiple innovative solutions. The possibilities are endless.

From that wide range of options, we then narrow down our choices ready for the next stage of the process. This is called convergent thinking, and it relies more on logic. We shall look at examples of both divergent and convergent techniques (Tips Box 12.1).

TIPS BOX 12.1

Practising Divergent and Convergent Thinking

- What often happens is that ideas generated during a divergent thinking exercise are shot down by the more logical, convergent thinkers. Set some ground rules at the start of the session to avoid this.
- Separate out the processes of convergent and divergent thinking by, for example, allowing 20 minutes where wild ideas are allowed and creativity can spark new trains of thought by one person building on the ideas of another.
- Then allow another 20 minutes to review all the ideas generated to come up with the most promising ones (convergent thinking).

Before you start problem solving, you and your team may want to clarify the external factors in which the problem exists. PESTLE stands for political, environmental, social, technical, legal and economic (Fig. 12.4) and it is a commonly used activity that is completed at the start of business planning or strategy development in the NHS and in wider business sectors.

Table 12.1 gives a worked example of the issues in relation to managing child asthma in primary care at the start of the COVID-19 pandemic. Having that shared understanding of your external environment will help your team to be realistic in what they propose to solve their problem.

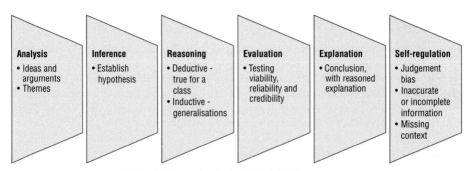

Fig. 12.2 Stages in a typical critical-thinking process.

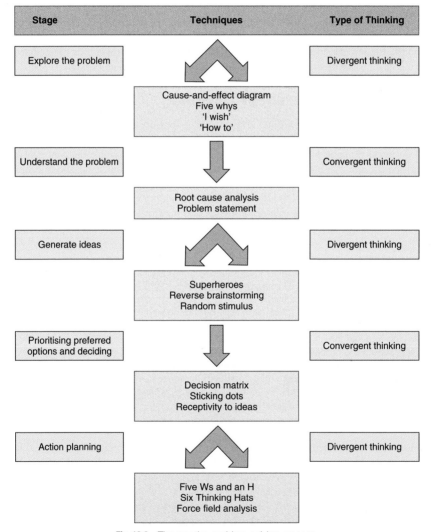

Fig. 12.3 The creative problem-solving process.

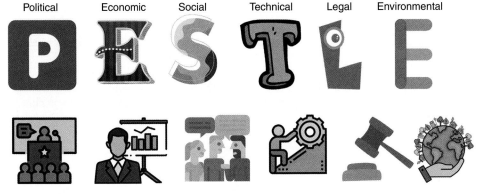

Fig. 12.4 PESTLE analysis.

TABLE 12.1 ▓ **PESTLE Analysis of Supporting Children With Asthma in Primary Care During the 2020 Pandemic**

Political	Economic	Social
Rapid shifts in health and care policy giving rise to uncertainty in the surgery and in the family. Increased globalisation of pandemic risks and plans.	Banking support to GP surgeries as small businesses. Government support to general practice transitioning to virtual consultations. Stress of redundancy and furlough puts pressure on family income, which may increase anxiety in children, triggering asthma symptoms. Increases in child poverty. Inhaler stockpiling by parents puts pressure on prescribing budgets.	Stress of school closures, home schooling and exam cancellation on the family triggers asthma. Increased community cohesion and volunteering. Potential fear and anxiety in families with asthma compounded by social isolation. Increases in family breakdown and domestic abuse. Problems maintaining a healthy lifestyle and regular exercise.

Technical	Legal	Environmental
Move to virtual communications, especially GP consultations, meetings and social media. Increase in electronic prescribing and online appointment booking. Lack of access to internet in low-income households may disadvantage online GP access. Hopes for a vaccine.	Government restrictions on travel, gatherings, events, etc. Designation of key workers.	Potential reduction in air pollution as an asthma trigger. Potential for reductions in exacerbations caused by circulating infections due to lockdown.

EXPLORE THE PROBLEM

'One day Alice came to a fork in the road and saw a Cheshire Cat in a tree. "Which road do I take?" she asked. His response was a question: "Where do you want to go?" "I don't know," Alice answered. "Then," said the cat, "it doesn't matter."'

LEWIS CARROLL, ALICE IN WONDERLAND

■ Time Out

What do you think Alice's problem is?

The first rule of problem solving is to understand the root cause of problem before you start, so you end up solving the right problem, otherwise you may end up solving the symptom rather than the cause.

Is Alice lost? Where does she want to go? Does she even know where she is?

■ Exercise 1: Five Whys

You have probably had the experience of a small child asking you lots of questions and then questioning the answer until they drill right down to the heart of the matter—such as 'why don't dinosaurs exist anymore?' or 'why is that man homeless'. This exercise involves asking the 'problem owner' (in this case, Alice) a series of questions starting with 'why':
- Pretend you are 5 years old again.
- Ask the problem owner 'why' questions.
- Avoid 'why don't you...'.
- Ask about:
  - The causes of problem
  - The consequences of problem

What 'why' questions would you ask Alice?

You might ask these questions and receive the following responses.
- Why are you lost? I can't find my way.
- Why can't you find your way? I've never been here before.
- Why have you never been here before? I fell down a rabbit hole by accident.
- Why did you fall down a rabbit hole? I was following a white rabbit.
- Why did you follow a white rabbit? I was curious.

This is an exercise in finding out more about the problem and possibly reframing it: is her problem that she is lost, or that she cannot find the white rabbit, or that she is insatiably curious and that leads her into trouble? Now think about the hierarchy of these problems: which one is the underlying cause and which is the effect? Which is the problem to be solved?

■ Exercise 2: 'I wish'

Here is another way to help surface what the problem is. This time, the problem owner generates as many statements as they can (sensible or crazy) in relation to the problem, starting with 'I wish'. This is good to do as a team so you generate lots of options. Do not censor any ideas. For this exercise think about the problem of overcrowded accident and emergency (A&E) departments.

Some examples might be:
- I wish we could close the doors!
- I wish we had more staff.
- I wish we could magic people better!
- I wish ambulances were operating theatres and could fix people before they arrive at hospital!

■ Exercise 3: 'How To'

For this exercise, you or your team generates a series of statements in the form of 'how to...'

Try to phrase the same problem in the form of 'how to' statements and generate as many of these statements as you can, no matter how silly. Again, do not censor your ideas.

Some examples might be:
- How to shorten waiting times
- How to stop inappropriate attendance
- How to prevent accidents
- How to help patients fix themselves
- How to say no to stupid requests

You can see from these statements that you can look at this problem in multiple ways. Then the team can start to debate which is the cause of the 'disease' (problem) and which is a symptom (or effect) of the disease.

■ Exercise 4: Cause-and-Effect Diagram

Cause-and-effect diagrams, sometimes called Ishikawa or fishbone diagrams due to their shape, are helpful when you want to understand the causes of a single event. They break down, in successive layers of detail, root causes that potentially contribute to a particular effect. It is often helpful to see what is going on in your/your team's heads set out in one diagram. You can use mind-mapping apps such as SimpleMind to help.

Fig. 12.5 gives an example of a cause-and-effect diagram created by a group of local fathers to try to understand the struggles that affect their wellbeing.

Here you can see that there are many reasons why fathers were struggling, and they could be grouped by the fathers into five main issues, which can then be further broken down into understanding the reasons for these issues. For example, they suffered from poor mental health because their relationship had broken down and they may have been asked to leave the family home. They suffered poor self-esteem, and one reason for this is that they were jobless. You can also see where the five issues interlinked, so joblessness was a major issue in itself with many factors affecting it, such as leaving school early and difficulties getting work because of a history of offending.

■ Time Out

Try drawing a cause-and-effect diagram for the problem of overcrowded A&E departments.

ROOT CAUSE ANALYSIS

These four exercises: cause-and-effect diagrams, five whys, 'I wish' and 'how to' (amongst many others) are used to help get to the root cause of the problem, as shown in Fig. 12.6.

If we take the fathers' wellbeing problem, we can see that the causes were multifactorial. The fathers could have addressed each factor—for example, they could have worked on their relationships or got help to secure a job.

Eventually, by going through the process of listening to each other to complete the cause-and-effect diagram, the fathers discovered that they were not alone with their problems. They realised that the root cause was not unemployment or being separated from their children, but that they bottled everything up due to pride and shame and did not feel that they could talk to anyone about it. This affected everything else: their mental wellbeing, their relationships, their drug use and so on. The root cause of the problem was the fathers' inability to be emotionally

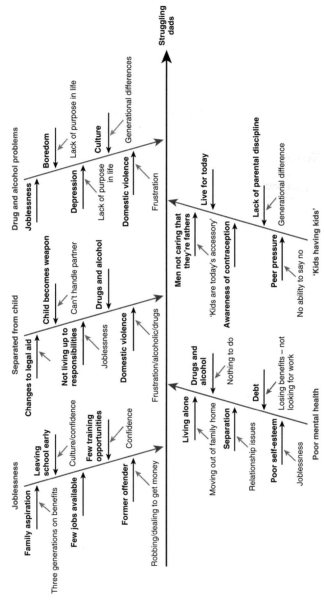

Fig. 12.5 Causes of poor wellbeing in fathers in one community.

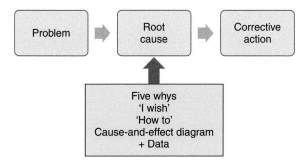

Fig. 12.6 The importance of root cause analysis.

open. They then set about looking for ways to share their worries, bearing in mind that this traditionally was difficult for men. Had they acted on the effects—such as family breakdown—they would have solved the wrong problem.

(Based on the work of Salford Dadz—Little Hulton, see Robertson et al. 2015)

THE IMPORTANCE OF DATA

At this stage of exploring the challenge and finding the root cause, you also need as much data as you can. Nusrat's example from earlier in the chapter shows the different types of data that she got from the GPs clinical system. Chapter 14 on improvement gives various examples on how to gather data.

CREATIVE PROBLEM SOLVING: PROBLEM STATEMENT

The next step after exploring the problem (divergent thinking) is to select the right problem to solve. This stage requires convergent thinking; that is, from the many ideas that have been generated about how to solve the problem, can the problem be phrased to summarise the issue? The best way to do this is to create a problem statement starting with 'how to' or 'how can we'.

Let us imagine that, with your help, a group of older people have undertaken a root cause analysis of their own wellbeing and have found that their lives have lost meaning because they do not feel in control of their lives. They phrase it as 'how to give older people in Anytown more control over their lives and more meaningful lives'.

CREATIVE PROBLEM SOLVING: GENERATING THE IDEAS

We shall now go on to looking at just a couple of creative and fun ways to generate potential solutions to this problem.

■ Exercise 5: Superheroes

This exercise is best done as a team, although you could do it on your own if you have lots of imagination! Each member of the team selects a superhero character, be that alive, dead or fictional.

They then take turns to explain how they, in the character of the superhero, would address the problem of giving older people greater control and more meaningful lives, using their character's special powers, characteristics or skills.

▨ Time Out

Take a few minutes now to choose a superhero, state their powers and jot down how they would solve this problem of 'how to give older people in Anytown more control over their lives and more meaningful lives'.

Again, the ideas should be creative so that they spark novel solutions when you come to the convergent stage of choosing a solution or solutions.

Take Spiderman: his superpowers are that, as a mutant, he can spin a web of any size, he can climb tall buildings and travel quickly by swinging on threads. Therefore:

■ He can catch isolated older people in Anytown in his web and deliver them to a local tea dance.
■ He can teach older people how to travel independently.
■ He is a mutant—an outsider—and he can share his knowledge on how he copes and has become a hero.

Do any of these ideas trigger any thoughts about a potential solution?

▨ Exercise 6: Reverse Brainstorming

For this exercise, you or your team reverse the problem statement, so it would read:
'How can we give older people in Anytown *less control and more miserable lives?*'

Then, once you get lots of silly solutions, you can think about what ideas are sparked when you reverse the solutions.

Here is an example: 'We can put fences around their homes so they can't go out and no one can get in.'

Reversing this: what is it about the built environment that stops older people connecting with others? Are there any natural places where older people congregate? How can we address this? Maybe we can invite older people to see the supermarket café as somewhere to mix and make friends every Wednesday afternoon, because they go there anyway and it is really easy to get to on the bus.

▨ Time Out

See how many creative ideas you can come up with for the problem of 'How can we give older people in Anytown *less control and more miserable lives?*'

Take your ideas and then see what happens when you reverse them.

▨ Exercise 7: Random Stimulus

This exercise is about using random words as a stimulus for creative solutions (von Oech 1986). For this you let your mind wander around ideas.

For example, you could look out of the window, open a book or a catalogue and choose two objects or words at random, such as 'ice cream' and 'taxi'. Now use free association to compare these objects or words to the problem 'how to give older people in Anytown more control over their lives and more meaningful lives'.

For example, an ice cream taxi sounds absolutely delightful. Fancy having your perfect sundae delivered to you just by clicking your fingers! Or maybe you get in the taxi to go for an ice cream with your friends. Maybe older people might want to make and sell their own ice cream by getting in a taxi with a freezer box and selling it in the park on a Saturday. That way they could get a bit of income as well as make new friends...

CREATIVE PROBLEM SOLVING: PRIORITISING AND DECIDING

Now that we have done a root cause analysis, developed a problem statement and generated a number of potential solutions, we shall look at how to prioritise them and then make a decision on the preferred option. This again is the convergent thinking stage.

■ Exercise 8: Receptivity to Ideas

This exercise helps your team to stay open-minded and to better understand what might seem at first to be a half-baked or naïve suggestion but might contain a seed of a good idea if you dig down hard enough. This can be the case, for example, when you have a nonexpert in the field, such a patient, a carer, a teacher, but remember that this person may be able to bring fresh eyes to the problem.

Paraphrasing Phase

Imagine that your group of older people like the idea of an ice cream taxi and you think it is a bit crazy, but you decide that you want to explore it some more in case there is something in it. Start the process by paraphrasing what the person has said, e.g., 'If I understand you rightly, you are suggesting that...'. Keep your language free from opinion or evaluation, as your purpose at this point is to mutual understanding. Evaluation will come later.

If the speaker agrees that what you have said is correct, you can move to the next stage. If not, come back with 'OK let me try this again. Am I correct in saying that the core of your idea is to...'. Continue to paraphrase until the speaker agrees that you have captured the idea correctly.

This stage is important because it signals that you are listening and it validates the speaker's ideas, showing that they are worthy of respect.

What you are left with may not resemble the original idea, but the developmental process avoids the rush to identify flaws. It is motivating for those involved and can develop ideas into transformational solutions.

Developmental Response

The next stage is responding to the idea. Start with listing the positive responses (pros) and explain how they would be useful, such as 'Well if isolated older people took a taxi to the supermarket on a Wednesday to have an ice cream together in the café, then that would generate income for local taxi drivers—or maybe we could find some volunteer drivers or use Ring and Ride?'. Be specific and genuine. When you have reached the end of the list, try to come up with at least one more pro. This process acknowledges the contribution of the speaker and helps create a better understanding.

Then start to list the cons, but phrase these so as to invite solutions by using 'how to' or 'how can we' as we did earlier. For example, rather than saying 'taxis are expensive', write down 'how can we make this less expensive?'.

Based on Harriman (1988).

■ Exercise 9: Sticking Dots

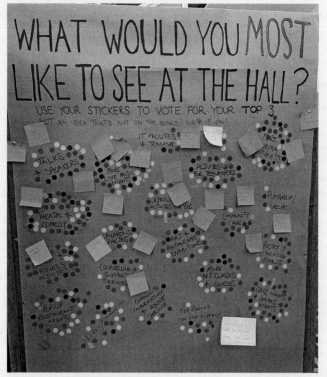

Dot voting for activities at Stretford Public Hall, Trafford, Greater Manchester.

A much simpler way of prioritising is by sticking dots against the preferred options. This helps a team, or even a large number of diverse groups, give an indication of their favoured option.

- List all the options on the left of a large sheet of paper, leaving plenty of space on the right and underneath each option for dots.
- Give each person the same number of dots. You could colour code them if you want to understand how certain groups, such as patients, view the options. Give any instruction, such as if someone has five dots, whether they can place more than one dot against a single option.
- Explain all the options, then allow time for people to decide how they want to 'vote' by distributing their dots against the option. Allowing everyone to vote at the same time means they are less likely to be influenced by each other than if you allow each person, or smaller groups, to vote in turn.

■ Exercise 10: Decision Matrix

In this exercise, let us go back to the example of managing demand in A&E departments. Your team has reframed the problem statement as 'How to reduce inappropriate attendance at A&E' and has identified three ideas:

1. GP station within the A&E department
2. Nurse-led walk-in centre
3. Telephone triage system

The team has also identified the key criteria on which the decision will be based: cost, staff availability, effectiveness (based on the current evidence base), how quickly it can be set up and the acceptability of the choice to all stakeholders, particularly to the local GPs who are wary of rising demand.

Next, the team scores each of the options together (although they could also score it separately and add the scores together) against the criteria from 1 (poor) to 5 (excellent); the results are shown in Table 12.2.

Having set the criteria, the team decides how important each of these criteria are from 5 (highly important) to 1 (little importance). This is called adding a weighting. They decide that effectiveness is weighted 5, cost second highest and the remainder are weighted 3. Then they add these weightings to the table and multiply the scores in Table 12.3 by the weightings to give a final score. For example, the initial score for the cost of a GP station is 3 and their weight given to cost is scored 4 so the final score is $3 \times 4 = 12$.

This weighted scoring shows that introducing telephone triage would be the preferred option.

Going back to the critical-thinking stages discussed earlier in the chapter, the team might now pause to go through the evaluation, explanation and self-regulation processes, and revisit whether they think that they have come to the right conclusion.

Voting this way gives a quick indication of the attitudes of a group and is useful as part of a wider decision-making process, but it is a poor way of making a carefully analysed final decision because of variations such as strongly heard views of minority groups, areas of expertise by certain group members, and so on.

CREATIVE PROBLEM SOLVING: ACTION PLANNING

Having analysed the solutions and prioritised them, we move now to the final section, which is about creating action plans. In Chapter 13 we can move on to implementation and managing change.

TABLE 12.2 ■ **Scored Options for Reducing A&E Attendance Using Criteria**

Factors	Cost	Staffing	Effectiveness	Speed	Acceptability	Total
Weights						
GP station	3	2	3	3	2	
Walk-in centre	1	3	3	1	3	
Telephone triage	5	5	4	3	4	

TABLE 12.3 ■ **Scored Options for Reducing A&E Attendance Using Weighted Criteria**

Factors	Cost	Staffing	Effectiveness	Speed	Acceptability	Total
Weights	4	3	5	3	3	
GP station	12	6	15	9	6	48
Walk-in centre	4	9	15	3	9	40
Telephone triage	20	15	20	9	12	76

■ Exercise 11: Five Ws and an H

'I keep six honest serving men
(They taught me all I know)
Their names are What and Why and When
And How and Where and Who.'

Rudyard Kipling, Just So Stories

Who, what, why, when, where and how, otherwise known as 'Five Ws and an H' form the basic checklist of questions in the English language. They can be used at any stage of the creative problem-solving process or as a personal checklist to keep in mind when discussing any situation.

The answer to these questions is usually a reductionist fact. For example, asking 'Who should undergo training on health beliefs to help address our problem with adherence to treatment' might result in the answer 'Mary and George.' To help with the problem-solving process, the follow-up question should by phrased 'In what way might...' (IWWM). For example, 'OK, so in what way might we make it easier to release Mary and George to attend the training without creating a backlog of work?'

■ Exercise 12: Six Thinking Hats

The Six Thinking Hats is a technique created by Edward de Bono (1985). It can be useful at the stage of action planning because it can help enhance the understanding of the idea to be taken forward.

It also helps when certain people are entrenched in a particular style of thinking, such as those who always think of the positives or someone else who is always thinking of the negatives. The six hats represent six artificial distinctions of thought, and each imaginary hat is put on in a certain order by the whole team, usually for a time-limited period of about 4 to 5 minutes (Table 12.4).

1. The team allocates a leader to wear the blue hat. Their role is to explain the process, keep the group to time, encourage contribution and move the group on from one 'hat' to the next.
2. Team members then all put on their imaginary white hat to state the facts relating to the discussion and ask, 'What data do we have or need?'
3. Next, everyone puts on their imaginary green hat to come up with ideas. No negative comments are allowed at this stage—this comes later. Questions like: 'Is there a different way to look at this?' and 'How could the plan be further developed?' are useful.
4. Once a number of ideas for implementing the plan have been generated, the team move on to wearing the yellow hat, and everyone lists the positives of the proposed plan.
5. The team then puts on the black hat to think about difficulties relating to any ideas. They ask themselves 'what could go wrong with this plan?' and 'what are the possible negatives?'
6. The red hat is the final hat to be worn. This is because people have to select a final idea, and this is often based on a gut feeling. Questions such as 'what do you feel about this?' and 'what is your gut feeling?' help.
7. The blue hat wearer will then ask the team 'could you summarise the findings so far? What needs to happen next?' before summing up the meeting and making sure that there is a clear action plan of who will do what.

TABLE 12.4 ■ De Bono's Six Thinking Hats and How to Remember Them

Hat colours	Calls for ...	Think of ...
White	Data, facts and information only	White paper
Red	Feelings and intuitions only	Fire and warmth
Black	Thinking about negatives, downsides, risks, cautions and warnings only	The black robes of a judge
Yellow	Thinking about positives, optimism, benefits and goodness only	Sunshine
Green	Creativity and new ideas	New growth and vegetation
Blue	Attention to the big picture, direction and management of thinking process	The sky above or a police officer directing traffic

Source: NHS Improvement, 2018. Six Thinking Hats. <https://improvement.nhs.uk/resources/six-thinking-hats/>.

■ Exercise 13: Force Field Analysis

The final technique is a force field analysis. This is a tool for summarising, in the form of a simple diagram, what the forces are that could drive the solution proposed and what the oppositional restraining forces are. It can be used both when exploring a problem or at the action-planning stage. For this exercise we shall use the example of a team of student nurse leaders at a university who are not getting their rosters in sufficient time to organise family life. Their solution is to ask the local NHS trust to introduce self-rostering software.

- The team brainstorms a list of factors that they think can drive through the proposed solution to the problem.
- They then brainstorm a list of factors that can restrain or oppose it.
- These factors are then drawn into a diagram such as the one in Fig. 12.7.
- The length of the arrow correlates to the strength of the driving or restraining force. For example, the longer the arrow, the more important that force is considered. Directly opposing forces are paired.
- In Fig. 12.7, student leadership is identified as both a driving force and a restraining force, as the student group is finding that their voices are not being listened to by both the trust and their university.
- The team then considers ways of tackling the restraining forces or increasing the power of the driving forces. By doing the latter, the team may antagonise the restraining forces and so:
  - The team organises a survey of students who have experienced self-rostering and collates the benefits. They do the same with staff in a clinical area who allow students to do this and summarise the positive impact this has had.
  - The team then explains the benefits to the trust in terms of being seen as 'student friendly' and the increased likelihood (with evidence) that students will not drop out of their course and will want to work at their trust, thus helping with workforce shortages.

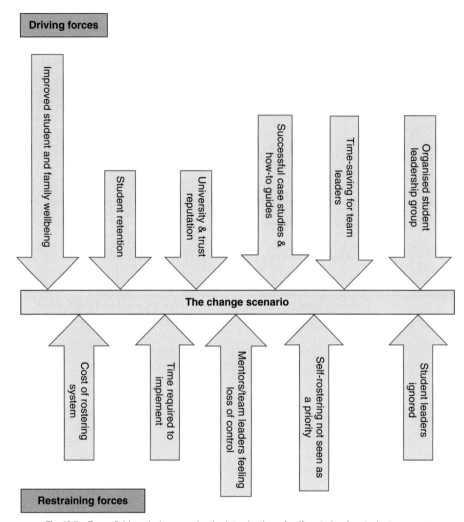

Fig. 12.7 Force field analysis example: the introduction of self-rostering for student nurses.

■ **Time Out**

You now have thirteen creative problem-solving techniques to practise with your own problem-solving project. Jot down a few ideas about how you might use any of these techniques in your current leadership activities.

Organisational Factors That Can Enhance Creativity

Having now looked at both critical thinking and the creative problem-solving process, we now move on to look at how to nurture creativity in your teams and share a couple of examples (Case Studies 12.1 and 12.2). There are six factors for you to nurture if you want to enhance your or your team's creativity (Amabile, 1998):

■ Challenge
  ■ Match the right people to assignments and give them sufficient stretch so they are neither bored nor overwhelmed.

- This means knowing people's strengths (and them knowing their own!) as we have previously discussed.
- Freedom
  - Give people autonomy about the means but not the ends. Once a goal or outcome has been decided, it is up to the person or team who you delegate to, to decide how to achieve it.
- Resources
  - The two main resources that affect creativity are time and money.
  - Time pressure can heighten creativity (such as what happened during the race to create a vaccine against SARS-CoV-2), but artificial deadlines can kill it.
  - Sometimes leaders need to allow time for incubation of ideas.
  - The 'right' physical space (open plan, potted plants, etc.) is a lower-order need.
- Team features
  - Take time to build the team chemistry and know what motivates them.
  - Creativity is built on diversity of perspectives and backgrounds.
  - The team shares their excitement over the team's goal.
  - They recognise the unique knowledge and perspective of other team members and are willing to help each other.
  - Beware homogenous teams that reach solutions quickly.
- Supervisory encouragement
  - Encourage intrinsic motivation by acknowledging innovative efforts and the importance in achieving the common goal.
  - Never ignore new ideas or foster criticism.
  - Encourage learning from failure and never criticise it.
- Organisational support
  - Creativity is enhanced best when it is part of the organisational culture.
  - Encourage information sharing and collaboration.
  - Take action to avoid in-fighting and internal politics.

Let us now look at an example of this in Case Study 12.1.

CASE STUDY 12.1 **Naomi Berry, Newly Registered General Practice Nurse and Nurse Lead for the Undergraduate Programme for Bradford Training Hubs**

'I'm the palliative care lead at our practice... we'd had a really bad death [of a patient]. When I first got there, the relationship between the practice nurses and the district nurses was strained due to increased workloads and low staffing levels. Coming from a community background as a healthcare assistant (HCA), I thought "Ooh we have to change this." We need them as much as they need us. And we're going to have to work together. So, I reached out to them and said "Look I know it's difficult, but I've been in your shoes and I've been in a team where we've had 15 palliative care patients a day—I get it. But we're here, we want to try to work with you." And that's when we had the idea of... if we met up at the patient's house we'd have that continuation of care and the patient wouldn't feel forgotten about.'

'So now anybody that's newly diagnosed with cancer will get a GP of their choice visit with me. We'll both go out with the district nurses. We'll sit down together, and we'll tell them what we can do, what the district nurses can do. And they have direct access to us and they have a name. That way then they can come back to us. And they know who they're taking to. Because talking to me over the phone about the cancer diagnosis is the worst thing ever. They want a face-to-face person. I think that helps with family as well. Working with the palliative care team, the district nurses, means that we have proper networks and it's not disjointed.'

■ Time Out

Which of Amabile's six factors enhanced Naomi's clinical practice and that of her team?

Naomi's challenge was well suited to her skills and experience as a health care assistant who had worked in a palliative care team. The practice she worked in gave her freedom to innovate and supported her to make the connection with the district nursing team. She adopted the role of a relationships manager—making all the cogs work together.

Naomi used empathy, understanding what the district nurses' problems were and emphasising the common ground. She stimulated collaboration and information sharing to get the best result both for the patient/family and the team.

CASE STUDY 12.2	Using Creativity to Help Peers to Learn

Let us have a look at using creativity to assist with the problem of student nurses who may feel overwhelmed by their studies and their first introduction to clinical practice.

In Section I, we looked at peer-assisted learning (PAL) at the University of Plymouth and the experience of two student nurses, Ellie Looker and Rebecca Hollobone, both senior PAL leaders.

Here, second- and third-year students volunteer to help first- and sometimes second-year student nurses with their learning. Part of the PAL leaders' training is to encourage an active learning style rather than a passive, lecture style. They also have an awareness of different learning styles: those who prefer visual, aural or kinesthetic or those who prefer the written word.

This encouraged Ellie and Rebecca to use their creativity to identify a variety of exercises to encourage group cohesion and engagement and help students learn in creative ways. The PAL leaders and students are drawn from different fields of nursing and may not know each other, so it is important to spend time early on getting to know each other and developing relationships and trust.

Laughter is a useful tool to help people relax. One activity that they came up with was a game where students were invited to bounce ping pong balls into paper cups and at the bottom of the cup was a question that students were invited to ask each other.

A second example is the tricky task of referencing correctly using the Harvard referencing system. Ellie's creative solution was to cut the elements of a reference into sections, like a jigsaw puzzle, and encourage students to put the parts in the right order (Fig. 12.8)

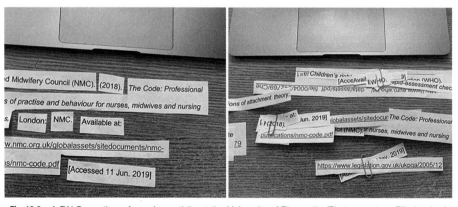

Fig. 12.8 A PALS creative referencing activity at the University of Plymouth. (Photo courtesy Ellie Looker.)

A Systems Perspective on Creativity

'As long as the idea or product has not been validated, we might have originality, but not creativity.'
MIHALYI CSIKSZENTMIHALYI

Amabile talks about organisational culture either fostering or killing creativity, and Csikszentmihalyi (1999) goes further, explaining that people or teams who are creative need to be supported by a field of practice. He explains that creativity occurs when a set of rules and practices are transmitted from the cultural domain to the individual person. The individual must then produce a novel variation in the content of the domain. The variation must then be selected by the field for inclusion in the domain. Ideas generated by the person are accepted or rejected by the field who act as gatekeepers. This is summarised in Fig. 12.9.

What this means for student nurses is that you need an awareness of the system that you are wanting to be creative within and an awareness of the field of nursing that you are practising in. When you act creatively, the field is there as a gatekeeper who can accept or reject the creativity.

Take for example Brian Dolan, who railed against the idea of patients staying in pyjamas and in bed. He sent his tweet at a time (which is still upon us) when hospital beds were at a premium and nurses knew that older people quickly lost mobility when left in bed too long. His field, hospital nurses, immediately took up his war cry, and a social movement #EndPJParalysis was born and then added to the field of practice.

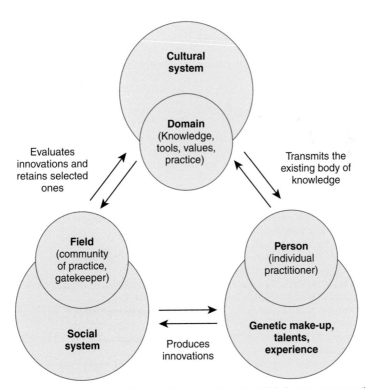

Fig. 12.9 A systems model of creativity. (Courtesy Csikszentmihalyi, M., 1999. A systems perspective on creativity. In: Sternberg, R. (Ed.), Handbook of Creativity. Cambridge University Press, Cambridge.)

Summary

The skills of critical thinking are essential throughout the process of creative problem solving, judgement and decision-making. When making judgements, student nurse leaders should avoid ignoring their gut feelings or intuition because they represent an accumulation of experience that we cannot always verbalise. However, when examining these gut feelings, leaders should use their critical thinking skills to look for bias. By working within diverse teams and encouraging constructive challenge, better decisions can be made.

The creative problem-solving process involves repeatedly going through a process of divergent followed by convergent thinking, allowing a range of ideas to be generated at each stage before they are narrowed down. The first stage is to use a number of prompting techniques, such as five whys and 'how to', to understand the root cause of a problem and to formulate a problem statement. This is then followed by generating ideas to solve the problem and prioritising the resulting ideas, before reaching a decision. Decision-making can be assisted by a range of tools such as dot voting and weighted scoring against criteria. Action planning can be assisted by techniques such Six Thinking Hats and force field analysis.

Creativity is an essential tool to help solve problems, and student nurse leaders can improve their creative thinking skills through practice. The culture of an organisation has a major bearing on whether it kills or nurtures creativity, as does the field of practice and the wider system within which the organisation sits.

Resources

Some resources in the field of creativity are classics. Digital Archive is an online open-source library service for archived older books. You can create a free account and borrow books for up to 14 days (such as Kuhn's book listed in the references) by creating an account at Digital Archive (https://archive.org/).

References

Amabile, T., 1998. How to kill creativity. Harvard Business Review. <https://hbr.org/1998/09/how-to-kill-creativity>.

Benner, P., 1984. From Novice to Expert. Addison-Wesley, California.

Berry, D., Deines, Z., 1993. Implicit Learning: Theoretical and Empirical Issues. Lawrence Erlbaum, Hove.

Claxon, G., 1997. Hare Brain Tortoise Mind: Why Intelligence Increases When You Think Less. Fourth Estate, London.

Claxon, G., 2006. Beyond cleverness: how to be smart without thinking. In: Henry, J. (Ed.), Creative Management and Development, third ed. Sage, London.

Csikszentmihalyi, M., 1999. A systems perspective on creativity. In: Sternberg, R. (Ed.), Handbook of Creativity. Cambridge University Press, Cambridge.

de Bono, E., 1985. Six Thinking Hats. Penguin, London.

Harriman, R., 1988. Techniques for fostering creativity. In: Kuhn, R. (Ed.), Handbook for Creative and Innovative Managers. McGraw Hill, New York.

Hochbaum, G.M., 1958. Public Participation in Medical Screening Programs: A Socio-Psychological Study. U.S. Department of Health, Education, and Welfare, Washington, D.C.

Miller, W.R., Rollnick, S., 2012. Motivational Interviewing: Helping People Change. Guilford Press, New York.

NHS Improvement, 2018. Six Thinking Hats. <https://improvement.nhs.uk/resources/six-thinking-hats/>. (accessed 17/03/2021).

Osborne, A., 1953. Applied Imagination: Principles and Procedures of Creative Problem Solving. Charles Scribner's Sons, New York.

Porter-O'Grady, T., Igein, G., Alexander, D., Blaylock, J., McComb, D., Williams, S., 2005. Critical thinking for nursing leadership. Nurse Leadership 3 (4), 28–31.

Price, B., Harrington, A., 2013. Critical Thinking and Writing for Nursing Students, second ed. Sage Publications, London.

Robertson, S., Woodall, J., Hanna, E., Rowlands, S., Long, T., Livesley, J., 2015. Salford Dadz: Year 2 External evaluation. Project Report. Unlimited Potential. <http://eprints.leedsbeckett.ac.uk/id/eprint/1728/>. (accessed 19/03/2021).

von Oech, R., 1986. A Kick in the Seat of the Pants. Harper and Rowe, New York.

Wallis, G., 1926. The Art of Thought. Harcourt Brace, New York.

Zori, S., Morrison, B., 2009. Critical thinking in nurse managers. Nursing Economics 27 (2), 75–79, 98.

CHAPTER 13

Leading Change

IN THIS CHAPTER

Managing the Emotions of Change

System Drivers

Kotter and Lewin's Change Models

Stakeholder Management

Communicating Change

OBJECTIVES

After reading this chapter and completing the activities, you should be able to:
- Describe the common emotions felt by people experiencing significant change
- Identify and engage stakeholders to deliver change
- Communicate the story of change
- Distinguish between changes that fall in the 'Identify how or whether people notice the need for change' and those that can be more easily planned.

Relevance to the Nursing and Midwifery Council (NMC) Code

Prioritise People
Paragraph 2:
Listen to People and Respond to Their Preferences and Concerns
To achieve this, you must:
2.1 Work in partnership with people to make sure you deliver care effectively

---

Life is full of change, and health and care is no different. Whether it is changes in education, in undertaking or implementing research findings or in delivering health and care services, student nurse leaders will be involved in change. The overarching message of this chapter is that change is something that we do with people, not to people. The role of a leader is not to have the answers, but to facilitate getting to the answers and recognise that all change is about understanding and coping with loss. Good leaders engage people in change right from the very start by developing a shared vision that meets organisational and staff priorities.

Most change is often done poorly, and the effect can be devastating and long lasting. So it is important that leaders understand the issues and equip themselves with techniques to support change-management initiatives.

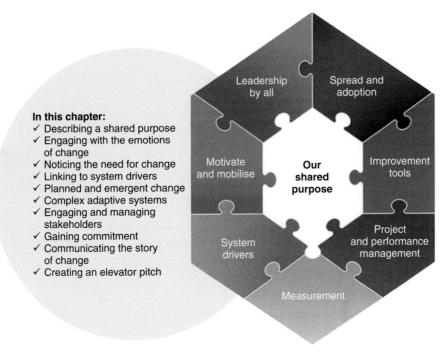

In this chapter:
- ✓ Describing a shared purpose
- ✓ Engaging with the emotions of change
- ✓ Noticing the need for change
- ✓ Linking to system drivers
- ✓ Planned and emergent change
- ✓ Complex adaptive systems
- ✓ Engaging and managing stakeholders
- ✓ Gaining commitment
- ✓ Communicating the story of change
- ✓ Creating an elevator pitch

Fig. 13.1 NHS Change Model. (Courtesy NHS England, 2018. The Change Model Guide (Version 5).)

Change is a necessary part of the growth and enhancement of organisations. When change occurs, people are asked to act in new ways, and this leads to a great deal of uncertainty and sometimes fear. However, just telling people that a certain change is a positive thing will not convince them that this will be a positive experience, so empathy is a really important skill to practise, remembering how change has affected you and putting yourself in the shoes of the people who you are leading.

This is the first of three chapters under the theme of managing change. This first chapter presents an overview of change, followed by Chapter 14 on improvement tools and techniques and then Chapter 15 on project planning. Because these are all huge subjects, consider these chapters as an introduction. The References and Resources sections will enable you to start to learn more.

One key reference to look for is the NHS Change Model, published in 2018, which is an online guide containing lots of downloadable tools aimed at senior managers embarking on transformational change. We shall be referring to some of the elements of this guide as we go through our next three chapters. The elements of the NHS Change Model are set out in Fig. 13.1, annotated with the change elements that we will cover in this chapter.

Reflecting on a Change Journey

■ Time Out

Choose a major change in the past that you were part of at work or in your studies, that you did not instigate. Use the experience to reflect on how you felt initially and in hindsight. Take out your journal and describe:
- ■ What was the situation?
- ■ What was the direct impact on you?

Continued

- How did you hear about the change?
- How did you initially react?
- How did your perceptions and feelings change over time?
- What triggered your revised view?
- Think about how you feel about the change now. Describe the process and the outcome again, but this time from your current vantage point.
- Note how you reacted then, compared with how you do now. What do you attribute this difference to?

Now that you have reflected on your own experience, you can start to see that many people often react warily and with some hostility initially to change. However, over time they may reflect on the outcome and often adopt a more positive viewpoint.

By working through this activity, you can start to realise how others may react to any changes that you propose and how you can respond with empathy to resistance and objections that you may encounter.

Response to Change

'Change is the only constant in life. One's ability to adapt to those changes will determine your success in life.'

BENJAMIN FRANKLIN

It may take up to 4 years to get used to a major change in our lives, and it takes on average around 2 years to become fully competent in a new job (Hay 2009). Our response to change can move through a series of phases, which appear similar to those experienced when someone is bereaved: denial and isolation, anger, bargaining, depression and acceptance. (Kübler-Ross 1969).

According to Hay (2009) (Fig. 13.2), the first phase of responding to change is when we seem *immobilised* for a while because we may lack information, may be afraid of feeling stupid by doing things wrong, feel paralysed by fear of the unknown or lack motivation to make the change work.

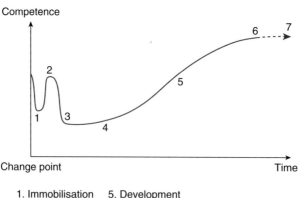

1. Immobilisation	5. Development
2. Denial	6. Application
3. Frustration	7. Completion
4. Acceptance	

Fig. 13.2 The competence curve. (Courtesy Hay, J., 2009. Transactional Analysis for Trainers. Sherwood Publishing, Watford.)

The second phase is *denial*. This is when we act as if our past behaviour patterns will still be appropriate (Tips Box 13.1). We then move into the third stage of *frustration*, where we now recognise the need to behave differently but we do not know how. In stage 4 we start to test out new ways of doing things and begin to *accept* the change. By stage 5 we move into the *development* phase of acquiring new skills and knowledge. In stage 6 we start to *apply* our new skills and consolidate our knowledge. The final stage, stage 7, is that of *completion*, where we feel comfortable and are no longer consciously aware of the change.

TIPS BOX 13.1

Some of the ways that you can address negative responses to change include:
- providing sufficient time to allow the implications to sink in,
- listening and acknowledging feelings,
- responding empathetically and encouraging support,
- addressing concerns and providing information, and
- explaining what you expect of staff and what training and support is available to aid transition.

Noticing the Need for Change

You will recall from the chapter on communication that storytelling is a device that helps people to engender emotions that can mobilise people to take action, so it is used a lot in change management.

Who Moved My Cheese is a famous fable written by Spencer Johnson (1998) to teach leaders in organisations to see, anticipate and adapt to change. A classic example of this is Kodak, who failed to notice that the future lay in digital images and not in the manufacture and development of photographic film. An example in the NHS is, until recently, the reliance on old-fashioned fax machines rather than more modern forms of communication, resulting in the Secretary of State for Health having to issue instructions to ban them (Department of Health and Social Care 2020).

In Johnson's story are two mice, Sniff and Scurry, and two little people, Hem and Haw, who exist in a maze. All four know the way to a pile of cheese, but one day the cheese is not there. The cheese is a metaphor for what we want in life or business. The mice work on their instincts (hence their names, Sniff and Scurry). They had already noticed changes at their cheese station and were not surprised to find no cheese. They decided, after visiting the cheese station for several days and finding nothing there, that they needed to find new cheese.

Hem and Haw keep returning to the station day after day hoping that the cheese will return. They are not instinctual like the mice, possessing more complex intelligence and differing attitudes to change. They both start by denying and resisting change; however, Haw learns to adapt to change when he envisages a better future. They are both uncertain, worried about getting lost and fear failure, but Hem posed the question to himself 'What would you do if you weren't afraid?' and he worked on envisioning himself being successful in finding new cheese, which he eventually did.

There are many messages in the story, but some key ones are:
- Expect change.
- Look for signs that change is coming. Spencer describes this as 'smell the cheese often so you know when it's getting old'.
- Adapt to change quickly.

■ **Time Out**

There are many animated summaries of *Who Moved My Cheese* on the internet. Find and watch one and then consider:
- Who do you know that share the characteristics of Sniff, Scurry, Hem and Haw?
- Which one are you?
- Are there any signs that change is coming, either at work or in your home life, at the moment?
- Which lessons from the story resonate most and will help you right now?

Acknowledging System Drivers

Change occurs within a system, so it is important when making a case for change, that you align what you want to achieve with what the wider organisation wants to achieve also. You can look for system drivers in:
- your organisation's strategic business plan (on the website or intranet)—what are your organisation's priorities?
- national standards, such as the NMC's standards of proficiency for registered nurses or the code;
- national strategies and policies, such as the NHS Long Term Plan or your local policies, say on tackling violence towards staff;
- incentives for change, for example in general practice there is the Quality and Outcomes Framework or there may be grants available to encourage research in particular areas;
- national targets, such as the 4-hour wait target in accident and emergency (A&E) departments; and
- national concerns, such as the rise in homelessness.

Based on NHS Change Model (2018).

Planned, Emergent and Spontaneous Change

Change does not always happen in the same way. Take for example:
- planned: moving a ward from one site to another;
- emergent: an intensive care unit understanding and developing the best treatment for a new infection such as COVID-19; and
- spontaneous: an A&E department responding to a train crash or a new-power change such as the #HelloMyNameIs movement.

There is no single best way to manage change. It will depend on the context, the people and the nature of the change. You will remember from Chapter 11 on systems that the more complex the change is, the more we practice in a systems leadership way—which is about building relationships and being the enabler of change rather than leading it.

PLANNED CHANGE: KOTTER'S EIGHT-STEP PROCESS FOR LEADING CHANGE

The predominant approach to managing change is the planned approach. One of the most used change-management models is John Kotter's Eight-Step Process for Leading Change. Like Spencer, he also wrote a fable called *Our Iceberg Is Melting* to illustrate the steps. The story, summarised in Table 13.1, is based on a group of penguins in the Antarctic who notice that their iceberg is melting and they have to convince the colony to move to find a new home.

TABLE 13.1 ■ **Summary of Kotter's Eight-Step Process for Leading Change**

Stage	Storyline
Create a sense of urgency	A penguin called Fred notices a big crack in the iceberg filled with water. He shows it to a couple of others, including the 'scientist' of the colony. Together they conduct an experiment to demonstrate to the colony why and how the iceberg is melting. They demonstrate the freeze-thaw mechanism that is splitting the ice using a glass bottle filled with water. Overnight, the water freezes and the glass breaks, just like frozen water is splitting apart their iceberg.
Pull together a guiding team	Fred convinces some of the leaders about the problem. Pretty soon they have a team consisting of people with the complementary talents and skills that are needed.
Develop the change vision and strategy	The team meets a seagull who scouts around to find the best place to live. The team develops a vision of a future where they move to a better and safer iceberg with plenty of fish. They tell the story of the seagulls and how they have scouts to help them find the best places to live. They suggest that the colony become nomadic just like them and have scouts constantly searching for a new place to live.
Communicate for understanding and buy in	The team appeals to the penguin's values: 'The iceberg is not who we are. It is only where we live. We are smarter, stronger and more capable than the seagulls. So why can't we do what they have done, only better? We are not chained to this piece of ice. We can leave it behind us.' Twenty penguins put up posters with slogans every day for a week, even under the sea, where the penguins fish.
Empower others to act	The team deals with negative troublemakers and invites others to get actively involved in supporting the cause. They come up with their own solutions, such as empowering the schoolteacher to tell positive stories to the children about how they could become heroes by helping in the cause. This allays the children's fears, which helps parents to accept the idea.
Produce short-term wins	The fittest birds are nominated to become scouts, and the team invents a 'Heroes Day' event to celebrate their role. The admission to the celebration event is two fish each, which are fed to the scouts, who have no time to fish for themselves when they are scouting. When the scouts return, they tell tales of what marvels they had seen.
Do not let up	Even though the scouts find a suitable new iceberg and the colony moves there, they repeat the exercise again and move to an even better iceberg.
Create a new culture	At first the colony wants to stay on this new iceberg, which could have led to the same problems as before. The nomadic culture is embedded by recruiting new members to the leadership team and by making the scout selection process even tougher, so raising their status. 'Scouting' is added to the school curriculum.

Adapted from Kotter, J., Rathgeber, H., 2006. Our Iceberg Is Melting. Macmillan, London.

■ **Time Out**

Read a precis of the story by searching on SlideShare (https://www.slideshare.net/) for *Our Iceberg Is Melting* or read the book itself. It is only a short story that will take about an hour to read.

Think of a planned change that you have been involved in, such as the introduction of a new procedure or technique, or the process of curriculum change for your course.
- Which steps of Kotter's model were used?
- Which were not used and would have helped?

PLANNED CHANGE: LEWIN'S MODEL

The second planned change model that is commonly used in nursing is Kurt Lewin's (1947) three-step model of unfreeze—change—refreeze. The model uses the analogy of melting a block of ice in one shape and then refreezing it into another shape.

TABLE 13.2 ■ Lewin's Three-Step Change Model

Stage	Tasks
Unfreeze	Identify those affected by the change (stakeholder analysis). Communicate with stakeholders about the change. Deal with questions, doubts and concerns.
Change	Keep communicating about the change. Emphasise how people will benefit from it. Allow time for people to get used to the idea.
Refreeze	The change becomes part of the culture. Check that change has happened and that people are using the new processes. Train and support people to help them stay on track. Celebrate everyone's hard work. This helps people to find closure and helps them to believe that future changes will also be a success.

Courtesy Lewin, K., 1947. Frontiers in group dynamics: concept, method and reality in social science; social equilibria and social change. Human Relations, 1, 5–41.

Imagine that you have a block of ice and you want to turn it into a cone of ice. The first task is to make the ice amenable to change by unfreezing it. Then you mould the iced water into the shape you want—you change it. Lastly, you want to solidify the new shape—you refreeze it.

By looking at the change process as three distinct stages, you can prepare yourself for the transition and plan for it. In many change processes, people fail to have a proper plan for each stage, which causes turmoil and, often, failure (Table 13.2).

CRITICISMS OF PLANNED CHANGE MODELS

A word of caution here: as we have seen with complexity theory, every organisation and every change is different in terms of people, culture, values and so on, so it is best to use change models as a guide rather than slavishly following them.

In Chapter 9 on power and influence we learnt about old-power and new-power models. Planned change is more often associated with old-power models. Change can also be initiated through new power in a spontaneous, cocreated way. Commentators like transformational change expert Helen Bevan (North West Leadership Academy 2020) observed that, during the COVID-19 pandemic, both old- and new-power changes were observed. Whilst there was of necessity a need for emergency planning—very much an old-power model of command and control—many others cocreated inventive solutions in interdependent ways. She estimates that about 80% of the conversations in the future will be new-power conversations focusing on this interdependence.

Creating a 'Shared Purpose'

In both Kotter's and Lewin's models, stakeholders accept that change is necessary and that people feel part of the change.

Mark Jaben, an emergency physician in Florida, has studied the neuroscience of resistance to change. This involves the prefrontal cortex interpreting the various thoughts and options that occur in the brain when faced with change options. What often happens is that a small group of change agents identify an issue. Options will be identified and then the group makes a choice and engages people at this point. What we actually need to do, he says, is to engage people at the stage of identifying an issue so that the desired outcome is a shared outcome. This allows the brains of stakeholders to work out the best option for themselves. This represents a shift in thinking from inviting stakeholders to 'buy in' to inviting them to 'invest' (Fig. 13.3).

The NHS Change Model describes this as developing 'our shared purpose'. These three words are broken down as in Fig. 13.4. This is about aligning stakeholders to a common goal and common values by involving them at the earliest stages in planning the change. At this stage the important thing is explaining *why* change is needed, rather than what changes are needed and how they will happen. There are three steps to create a shared purpose:

1. Create a shared space to listen and allow genuine communication with stakeholders.
2. Look for commonalities—the things that people agree on, despite their differences—like good patient care or a commitment to improving educational provision.
3. Design together—translate that shared understanding into an action plan that will involve stakeholders.

NHS England (2018).

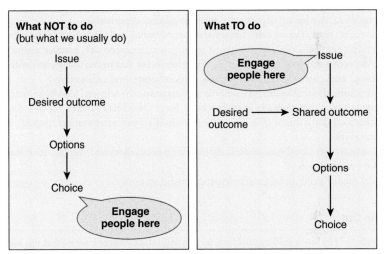

Fig. 13.3 Engage people early in change. (Courtesy Jaben, M., 2019. Free the Brain: Overcome the Struggle People and Organizations Face with Change. Egbert Publishing.)

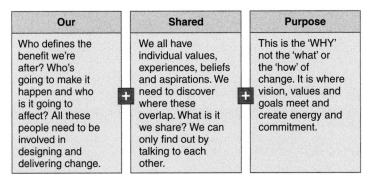

Fig. 13.4 NHS Change Model: Our Shared Purpose. (Courtesy NHS England, 2018. The Change Model Guide (Version 5). <https://www.england.nhs.uk/publication/the-change-model-guide/>).

Engaging and Managing Stakeholders

Think about the different types of people that you might need in the following scenario.

■ Time Out

You are part of a student-led movement leading a new joint NHS trust and university effort to promote careers in health care to pupils in years 8 and 9 (aged 12–14 years) in local secondary schools. You want 80% of career education curricula in those schools in the hospital catchment area of Anytown to include careers in health care in 12 months' time. There may be other opportunities, like shadowing opportunities or empowering secondary school pupils themselves to come up with their own ideas to boost enrolment in access courses and higher education.

List all the stakeholders for this change scenario—any person, group or institution, inside or outside the organisation, who has a stake or interest.

Here is who you may have mentioned (and you may have identified others):

- NHS Trust: human resources (HR) team, director of nursing, clinical director, education department, marketing department, relevant clinical department
- University: dean, faculty staff, library staff, recruitment and marketing team, curriculum development leads, placement support team, practice supervisors, practice assessors, all the departmental heads for each discipline (which for this university are midwifery, nursing, medicine, occupational therapy, physiotherapy and radiography)
- Education: all local secondary schools in Anytown, the 'cluster' lead head teacher for those schools, careers leads at each school, local OFSTED (Office for Standards in Education) department (the regulator for schools), parent governors, pupils themselves
- Local authority: local education authority, ward councillors and the executive lead councillor for education
- Local media: print and online newspapers, radio stations

■ Time Out

Kotter talks of creating a guiding coalition, so it is helpful, as student leaders, that you identify the right people to be part of that guiding coalition. Make a list of who could be on a guiding coalition for this project:
- Do you need a senior sponsor from management, to champion the cause?
- What about someone technical, good at numbers or good at measuring outcomes?
- Good spokespeople? Perhaps someone who people can relate to easily?
- Someone who can plan and keep you on track?
- Someone representative of your target audience?
- What other skills might you need?

You might want:
- Senior leaders from both the university and the NHS trust, such as a senior tutor and HR manager, so the change project fits in with workforce planning and university recruitment
- A local teacher and high school pupil, or former pupil, to advise you
- Health care students—perhaps one drawn from a discipline where there are national shortages, such as therapeutic radiography, and another where you want to address image

issues, such as nursing. They will liaise with all the other disciplines (midwifery, medicine, etc.).

- Someone who will draw up a project plan and keep you all on track
- Another who can keep an eye on numbers of schools and young people engaged and any other outputs or outcomes—someone who can present figures well on charts and graphs
- You might also want someone to liaise with the NHS Ambassador scheme at the national level (a group of volunteer nurses who promote nursing careers in schools) to advise you if you get stuck and someone locally who can link into the local education authority of the borough council

Look back at Chapter 6 on effective teams to help guide you towards building the most diverse and effective team.

Strong and Weak Ties

When we are leading teams to make improvements, we often seek to work with peers, 'people like us' who understand what it is like to work in health care and what it is like to be a nurse. We trust each other, know what each other does and exchange information and build networks to share ideas. Hospitals scale improvements by working with hospitals, universities with universities and so on. These are called 'strong ties' and they have dominated the way that the NHS leads and makes improvements for many years. When we are uncertain and situations are complex, we often revert to these strong ties.

Over the last decade or so, the NHS has started to learn from how citizens start and lead social movements (Bevan 2010). It is important that we learn to engage wider partners to accelerate innovations and improvements, especially where there is no real path to follow. This is where we actually need not strong ties, but 'weak ties'—people from other walks of life who may have ideas and resources to help us solve our problems.

The number of connections we can maintain is often limited by time and cost. We reach for strong ties, which are the strong connections that we have with family and close coworkers, that can sustain us. But we also need weak ties—people we reach out to, to act as bridges to new resources and ideas. Our use of social media to find out information and make connections is an example of this. The links that we have with people with whom we have weak ties are utilised less frequently and do not need a lot of management. Take, for example, the person who heard of a job through a friend of a friend, or a new idea that you heard over coffee when you attended a conference. The professional business social network LinkedIn is a network of both strong and weak ties: you are able to see people who are connected to your contacts who may be able to help you.

So as you make your change, think of both the people you have strong ties with and also how you can harness the weak ties—for example, do you need someone well connected in education to help make further connections in schools?

Commitment Mapping

As a change leader, you need to ensure that you have engaged all your important stakeholders, listened with empathy to what they say and gauged their interest. Commitment mapping is a simple technique for mapping each stakeholder's current commitment. There are four levels (see Fig. 13.5):

1. Not committed or opposed
2. Will let the change happen
3. Will help the change to happen
4. Will make the change happen

Stakeholder	Not committed (opposed?)	Let	Help	Make
Director of nursing	O ———→ X			
Cluster lead head teacher		O ————————————→ X		
School careers leads	O ————————→ X			
Faculty representative: nursing			O ———→ X	
Faculty representative: radiography	O ——————————————————————→ X			

Fig. 13.5 Example of a commitment map.

Add the symbol 'O' for their current position and an 'X' for where you would like them to be, adding an arrow between the two. Some stakeholders of course just need to be informed, so they give you advice early and do not say 'why wasn't I told!'

So, for example, currently the clinical director is not committed (you have not approached her yet) and you want her to *let* the change happen, but you need your fellow students to *make* it happen.

Then you plan how you will engage each stakeholder so they let, help or make it happen. Remember that this is an invitation to get involved and shape the shared purpose and not to bulldoze your ideas through, so every meeting is an opportunity to listen and maybe make changes to your ideas based on what people say.

Communicating the Story of Change in the Best Way

You will notice in Kotter's story how emotive the language was from one of their leaders:

> 'The iceberg is not who we are. It is only where we live. We are smarter, stronger and more capable than the seagulls. So why can't we do what they have done, only better? We are not chained to this piece of ice. We can leave it behind us.'

Public narrative is a storytelling technique that enables you to succinctly present yourself to an audience, connect hearts and minds and call upon them to take action (often termed a 'call to action'). The key to motivating people intrinsically is being able to communicate your values, and this will inspire action through emotion (Fig. 13.6).

Take for example the story of the little girl Ella Kissi Debra who died of an asthma attack and how her mother told her story for many years until a coroner ruled that air pollution was a material cause in her death. This has now strengthened the calls for a health protection plan to protect the public from toxic air. Public narrative is part of something called social movement theory—how to create a movement of people who collectively share a dissatisfaction with the current state and want to work towards a shared vision for something better.

The Story of Self, Us and Now

There are three parts to communicating your public narrative (Ganz 2009):
1. *Story of self:* In the story *Our Iceberg Is Melting*, a likeable penguin called Buddy starts by talking about himself. He explains that he is a scout for the colony and how he met the

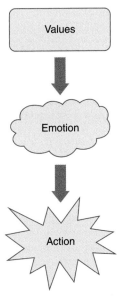

Fig. 13.6 Sharing values inspire action through emotion.

seagull who talked about how seagulls are free to go anywhere they want to. Your story of self is about 'revealing your values that lead you to act' (Ganz 2009). Buddy is seen as a pioneering scout seeking a positive future for the colony.

2. *Story of us:* Another penguin called Louis then takes up the story from Buddy. Here the element of the story is about the penguin's shared, current experience, and he talks about the iceberg '...not being who we are...' and is only where the penguins live. This part of the story emphasises the shared values and experiences of people present. Louis says, 'We are smarter, stronger and more capable than the seagulls.'

3. *Story of now:* In this third stage, it is about setting out:
   - The challenge: Our iceberg is melting.
   - The choice: Stay and put families at risk or find better a safer place to live.
   - The outcome: Louis says, 'We will never have to put our families at risk from the sort of terrible danger we face today. We will prevail!'

■ **Time Out**

Watch 'The speech that made Obama president' on YouTube. Identify the three parts of public narrative: story of self, story of us and story of now.

Practice creating your own public narrative. It will not seem natural at first, especially if you are not used to talking about yourself, so try it out in front of a friend or partner first. Include little details in your story that people can engage with, like names of places or experiences that people can relate to.

To show you how possible it is to use public narrative effectively to engage people to support your cause, check out 'Salford Dadz in their own words' on YouTube. Salford Dadz—Little Hulton, whom I worked with, are working together to improve their children's wellbeing by improving their own wellbeing. The video shows a group of actors at the local high school acting the fathers' own words, with a view to having their story told. The fathers explain to their community that they do not want their children growing up to have the same experience as themselves.

I did not teach the fathers to carry out a public narrative, or told them what to say, I just told them to speak from the heart. During general discourse, people naturally tell stories and this is exactly what the dads did. In doing so they revealed some of the emotional details of their lives. This helped them to engage the support of local people to help them to improve the lives of their children. (Written consent for this video was obtained from the fathers and the actors' parents.)

Create an Elevator Pitch

Once you have debated and distilled the essence of the project with stakeholders, an elevator pitch will help you to give a short explanation of what your change project is about. It is called 'elevator' because it is designed to be short enough to be explained in a short ride in an elevator (30–90 seconds). It is important that the 'guiding coalition' agree to the common elements of the elevator pitch so the message remains clear and consistent.

Typically, it will follow this simple four-part formula:
1. 'Here's what our project is about...'
2. 'Here's why it's important to do...'
3. 'Here's how it will help with your priorities ...'
4. 'Here's how you might want to be part of this...'

The message must resonate with its recipient, so you can create more than one version if stakeholder priorities are different. So, in our example change project of encouraging pupils to consider careers in health care, a careers teacher will be interested in how this will help them to pass their OFSTED inspection, whereas an NHS Trust HR manager will be more interested in lowering their job vacancy rates.

Based on GE Change Acceleration Process (2014).

■ **Time Out**

Create your elevator speech for the Dean of Anytown University to move her from 'not committed' to approving the change project and offering her marketing team's support, by completing the sentences:
  1. Here's what our project is about...
  2. Here's why it's important to do...
  3. Here's how it will help with your priorities
  4. Here's how you might want to be part of this...
Think about what the benefits will be to her. You have 90 seconds to deliver your pitch and 15 minutes in total to convince her!

Your pitch might look something like this:

'Hi, I'm Patrick, a second-year student nurse. I'm part of a student-led movement to promote careers in health care in local secondary schools.

This could be important to you as dean because I know that this university faces stiff competition from Norbrook and DeClancy Universities to meet its enrolment targets in nursing and physiotherapy courses. This project could present a positive marketing image of the university because we will focus on raising career aspirations in high school students in disadvantaged areas.

In 12 months' time, we want to see 16 of the 20 schools in our area promoting careers in health care.

We'd like to invite you to help us by engaging the university's marketing team so positive stories of student aspiration can be shared over the next 12 months with local media.'

That took me 50 seconds to read out!

Summary

Change is part of our lives and on the one hand it represents positive growth and development, but on the other it can bring anxiety and fear. The stages of responding to change have been described like the stages of bereavement that people work through. By recognising our own responses to change we can support others through change with more empathy.

As we consider the need for change, we should link this to factors that are driving the system that we are in. We must also notice signs that change is forthcoming and remain open to the need for change.

Whilst some changes are relatively straightforward and can be handled in a logical and linear way, many changes occur in a complex and dynamic environment, requiring leaders to be the enablers of change rather than leading the change itself.

Listening and responding to stakeholder concerns is a critical process. Involving them at the earliest opportunity encourages them to invest in the change rather than have to buy into it later. When we speak about the change we seek, we should lead with our values, weaving these into a story of self, of us and of now. This will help motivate others to follow the 'call to action'.

Resources

NHS Leadership Academy Horizon's team run a school for change agents that you can join. They have a free course on the FutureLearn platform, part of the Open University, which can be found at https://www.futurelearn.com/courses/school-for-change-agents. The format of FutureLearn is what is known as a 'MOOC', which stands for massive open online course. The format for delivery is open learning, where you will be interacting with an educational organisation and also a cohort of other learners.

The Institute for Healthcare Improvement has a range of tools and techniques for managing change and improvement, which can be found at http://www.ihi.org/.

The National Institute for Health and Care Excellence has a great 'How to Change Practice' guide (2007). Just search 'How to Change—NICE'.

The NHS Change Model is a framework for any project or programme that is seeking to achieve transformational, sustainable change. It is available online at https://www.england.nhs.uk/sustainableimprovement/change-model/. Be aware that this covers large-scale change. The webinar explaining the model can be viewed at https://www.youtube.com/embed/vTv4FbCQlag.

References

Bevan, H., 2010. Community organising, leading change and shifting power: why the NHS needs to build weak ties now. Health Service Journal. <https://www.hsj.co.uk/the-nhs-change-agent/community-organising-leading-change-and-shifting-power-why-the-nhs-needs-to-build-weak-ties-now/5020333.article>. (accessed 08/01/22).

Department of Health and Social Care, 2020. Health and Social Care Secretary Bans Fax Machines in NHS. <https://www.gov.uk/government/news/health-and-social-care-secretary-bans-fax-machines-in-nhs>. (accessed 21/02/2021).

Ganz, M., 2009. Why stories matter: the arts and craft of social change. Sojourners, March 2009, 16–21. <https://friendsofjustice.blog/2009/02/18/marshall-ganz-why-stories-matter/>. (accessed 23/03/2021).

GE Change Acceleration Process, 2014. Slideshare. <https://www.slideshare.net/HomerZhang/ge-change-managementcap>. (accessed 14/06/2021).

Hay, J., 2009. Transactional Analysis for Trainers. Sherwood Publishing, Watford.

Jaben, M., 2019. Free the Brain: Overcome the Struggle People and Organizations Face with Change. Egbert Publishing.

Johnson, S., 1998. Who Moved My Cheese. Vermillion.

Kotter, J., Rathgeber, H., 2006. Our Iceberg Is Melting. Macmillan, London.

Kübler-Ross, E., 1969. On Death and Dying. Scribner, New York.

Lewin, K., 1947. Frontiers in group dynamics: concept, method and reality in social science; social equilibria and social change. Human Relations, 1, 5–41.

NHS England, 2018. The Change Model Guide (Version 5). <https://www.england.nhs.uk/publication/the-change-model-guide/>. (accessed 15/09/2021).

North West Leadership Academy, 2020. Webinar: Leadership Masterclass: Taking the Power to Make Change Happen, with Helen Bevan. <https://youtu.be/0kW09gS0J98>. (accessed 09/05/2021).

Leading Quality and Improvement

OBJECTIVES

After reading this chapter and completing the activities, you should be able to:
- Describe the three components of quality
- Explain the difference between clinical audit, research and improvement
- Name the common improvement approaches used in health and care and outline how they work
- Undertake a simple plan-do-study-act cycle
- Draw a high-level process map
- Identify common statistical process control approaches in nursing.

Relevance to the Nursing and Midwifery Council (NMC) Code

Preserve Safety
Paragraph 8:
Work Cooperatively
  8.4 work with colleagues to evaluate the quality of your work and that of the team

Paragraph 19:
Be Aware of, and Reduce as Far as Possible, any Potential for Harm Associated with Your Practice
  19.1 take measures to reduce as far as possible, the likelihood of mistakes, near misses, harm and the effect of harm if it takes place
  19.2 take account of current evidence, knowledge and developments in reducing mistakes and the effect of them and the impact of human factors and system failures

All nurses must:

act as change agents and provide leadership through quality improvement and service development to enhance people's wellbeing and experiences of healthcare.
STANDARDS FOR COMPETENCE FOR REGISTERED NURSES, NMC (2018)

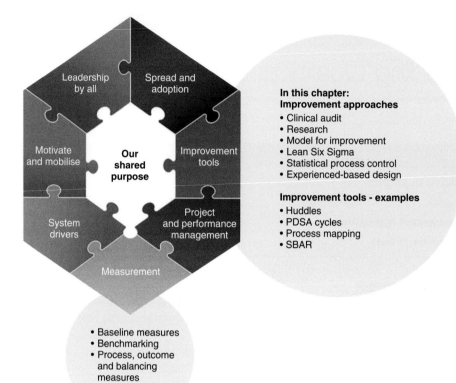

In this chapter:
Improvement approaches
• Clinical audit
• Research
• Model for improvement
• Lean Six Sigma
• Statistical process control
• Experienced-based design

Improvement tools - examples
• Huddles
• PDSA cycles
• Process mapping
• SBAR

• Baseline measures
• Benchmarking
• Process, outcome and balancing measures
• Run charts

Fig. 14.1   Improvement approaches and tools as part of the NHS Change Model. (Courtesy NHS England, 2018. The Change Model Guide (Version 5).)

In Chapter 13 we discussed ways to manage change, and in this section we go on to the more practical matter of techniques and tools to change things for the better: improvement. Improvement approaches and measurement are part of the NHS Change Model (Fig. 14.1).

'Everyone in health care should have two jobs: to do the work and to improve how the work is done.'
MAUREEN BISGNONO, CHIEF EXECUTIVE,
INSTITUTE FOR HEALTHCARE IMPROVEMENT

The aim of this section is to introduce some fundamental concepts around the importance of quality in organisations, give a broad overview of the main improvement approaches that you may come across and then introduce you to some commonly used tools and techniques.

This will just be an introduction, and the Resources section can then signpost you on the more detailed resources.

Leadership Qualities Needed for Improvement

Leaders play a key role in creating the right conditions for quality improvement. They need to build board-level commitment, because, as we shall see, the board has a legal duty not only to just 'assure' quality but to improve it too.

Good leaders should:

- Engage with clinical staff directly.
- Empower their staff to act and make decisions.
- Avoid imposing quality initiatives from the top down.
- Offer a systematic approach to supporting teams using proven improvement methodologies.
- Offer learning programmes and facilitation.
- Encourage ways to help evaluate and share learning across the organisation and beyond.

Student Nurses Are Ideally Placed to Support Improvement

'Sometimes when nurses are fatigued they don't have the energy or time to follow through on their passions... whereas student nurses come in with fresh eyes and fresh passion... it helps to have that drive... and this can be infectious.'

JOY O'GORMAN, STUDENT NURSE, UNIVERSITY OF PLYMOUTH

Through the concept of distributed leadership, every student can make a difference to the quality of care. Leaders strive for a workplace that supports continually improving, high-quality, safe and compassionate health and care. Students are ideally placed to identify improvements because they come to situations with fresh eyes and wider life experience. Students are generally not institutionalised and so can challenge 'this is the way it is'. Students work on the front line where they can identify small improvements that may lead to bigger effects. Here are three examples in Case Studies 14.1 to 14.3.

CASE STUDY 14.1   **Supporting Students Who Are Parents**

Student nurse Nathan Harrison was chairing the University of Salford's Nursing Society when he noticed that a number of student nurses were having a tough time supporting their families whilst on placement. The need for improvement was identified during feedback sessions between students and their personal tutors after placements, where students who were parents reported that they felt like their children were suffering because they were not seeing their parents as often. Some students also admitted that they were struggling financially.

Nathan initiated the development of a parent and carers student support network, accessed via a private Facebook page. The Facebook page was launched in January 2020 and 9 months later had over 100 members.

The move towards online learning for the students and home schooling for children during the COVID-19 pandemic brought additional difficulties in balancing caring and learning, but it also offered the opportunity for students to offer each other peer support. They helped each other to access parental support dependency allowances and signpost people to things like counselling support.

The initiative was noticed by the University of Bradford, and Nathan gave them help to set up their own parent and carer support network.

CASE STUDY 14.2   **Improving Injection Technique**

A student observing an intramuscular injection given by a registered nurse noticed that it was administered by the registered nurse at a 45-degree angle. She mentioned that she thought that it should be 90 degrees. The ward researched it and as a result implemented the student's evidence-based practice.

CASE STUDY 14.3   **Improving Communication Between Doctors and Nurses**

Sometimes improvements can start small, perhaps as an unintended consequence of a question from a student who strives to do things better. Gloria Sikapite, a third-year student nurse, reflected on how she was summarising the current condition of her patient over the phone to a foundation year 2 doctor. She was taking care to offer a holistic assessment and yet she felt that she was not getting to the nub of what he wanted to hear.

This doctor would always say hello to her, listen to her, sit at the nurse's station and asked nurses for their opinions. This emboldened Gloria to speak to him about her concerns about how to better communicate with him about her patient, knowing that he would listen. She initiated an open conversation that helped them both. As a result, the doctor went on to develop a project at the hospital on improving doctor—nurse communication, sharing what they had learned by working together.

It Starts With Clinical Governance

'Clinical governance is a system through which NHS organisations are accountable for continuously improving the quality of their services and safeguarding high standards of care by creating an environment in which excellence in clinical care will flourish.'

SCALLY AND DONALDSON (1998)

Clinical governance is a systematic approach to maintaining and improving the quality of patient care within NHS. It rose to prominence following a series of care scandals, most notably the Bristol heart scandal in 1995, where an anaesthetist, Dr Stephen Bolsin, exposed the higher-than-expected mortality rate for paediatric cardiac surgery at the Bristol Royal Infirmary.

Prior to 1999, the principal statutory responsibilities of UK NHS Trust Boards were to ensure proper financial management of the organisation and an acceptable level of patient safety. Trust Boards had no statutory duty to ensure a particular level of quality, which was seen to be the responsibility of the relevant clinical professions. In 1997 a government White Paper mandated that Trust Boards in England would assume a legal responsibility for quality of care and clinical governance. The other nations of the United Kingdom followed.

The term clinical governance was used to echo the term 'corporate governance'—the structures, systems and processes needed for the operational ability of a trust.

There is no mandated way that trusts are required to implement clinical governance, so it can be interpreted in different ways. It is viewed as both:

- Positive and developmental
- A way of addressing concerns

QUALITY ASSURANCE

So, the boards of organisations must assure themselves that their organisation maintains and improves quality, and the chief executive is the individual accountable for it. Quality assurance has been defined in many ways. The World Health Organisation (1983) divides quality into four aspects:

- Professional performance (technical quality)—the responsibility of clinical leads in organisations, backed by regulators such as the NMC
- Resource use (efficiency)
- Risk management (risks of injury or illness)
- Patient satisfaction

REGULATION ACROSS THE UNITED KINGDOM

The Care Quality Commission (CQC) regulates and inspects health and social care in England. In Wales it is the Healthcare Inspectorate, in Northern Ireland the Regulation and Quality Improvement Authority (RQIA) and in Scotland it is Healthcare Improvement Scotland (HIS).

WHAT DO WE MEAN BY QUALITY IMPROVEMENT?

Quality improvement is a systematic approach to improving health services, based on iterative change, continuous testing and measurement, and empowerment of frontline teams. Some organisations try out improvement in discrete projects, but what really makes a difference is having a systematic approach throughout an organisation. It does not really matter which improvement approach you use; what is more important is that you use an approach consistently (Ross and Naylor 2017). Whilst much of the focus for quality improvement has been in hospitals, quality-improvement approaches are transferrable to other settings, such as mental health (Ross and Naylor 2017) and home care (Chadborn et al. 2021). Quality is defined as:

> '...care that is effective, safe and provides as positive an experience as possible'.
> DEPARTMENT OF HEALTH (2013)

This can be further broken down (Fig. 14.2) into the following elements, more easily remembered using the mnemonic TEPEES (Health Foundation 2013):
- Timely—reducing waits and delays
- Effective—providing services based on evidence and that produce a clear benefit
- Person-centred—establishing a partnership between practitioners and patients to ensure care respects patients' needs and preferences
- Efficient—avoiding waste
- Equitable—providing care that does not vary in quality because of a person's characteristics
- Safe—avoiding harm to patients from care that is intended to help them

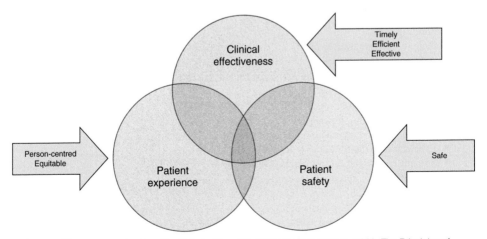

Fig. 14.2 The components of quality. (Adapted from World Health Organisation, 1983. The Principles of Quality Assurance. WHO, Copenhagen. Health Foundation, 2013. Quality Improvement Made Simple. WHO, Copenhagen.)

■ **Time Out**

From your experience so far on placement, write down some positive examples of high-quality care, for example:
- What work has been done to reduce waiting times?
- What processes are in place to avoid harm?

If you can, enquire how these improvements were accomplished

One technique that has been used in various specialisms, such as day surgery, is to map the patient journey along a clinical pathway and measure delays. Then teams work together to try to streamline the pathway and avoid waits.

THE INVOLVEMENT OF PEOPLE AND COMMUNITIES IN IMPROVING CARE

Patient experience is one of the three components of quality (see Fig. 14.2). In education, this applies equally to students too. Today's modern ethos of person- or community-centred care and 'no decision about me without me' (Department of Health 2012) means that it is essential for patients, carers, communities and service users to be involved in quality improvement. Likewise, universities and national bodies involve student nurses in their own improvement activities.

■ **Time Out**

In what ways have you seen organisations such as universities, NHS Trusts, care homes and voluntary sector services such as hospices and learning disability charities involve people and communities in improvement activities?

Methods include:
- Patient representation at organisational quality committees
- Shadowing the patient journey to identify quality shortfalls
- Patient-led assessment of the health care environment
- Completion of patient satisfaction surveys
- Review of patient information materials
- Patient networking to share self-care strategies
- Analysis of patient complaints, concerns and claims
- Patient involvement in quality-improvement focus groups
- Student representation in curriculum planning and course delivery
- Student voice in developing national strategy and policy

Adapted from Health Quality Improvement Partnership (2015).

There may be regional or local clinical networks operating, and these are important for sharing experiences, techniques and learnings about quality. Such networks encourage collaboration between peers and offer a good sounding board. So, if you are interested in quality improvement in a particular clinical area, such as cancer for example, it is worth finding out if a local network exists.

VARIATION IN QUALITY

One of the main philosophies behind quality improvement is to reduce variation in the quality in health organisations (Secretary of State for Health, 2017). As a student nurse, you have the opportunity to work in a variety of settings and organisations and may have experienced that variation for yourself. For example, you may have noticed that in one placement patients are fully involved in decisions about their care, but in another it feels more like things are 'done to' patients. Family and friends may tell you that all their preoperative tests and investigations were completed at one appointment, and others tell you that they had to make two or more visits to get everything done.

Generally, organisations fall along a distribution curve from low quality to high quality, with most falling somewhere in the middle (Fig. 14.3). The challenge for organisations is to learn from excellence and to move the mean of this distribution curve to the right. Much effort has been expended over recent years to encourage organisations to spread and adopt effective practice. We shall discuss the challenges of spread and adoption in Chapter 15 on implementing projects and programmes.

Methods to Improve: Approaches and Techniques

So, the drive for improvement came from failures in care, resulting in legislation to mandate NHS organisations to improve quality. Let us start to look at the ways that health and care organisations—and indeed universities too in their education and research agendas—can work to improve care.

Improvement science includes (see Fig. 14.1):
- approaches to improvement: different ways of looking at it, such as audit and research;
- tools and techniques such as plan-do-study-act (PDSA) cycles; and
- ways to measure improvements, such as run charts.

We shall start with looking at some of the major approaches and then go on to look at some common tools and measurement methods that you might come across.

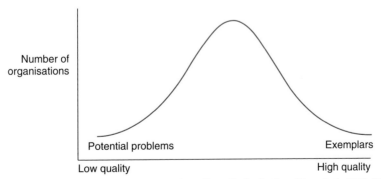

Fig. 14.3 Variation in the quality of health organisations. (From Scally, G., Donaldson, L.J., 1998. Clinical governance and the drive for quality improvement in the new NHS in England. British Medical Journal, 317, 61–65.)

The science of improvement originated outside health care, and their principles have subsequently been adapted and applied to it. Some of the main approaches used in health and care are:

- The **Institute for Healthcare Improvement's (IHI) model** for quality improvement (IHI-QI) is characterised by completing PDSA small tests of change.
- **Lean,** which emerged from car manufacturer Toyota, is about making processes better, faster and cheaper by the elimination of waste.
- **Six Sigma** emerged from Motorola's manufacturing processes and is a set of tools and techniques designed to eliminate defects. Sometimes Lean and Six Sigma processes are combined and termed 'Lean Six Sigma'.
- **Statistical process control** (SPC) is about examining a series of data and identifying, explaining and eliminating variation. Charts are used to visualise performance over time. A simple clinical example might be the monitoring of peak expiratory flow rate. SPC is also described as a tool.
- **Experience-based codesign** (which we covered in Section 2) is about involving patients or service users to codesign services.
- **Clinical audit** was the predominant method used to improve quality in the NHS in the 1990s. Audit is a process to check that clinical care meets defined quality standards and monitors improvements to address shortfalls.
- **Research** is concerned with generating hypotheses and verifying scientifically a predicted, but not necessarily proven, relationship between or among variables such as clinical processes and outcomes.

There is often confusion between audit, research and improvement. In brief:

- Audit is about checking that care meets quality standards, for example auditing door-to-needle times for thrombolysis for people having a stroke.
- Improvement is about learning what will improve care by undertaking cycles of testing, for example by doing PDSA cycles to improve the care pathway.
- Research is about trying to demonstrate the effectiveness of an intervention, for example researching if a new clinical pathway for stroke reduces mortality rates.

Based on Institute for Healthcare Improvement (2015).

Let us explore audit, improvement and research in more detail.

CLINICAL AUDIT

Audit measures current practice against a defined (desired) standard. Doctors are required, as part of their 5-year revalidation, to take part in audits, but it is not part of nurse's revalidation, although nurses often work as part of audit teams.

In simple terms, audit is:

- Viewing what is happening now—the real situation
- Comparing this with what should be happening—the ideal situation
- Taking action to close the gap

The standard audit cycle is given in Fig. 14.4

For effective audit there should be:

- A quality issue of interest
- Local standards, which could be based on national standards
- Recent data
- Involvement for everyone (and keep them informed all the time)
- Brevity and simplicity ('keep it short and simple'—KISS)

Based on Kinn (1995).

Example: Learning Disability Audit

'It remains a considerable concern that most mainstream health care professionals including General Practitioners (GPs) lack confidence in caring for people with a learning disability.'

EMERSON AND TURNER (2011)

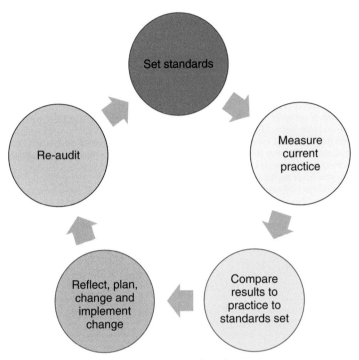

Fig. 14.4   The audit cycle.

A common audit undertaken as part of the GP's contract is that people with a learning disability have an annual health check because of the significant health inequalities they experience. General practice nurses are often involved in such audits.

Practices are required to:

- establish and maintain a learning disabilities 'health check register' of patients aged 14 years and over with learning disabilities;
- attend a multiprofessional education session; and
- invite all patients on the register for an annual health check and produce a health action plan.

GP surgeries are assisted in their audit activities by a range of toolkits. They are given a detailed description of the standards, which are nationally set. Standardisation of coding on their clinical systems helps them measure current practice, meaning that they can produce data on how they are doing against the standards by conducting a search on those codes. This allows them more easily to compare their results to the standards and think about changes that they may need to make (see Royal College of General Practitioners 2017).

RESEARCH

Research has an important role in improving quality and is something that student nurses can engage in. Students can both critically appraise research and help introduce evidence into practice and also, as one student found, help to develop and undertake research and develop research-based improvements (Case Study 14.4).

| CASE STUDY 14.4 | **Improving Dementia Awareness and Perception in Northern Ireland** |

In 2019, Victoria McTurk, an adult nursing student at Queen's University Belfast, was invited by her tutor Dr Gary Mitchell to become part of a research team investigating and exploring public perceptions, facilitators and barriers to living well with dementia in Northern Ireland.

During her first year as an undergraduate adult nurse at Queen's University Belfast, she was asked by Gary to assist him and other colleagues in two pieces of work.

The first was a series of workshops with stakeholders such as undergraduate students, health professionals and members of Dementia Northern Ireland (Dementia NI) to codesign an online 'dementia awareness game' to raise awareness and perception of the public about people with dementia. The idea of gamification as an interactive and kinaesthetic process offered the exciting possibility of an improvement designed to change perceptions. The 'Dementia Game' that was subsequently developed and tested is now freely available (Focus Games and Queen's University Belfast, https://www.dementiagame.com/) and involves members of the public answering multiple-choice questions about dementia correctly to proceed through a virtual journey of everyday life, against the clock.

The second role was about joining the research team who was undertaking a piece of qualitative research to explore current public perceptions of dementia and identifying the facilitators and barriers to living well from the perspective of people living with the condition in Northern Ireland.

Victoria was initially chosen to be a part of the workshops developing the online game due to her own experiences of supporting family members with dementia.

Gary comments 'At such an early stage in her nurse training Victoria demonstrated empathy, compassion and person-centredness. I was keen to work with her on this project and hence why I selected her.'

She also had the advantage of her fresh eyes, observing how people with dementia are perceived, as a student working in various wards throughout Northern Ireland. However, she was quickly talent spotted and invited to be part of the academic team itself:

'Throughout the workshops, it became apparent to Gary that I was very invested and outspoken about the topic and engaged actively with the Dementia NI members and the other members of the academic research team. During discussions I would take the lead and encourage everyone to participate and give their thoughts and opinions. I'd stimulate people's own ideas and encourage them to vocalise any fears that they may have about the topic. Then Gary asked me if I could help with both pieces of work: to become part of the research team into public perceptions about people with dementia and help to identify questions to be included in the game.'

When it came to the research into the perceptions of the public, Gary and Victoria assigned themselves roles in the research according to their strengths. Four focus group interviews had been conducted with 20 people living with dementia across three Northern Irish counties. These interviews were audio recorded, transcribed verbatim and then underwent thematic analysis. Victoria's role was to transcribe the recorded focus groups ready for thematic analysis:

'Any piece of work I completed I would let Gary read and critique so that I could understand areas that needed improvement or expanding on, as I had no experience in writing a research article. So I listened to his advice and guidance on everything I completed.'

'Once the research article was drafted Gary sent it to his academic peers to get their thoughts and opinions. Then the research was accepted for publication by BMC Geriatrics (Mitchell et al. 2020). I am so proud of this achievement as it was something I never thought I could have accomplished, and I hope it inspires other student nurses to pursue their passion for research and make it a reality.'

What Victoria and Gary's team reveals from their improvement research is that society focuses on the disability element of a diagnosis of dementia rather than supporting people's capabilities. It uncovers ways that the public could encourage people living with the condition to enjoy greater independence. This paves the way for the research to be used to make improvements in public perceptions and meaningful behavioural change so that people can live well with dementia in their local communities.

Further research conducted by Queen's University Belfast on the impact of the 'Dementia Game' shows that after playing the game, a person's attitudes to people living with dementia improve. The game has now been played over 5000 times and continues to be a feature as a learning tool in year one of the undergraduate nursing curriculum. The university has also received some funding to develop a children's version of the 'Dementia Game'. The game was also a runner-up in the innovation category of the National Dementia Awards.

Gary describes Victoria's leadership as transformational: formulating a plan of what needed to change and cocreating a vision to guide the change. She inspired and supported the codesign of the game with the other members of the team.

Model for Improvement and PDSA Cycles

Let us go on to some more detail on some of the most common improvement approaches that you as student nurses might come across and try out some of the tools used.

'Model for improvement' was developed by the IHI and is based on systematically testing ideas for making improvements (Fig. 14.5). The model is based on three fundamental questions that can be answered in any order:

- What are we trying to accomplish?
- How will we know that a change is an improvement?
- What change can we make that will result in improvement?

The questions are answered by testing change ideas using PDSA cycles. This means taking ideas, trying them out in practice at the smallest level, learning what works (or does not work), making small changes, testing again and then repeating the cycle until you have the improvement you want.

Model for improvement

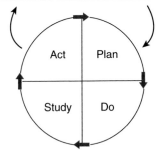

What are we trying to accomplish?

Setting aims
The aim should be time-specific and measurable; it should also define the specific population of patients or other system that will be affected.

How will we know that a change is an improvement?

Establishing measures
Teams use quantitative measures to determine if a specific change actually leads to an improvement.

What change can we make that will result in improvement?

Selecting changes
Ideas for change may come from those who work in the system or from the experience of others who have successfully improved.

Act | Plan
Study | Do

Testing changes
The Plan-Do-Study-Act (PDSA) cycle is shorthand for testing a change in the real work setting – by planning it, trying it, observing the results, and acting on what is learned. This is the scientific method adapted for action-oriented learning.

Fig. 14.5 The model for improvement. (Langley, G.L., Moen, R., Nolan, K.M., Nolan, T.W., Norman, C.L., Provost, L.P., 2009. The Improvement Guide: A Practical Approach to Enhancing Organizational Performance, second ed. Jossey-Bass Publishers, San Francisco.)

Tip—Remember Shared Purpose!

As we discussed in the previous section, we might begin, however, with a discussion on who has a stake in this proposed improvement and then engage them to create a shared or common purpose before setting an aim. This will help reduce change resistance.

Let us break down these four steps:

Step 1: Plan

Plan the test or observation, including a plan for collecting data:

- State the objective of the test.
- Make predictions about what will happen and why.
- Develop a plan to test the change (Who? What? When? Where? What data need to be collected?).

Step 2: Do

Try out the test on a small scale:

- Carry out the test.
- Document problems and unexpected observations.
- Begin analysis of the data.

Step 3: Study

Set aside time to analyse the data and study the results:

- Complete the analysis of the data.
- Compare the data to your predictions.
- Summarise and reflect on what was learned.

Step 4: Act

Refine the change, based on what was learned from the test:

- Adapt (make modifications and run another test), adopt (test the change on a larger scale) or abandon (do not do another test on this change idea).
- Prepare a plan for the next test.

■ Time Out

Design your own simple PDSA cycle. Write down:

- What are you trying to accomplish?
- How will you know that a change is an improvement?
- What change can you make that will result in improvement?

This can be, for example, something as simple as:

- What are you trying to accomplish? Teach your new puppy to sit on command tonight between 8.00 and 8.30 pm.
- How will you know that a change is an improvement? He will sit when prompted (outcome).
- What change can you make that will result in improvement? You will use the technique of holding a treat in front of his nose whilst he is standing and raise the treat so that his bottom starts to go down (process), then reward him with the treat and praise. Whilst doing that you will say 'sit' so that he begins to associate the process with the reward.

Now complete your first PDSA cycle and record what happens. Remember that this first cycle is just a small test of change. In my example, maybe your puppy was distracted by your youngest child and fails to sit. So, your next test tomorrow night will be just you and the puppy. And maybe you will do the test earlier and before you have fed the puppy, so he is alert and hungry.

It is important that you record what methods you use and what the result is, so that you have a record for others to follow.

MEASURE WHAT'S IMPORTANT

Consider what you trying to achieve. What would tell you that you had achieved it? What would you need to have in place to know you were making progress towards that aim? These questions should help you identify what you need to measure and therefore what data you will need. You do not need lots of complicated data—just enough to tell you whether you are making progress or not (Tips Box 14.1). So for example, if you want to encourage people with depression to exercise to improve their wellbeing, you will need to use a valid and reliable tool to measure their current wellbeing score and possibly a depression score too.

TIPS BOX 14.1

Try to avoid the ICE approach:
* Identify everything that is easy to measure and count.
* Collect and report the data on everything that is easy to measure and count.
* End up scratching your head thinking 'What are we going to do with all this data?'

———

Courtesy NHS Improving Quality (2014).

If you want to use routinely collected data, such as admissions data, then contact the information department or ask someone senior in the organisation who supports your project (this person is usually called a 'sponsor') to do it on your behalf. Think also about who will be responsible for collecting and analysing the data.

BASELINE MEASURES

It is important that you measure the starting point so that you know whether any change is an improvement or not. So, in our example of relieving depression with exercise, you would administer baseline scores for both depression and wellbeing using questionnaires. As you do these baseline measures, make sure that you consider the person's experience so they do not end up feeling like they are just filling in forms like laboratory rats!

Benchmarking

Benchmarking has been described as:

> 'A systematic process in which current practice and care are compared to, and amended to attain, best practice and care.'
>
> DEPARTMENT OF HEALTH (2010)

Benchmarking is like a measuring stick: it allows comparison between you, your organisation's or team's performance and best practice standards. It is used to:
- identify strengths and weaknesses within organisations;
- identify the level of performance possible by looking at the performance of others, and how much improvement can be achieved;
- promote changes and deliver improvements in quality, productivity and efficiency; and
- help to better satisfy the need for quality, cost, product and service by establishing new standards and goals.

Courtesy Royal College of Nursing (2017).

The common steps that are taken in benchmarking mirror the nursing process—assess, plan, implement and evaluate:

- Establish priorities for improving practice and care within the environment or organisation.
- Establish and agree on best (evidence-based) practice and care for people within the organisation.
- Ascertain current practice and care.
- Compare the differences and identify the gaps and barriers between current and best practice and care, and identify achievements.
- Develop a plan of what goals need to be met to achieve best practice and care (i.e., working out what needs to be done and how).
- Implement the plan (i.e., change things, for example, activity, perspective, approach, culture, education and training, or environment) to meet the goals.
- Evaluate practice and care by assessing and measuring whether goals have been met.
- Establish improved practice and care across a team or organisation(s).
- Establish priorities and further goals to continuously improve quality of practice and care (i.e., go through the steps again).

Department of Health (2010).

To compare yourself, you need to identify best practice. To do this:

- Look at research findings.
- Compare examples of clinical practice between peers (often by setting up benchmarking networks).
- Use professional consensus.

The NHS has its own benchmarking network, acting as a central reference point for publicly funded health and care services (see the Resources section).

■ Time Out

In 2010 NHS England produced its 'Essence of Care' guidelines (see Resources section), which is a set of 12 benchmarks that aim to support localised quality improvement and frontline care across care settings at a local level. These benchmarks were identified by asking people, staff and carers what they were unhappy with. They are:

- Bladder, bowel and continence care
- Care environment
- Communication
- Food and drink
- Prevention and management of pain
- Personal hygiene
- Prevention and management of pressure ulcers
- Promoting health and wellbeing
- Record keeping
- Respect and dignity
- Safety
- Self-care

Think of an area covered by Essence of Care where you have seen most dissatisfaction during your placements—maybe because of patient, service user or carer complaints. On the NHS England website, find the benchmark for the relevant area of care.

Working with your mentor or personal tutor, identify good practice locally or nationally, by looking at research or tapping into clinical networks.

Make some notes on how you, as a future leader, would go about making an improvement, based on your learning so far from this book.

Like many other leadership issues that we have covered, success in establishing routine benchmarking activities to make a difference to what matters to people lies in influencing the culture of the organisation, which comes down to role modelling good leadership at every level, including the board level.

PROCESS, OUTCOME AND BALANCING MEASURES

Measures are critical for a team because they tell the team whether the changes are actually leading to an improvement. The IHI uses the analogy of a coach advising a golfer on how to improve her swing to explain the difference between process, outcome and balancing measures.

The golfer keeps slicing the ball, and the coach is advising on ways to improve her grip. As she does this, the ball goes straight, and this is a measurement of outcome. The coach notices her grip, which is a measurement of process. To improve, she and her coach need to record which grip is used with each swing and what the outcome was—straight or sliced—to learn how to improve. It is helpful here to graph each swing on what is called a 'run chart', which is a sequence of data that presents as a pattern, much like you would see on a temperature chart, so that you can keep track of which grip produces each result.

Whilst practising the swing with the correct grip, the golfer notices that her back twinges. This is called a balancing measure or 'side effect measure'—things that are inadvertently or undesirably affected by the change. These too need recording in the run chart—which grip and swing cause back twinges. An example of a balancing measure might be that when you are improving hand hygiene through handwashing, you measure the number of skin rashes that may be triggered. The prevalence of this balancing measure needs to be recorded and reported alongside the process and outcome measures.

Lean/Six Sigma

These two improvement processes are often used together. 'Lean' focuses on improving system flow and reducing waste. 'Six Sigma' focuses on understanding the root causes of variation and reduce them. Let's start with Six Sigma.

Six Sigma is a continuous improvement philosophy, methodology and toolkit that focuses on what the customer (in our case, the patient or community) wants. It involves improving process performance, decrease variation and maintaining consistent quality of the output of the process and in so doing, reducing costs. It focuses on eliminating unnecessary procedures and delays (or wastes) to help organisations to improve performance. The methodology includes the following stages: Define, Measure, Analyse, Improve and Control (DMAIC).

Six Sigma projects focus on the identification of root causes of problems rather than focusing on the symptoms of the problem and focus on facts and hard data, that is measured and analysed, rather than on opinion. It is called Six Sigma because it is a process to reduce variation so that acceptable performance is within six standard deviations. A 'standard deviation' is a measure that is used to quantify the amount of variation or dispersion of a set of data values and is represented by the Greek letter sigma (σ). The aim is to avoid defects; in case of nursing, a 'defect' may refer to the development of a pressure ulcer, delays in commencing antibiotic treatment or a patient fall.

Introducing Six Sigma improvement methods into health and care usually follow significant investment and training of staff. Presented here are the basic steps followed by some of the most common tools used so that you will be able to recognise them if you come across them on placement. You may be using some of the principles of Six Sigma every day at home: such as finding more efficient ways for you and your children to get to school and work on time, by streamlining everyone washing, dressing, breakfasting and travelling.

DMAIC

There are 5 steps to the DMAIC method which are shown in Fig. 14.6.

Let's now turn to some of the most common tools used in Lean Six Sigma.

PROCESS MAPPING

A 'process map' is a flow chart that visually describes the flow of work. A team, working together, identifies and maps the sequence of steps, components and/or activities that are needed to deliver any result or outcome. Once you know what the process is to deliver a result, it can be measured. Once it is measured, it can be improved.

Process maps normally start as a high-level map and then drill down to more detail. They are usually done by the team involved in care delivery to ensure no steps are missed and to build in ownership of the process.

Define
What is important?
- Identify the improvement opportunity, e.g., reducing pressure ulcers.
- Define the problem.
- Define the project's purpose and scope.
- Collect background information.
- Listen to the patient, carers, team etc.
- Map the existing process that is currently followed.

Measure
How are we doing?
- Understand the baseline position and current levels of performance.
- Identify the measures to be used, e.g., pressure ulcer classification system to be used.
- Develop operational definitions such as 'blanching' or 'partial thickness'.
- Develop and implement a measurement plan.

Analyse
What is wrong?
- Establish the problem's root causes and understand their effect on process, e.g., low staffing? Lack of equipment? Are these the root causes or does somethng lie behind them?
- Validate the root causes.
- Determine the true sources of variation.
- Analyse detailed process maps (see Figs 14.7 and 14.8) and identify improvement opportunities.
- Plot and analyse the data (see Fig. 14.9).
- Determine the amount of variation in the process.

Improve
What needs to be done?
- Develop, select and implement the best solutions.
- Generate solution ideas.
- Develop a process map for the solution.
- Initiate, measure and evaluate the pilot.
- Share and evaluate the results with the team.

Control
How to sustain improvement?
- Embed and maintain the gains.
- Verify the reduction in variation.
- Monitor performance.
- Integrate lessons learned.
- Identify new opportunities.

Fig. 14.6   The five steps of DMAIC. (Based on NHS Improvement (2011) An overview of Six Sigma.)

■ Time Out

Draw a high-level process map for how you prepare a slice of buttered toast, showing all the steps along the way.

Your process map might look like Fig. 14.7. But these are not all the steps you might take. Adding more detail identifies further steps in the process (Fig. 14.8).

If we were to **improve** (DMAIC) by 'adding value' to our toast making, by making sure that there are no delays (we need to have a quick breakfast!) and it is 'safe', we might do things like:

- Stack all the things we need (bread, butter, plate, knives, etc.) by the toaster the night before, so we do not have to get everything together in the morning.
- Switch to margarine so it spreads quickly and evenly rather than try to spread cold butter out of the fridge (because it is high summer and the butter will melt if we leave it out).
- Make sure all equipment is clean and safe—we have the toaster portable appliance tested so it is not a fire risk and we clean the dishwasher monthly so we know that plates and knives are clean.

LEAN

Having completed a process map and identified value, teams often identify what are called in Lean improving the 'seven wastes' (Table 14.1). An everyday example of reducing waste might be to plan what you want to eat during the week and doing a shopping list so that you don't either run short of food or over-buy. This is an example of what is called reducing 'inventory waste'.

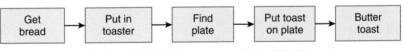

Fig. 14.7   High-level process map—buttered toast.

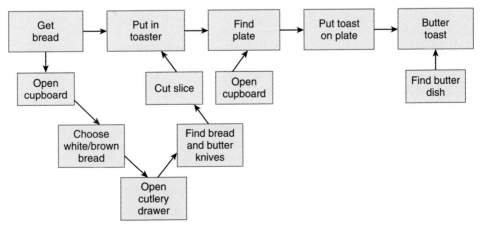

Fig. 14.8   Detailed process map—buttered toast.

TABLE 14.1 ■ The Seven Wastes of Lean, With Examples

Waste	Description	Example
Correction	Rework due to faulty processes	Readmissions due to poor discharge procedures Repeating things incorrectly done Adverse drug reactions Iatrogenic illness Wound breakdown
Waiting	People waiting for information, equipment or other people	Waiting for: Patients Results Dispensing Team members' actions
Transportation	Moving materials unnecessarily	Frequently used items stored at the end of corridors rather than close to hand One central vaccine fridge instead of local fridge
Overprocessing	Performing unnecessary processes that do not add value	Repeated history taking Duplicated record keeping
Inventory	Keeping too much stock Too much work in progress Information or patient queues	Waiting lists Overstocking items Patients waiting to be discharged
Motion	Unnecessary travel, walking, searching or motion Things not accessible or within easy reach	Not having basic equipment in each examination room Storing syringes and needles in different parts of the room Using cupboards that need opening rather than shelves that can avoid searching for items
Overproduction	Producing more than is needed, or earlier than needed	Ordering unnecessary tests Inviting too many patients to outpatient appointments at the same time

Based on NHS Institute for Innovation and Improvement (2007).

■ **Time Out**

Identify a process at work that you know, such as admitting a patient, doing a drug round or preparing a person or group of people with a learning disability for a day out. Try to identify any of the seven wastes in these processes.

For the second part of this activity, identify a process that has undergone significant change, perhaps brought about by the COVID-19 pandemic. For example, which of the seven wastes have been eliminated by switching to remote consultations, mass vaccination and testing processes and finding ways of catching up with routine screening and treatment?

STATISTICAL PROCESS CONTROL

SPC is a tool for measuring and controlling the quality of a process against predefined parameters. This is the 'C' of **control** in DMAIC, and this enables project teams to have a monitoring plan.

Outputs from a process are charted (Fig. 14.9) on what is termed a 'run chart' so that users can see variations. Lower and upper control limits (in red) are set using standard deviations from the historical mean (in grey) or from baseline measurements. The chart is then used to analyse when variation has occurred and why. Next, corrections to the process are made, followed by checking to see that the variance is corrected.

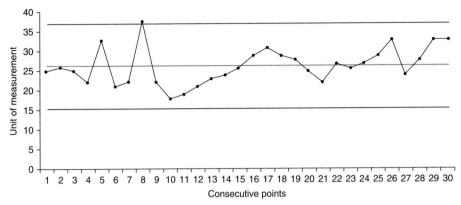

Fig. 14.9 A run chart used in statistical process control. (Source: NHS Institute for Innovation and Improvement, 2008. Statistical process control.)

■ Time Out

Can you think of a simple SPC process that is commonly used in nursing? What do the variances tell you and what do you do about them?

As nurses, we are trained to look out for variation from the norm and investigate the cause and take action. Some typical examples include charting temperature, pulse, respiratory rate, ECG and peak flows. For example, a temperature above 37°C may indicate a need to investigate for infection. Charting continues to assess whether, for example, antibiotics are taking an effect.

Improvement Tools for Patient Safety

HUDDLES

You may already be familiar with huddles, which are 10-minute stand-up meetings, usually at the start of the day, where teams identify quality and safety issues. Typical huddles will have an agenda that includes:

1. Sharing successes and concerns from the last shift
2. Marking issues on a huddle board
3. Discussing today's safety and quality issues
4. Reviewing previously identified issues
5. Making announcements and sharing any further information that may affect quality

See the Resources section for further information from the Institute for Healthcare Improvement on how to establish huddles.

SBAR

At the start of the chapter, we saw Gloria Sikapite recognising that she and her doctor colleague needed to improve the quality of their communications so that Gloria could better communicate what was happening with her patient and why she was concerned. The purpose of the SBAR tool is to provide a structure for doing just that. SBAR stands for situation, background, assessment and recommendation, and it is a well-known tool for communicating safely, assertively and effectively (Fig. 14.10).

SBAR can be used anywhere, including:

- Shift handovers
- Escalating a concern
- Between difference disciplines (e.g., Nurse to occupational therapist)
- Between different settings (e.g., sheltered housing manager to learning disability nurse or ward manager to district nurse liaison)

See the Institute of Healthcare Improvement (details in the Resources section) for more information on using SBAR.

S
Situation:
I am (name), (X) nurse on ward (X)
I am calling about (patient X)
I am calling because I am concerned that...
(e.g., BP is low/high, pulse is XX, temperature is XX, Early Warning Score is XX)

B
Background:
Patient (X) was admitted on (XX date) with...
(e.g., MI/chest infection)
They have had (X operation/procedure/investigation)
Patient (X)'s condition has changed in the last (XX mins)
Their last set of obs were (XX)
Patient (X)'s normal condition is...
(e.g., alert/drowsy/confused, pain free)

A
Assessment:
I think the problem is (XXX)
And I have...
(e.g., given O_2/analgesia, stopped the infusion)
OR
I am not sure what the problem is but patient (X) is deteriorating
OR
I don't know what's wrong but I am really worried

R
Recommendation:
I need you to...
Come to see the patient in the next (XX mins)
AND
Is there anything I need to do in the meantime?
(e.g., stop the fluid/repeat the obs)

Ask receiver to repeat key information to ensure understanding.

The SBAR tool originated from the US Navy and was adapted for use in health care by Dr M Leonard and colleagues from Kaiser Permanente, Colorado, USA

Fig. 14.10 SBAR tool. (From Quality, Service Improvement and Redesign Tools: SBAR communication tool - situation, background, assessment, recommendation.)

Improvement Programmes Across the United Kingdom

Each country of the United Kingdom has initiated a range of improvement programmes to support specific improvement campaigns across the four nations. They are accessible for student nurses so that you can understand more about improvement methods and priorities in the country in which you are based (see Resources section). These campaigns often focus on the three components of quality: patient experience, safety and clinical effectiveness.

Examples include:

- Essentials of Safe Care (Scotland)
- Care Home Cymru (Wales)
- Always Events (England)

■ Time Out

Discover your organisation's quality-improvement strategy by visiting the website or intranet of the current or last organisation in which you have had a placement.

- Do they have a quality-improvement strategy?
- Which of the three elements of quality (patient experience, safety and clinical effectiveness) are incorporated in the strategy?
- Is the organisation part of any national improvement campaigns?

Summary

Clinical governance rose to prominence because of high-profile care failings in the NHS. Trust boards are now accountable for the quality of care they provide. Patient experience, safety and clinical effectiveness are the three key components of quality. Improving care by adopting appropriate approaches and tools and by measuring improvements form a central part of an organisation's clinical governance strategy.

There is a long history of improvement science that originated in industry and has been subsequently adapted and adopted by the NHS. To be successful, organisations need to consistently choose and use one improvement model, embedding it into their culture and empowering leaders at all levels to act.

Improvement resources are easily accessible via a range of websites both nationally and internationally. These have enabled a wider range of care settings to benefit from improvement science, which started in the hospital sector and is now spreading across all sectors and disciplines.

Student nurse leaders are ideally placed to notice where improvements may be needed because they can bring fresh eyes and life experience into health and care settings. Many have been successful in making small improvements, including in health care, research and educational settings.

Resources

UK NHS Improvement Websites

Essence of Care. <https://www.gov.uk/government/publications/essence-of-care-2010>.
Health Improvement Scotland's ihub. <https://ihub.scot/>.
Improvement Cymru. <https://phw.nhs.wales/services-and-teams/improvement-cymru/>.
NHS Benchmarking. <https://www.nhsbenchmarking.nhs.uk/>.
NHS England's site. <https://www.england.nhs.uk/quality-service-improvement-and-redesign-qsir-tools/
quality-service-improvement-and-redesign-qsir-tools-by-type-of-approach/>.
Quality 2020 Northern Ireland. <https://www.health-ni.gov.uk/topics/safety-and-quality-standards/quality-2020>.

Non-NHS Improvement Agencies

The Improvement Academy. <https://improvementacademy.org/>.
The Institute for Healthcare Improvement. <http://www.ihi.org/>.

Specialist Resources

Hospice UK, Hospice care. <https://www.hospiceuk.org/what-we-offer/clinical-and-care-support/
quality-assurance>.
NHS England, General practice. <https://www.england.nhs.uk/gp/gpfv/redesign/gpdp/capability/>.
NHS England, Learning disabilities and autism. <https://www.england.nhs.uk/learning-disabilities/about/
resources/the-learning-disability-improvement-standards-for-nhs-trusts/>.
NHS Improvement, Learning disabilities and autism. <https://improvement.nhs.uk/improvement-hub/
learning-disabilities/>.
The National Collaborating Centre for Mental Health, Mental health patient safety. <https://www.rcpsych.
ac.uk/improving-care/nccmh/quality-improvement-programmes>.
The National Institute for Health and Care Excellence (NICE), Adult social care. Although aimed at commissioners, it may also be useful to provider organisations and people who fund their own care. <https://
www.nice.org.uk/about/nice-communities/social-care/quality-improvement-resource>.
The Royal College of Paediatrics and Child Health. <https://www.rcpch.ac.uk/work-we-do/quality-
improvement-patient-safety and https://qicentral.rcpch.ac.uk/>.

References

Canadian Health Services Research Foundation, 2007. Turning the tide on chronic disease: how a province
is using evidence to build quality improvement capacity. Healthcare Policy 3 (2), 67–70.
Chadborn, N.H., Devi, R., Hinsliff-Smith, K., Banerjee, J., Gordon, A.L., 2021. Quality improvement in
long-term care settings: a scoping review of effective strategies used in care homes. European Geriatric
Medicine 12, 17–26.
Department of Health, 2001. The report of the public inquiry into children's heart surgery at the Bristol
Royal Infirmary 1984-1995: learning from Bristol (Cm 5207(II)). <https://webarchive.nationalarchives.
gov.uk/ukgwa/20100407202128/http://www.dh.gov.uk/en/Publicationsandstatistics/Publications/Publica-
tionsPolicyAndGuidance/DH_4005620>. (accessed 09/01/2022).
Department of Health, 2010. How to Use Essence of Care. <https://assets.publishing.service.gov.uk/gov-
ernment/uploads/system/uploads/attachment_data/file/216690/dh_119970.pdf>. (accessed 08/01/2022).
Department of Health, 2012. No Decision About Me Without Me. Liberating the NHS: No decision about
me without me. <https://webarchive.nationalarchives.gov.uk/ukgwa/20130104181152/http://www.dh.
gov.uk/en/Consultations/Liveconsultations/DH_134221>. (accessed 08/01/2022).
Department of Health, 2013. Quality in the New Health System – Maintaining and Improving Quality
From April 2013. <https://www.gov.uk/government/publications/quality-in-the-new-health-system-main-
taining-and-improving-quality-from-april-2013>. (accessed 08/01/2022).
Emerson, E., Turner, S., 2011. Health checks for people with learning disabilities: an audit tool. Improving
health and lives learning disability observatory. Advances in Mental Health and Intellectual Disabilities,
6(1), 26–32.
Focus Games and Queen's University Belfast. The Dementia Game. <https://www.dementiagame.com/>.
(accessed 01/04/2021).

Health Foundation, 2013. Quality Improvement Made Simple.

Health Quality Improvement Partnership, 2015. A Guide to Quality Improvement Methods. <https://www. hqip.org.uk/wp-content/uploads/2018/02/guide-to-quality-improvement-methods.pdf>. (accessed 09/01/2022).

Institute for Healthcare Improvement, 2015. What's the Difference Between Research and QI? YouTube. <https://youtu.be/hyWJLhyKWjQ>. (accessed 28/03/2021).

Jones, D., Mitchell, A., Lean Enterprise Academy, 2006. Lean Thinking for the NHS. NHS Confederation.

Kinn, S., 1995. Clinical audit: a tool for nursing practice. Nursing Standard, 9 (15), 35–36.

Langley, G.L., Moen, R., Nolan, K.M., Nolan, T.W., Norman, C.L., Provost, L.P., 2009. The Improvement Guide: A Practical Approach to Enhancing Organizational Performance, second ed. Jossey-Bass Publishers, San Francisco.

Leonard, M., Graham, S., Bonacum, D., 2004. The human factor: the critical importance of effective teamwork and communication in providing safe care. BMJ Quality & Safety in Health Care, 13, 85–90.

Mitchell, G., McTurk, V., Carter, G., Brown-Wilson, C., 2020. Emphasise capability, not disability: exploring public perceptions, facilitators and barriers to living well with dementia in Northern Ireland. BMC Geriatrics, 20, 525.

NHS Improving Quality, 2014. First Steps Towards Quality Improvement: A Simple Guide to Improving Services. <https://www.england.nhs.uk/improvement-hub/publication/first-steps-towards-quality-improvement-a-simple-guide-to-improving-services/>. (accessed 09/01/2022).

NHS Institute for Innovation and Improvement, 2007. Going Lean in the NHS. <https://www.england.nhs. uk/improvement-hub/wp-content/uploads/sites/44/2017/11/Going-Lean-in-the-NHS.pdf>. (accessed 09/01/2022).

NMC, 2018. Standards for Competence for Registered Nurses.

Ross, S., Naylor, C., 2017. Quality Improvement in Mental Health. King's Fund, London.

Royal College of General Practitioners, 2017. Health checks for people with learning disabilities toolkit. <https://www.rcgp.org.uk/clinical-and-research/resources/toolkits/health-check-toolkit.aspx>. (accessed on 02/04/2021).

Royal College of Nursing, 2017. Understanding Benchmarking. RCN, London.

Scally, G., Donaldson, L.J., 1998. Clinical governance and the drive for quality improvement in the new NHS in England. British Medical Journal, 317, 61–65.

Secretary of State for Health, 1997. The New NHS. Stationery Office, London. <https://assets.publishing. service.gov.uk/government/uploads/system/uploads/attachment_data/file/266003/newnhs.pdf>. (accessed 09/01/2022).

World Health Organisation, 1983. The Principles of Quality Assurance. WHO, Copenhagen.

Leading Projects and Programmes

OBJECTIVES

After reading this chapter and completing the activities, you should be able to:
- Define the characteristics of a project
- Write SMART project aims and objectives
- Identify roles within a project team
- Describe the components of a project plan
- Develop a simple risk register
- Develop a logic model to identify project inputs, outputs and outcomes
- Identify the dos and don'ts of spreading improvements.

Relevance to the Nursing and Midwifery Council (NMC) Code

Practise Effectively
Paragraph 8:
Work Cooperatively
  8.1 respect the skills, expertise and contributions of your colleagues, referring matters to them when appropriate
  8.2 maintain effective communication with colleagues
  8.3 keep colleagues informed when you are sharing the care of individuals with other health and care professionals and staff
  8.4 work with colleagues to evaluate the quality of your work and that of the team
  8.5 work with colleagues to preserve the safety of those receiving care
  8.6 share information to identify and reduce risk

Promote Professionalism and Trust
Paragraph 25:
Provide Leadership to Make Sure People's Wellbeing Is Protected and to Improve Their Experiences of the Health and Care System
  25.1 identify priorities, manage time, staff and resources effectively and deal with risk to make sure that the quality of care or service you deliver is maintained and improved, putting the needs of those receiving care or services first

Now that we have looked at how to solve problems creatively, implement change and make improvements, the next steps are to use project-planning methods to deliver improvements.

Project management is the process of planning, organising, leading and controlling resources to achieve specific goals. Project management is a discipline, with specific qualifications for those who specialise in the field, and quite a lot of jargon too. This chapter will present a broad overview to allow student leaders to be able to plan and deliver small projects.

Nurses often make good project managers because of the transferrable skill of discipline required in nursing and the ability to understand the needs of a wide range of people.

Characteristics of Projects and Programmes

Projects deliver changes. Good project management, measurement and spread of changes are an intrinsic part of the NHS Change Model (Fig. 15.1). Projects often share the following characteristics:

- A series of tasks, many of which need to be carried out in sequence
- A timescale with a clear beginning and end
- A fixed project budget
- A specific deliverable
- The involvement of stakeholders—both those with a specific function and those within the organisations involved in delivery

A project is a single, focused endeavour. A programme, by contrast, is a collection of projects that form a connected package of work. The different projects complement each other to assist the programme in achieving its overall objectives. For example, there are NHS leadership programmes that include a series of projects that together deliver a comprehensive leadership initiative.

Elements of Project Working

Some of you may already have planned and delivered projects in previous jobs before you entered nursing. The process is just the same. The elements of good project work include:

- Creating a shared purpose
- Developing your project aims and objectives
- Establishing a project team
- Having a solid project plan
- Developing a robust communication plan
- Assessing and mitigating risks
- Having a plan for measuring and evaluating your project
- Considering how successful improvements can be spread and adopted by others

Project Seacole

For this chapter, we shall look back to the example we used in the chapter on managing change, which was a project about undergraduate health care students raising the career aspirations of secondary school pupils. The student leaders have named the project 'Project Seacole' after the pioneering Jamaican nurse Mary Seacole, who tended soldiers during the Crimean War.

PROJECT SPECIFICATION

You are part of a student-led movement leading a new joint NHS trust and university effort to promote careers in health care to pupils in years 8 and 9 (12–14 years of age) in 20 local secondary

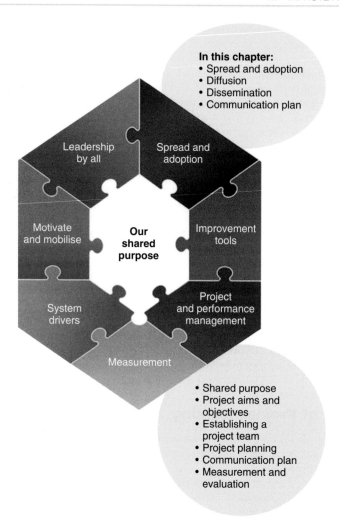

In this chapter:
- Spread and adoption
- Diffusion
- Dissemination
- Communication plan

- Shared purpose
- Project aims and objectives
- Establishing a project team
- Project planning
- Communication plan
- Measurement and evaluation

Fig. 15.1 Project planning as part of the NHS Change Model. (The central part of the figure is 'NHS Change Model'; the two circles and their text have been added by the author. The NHS Change Model is available at <https://www.england.nhs.uk/sustainableimprovement/change-model/>.)

schools in the hospital catchment area of Anytown. In 12 months' time you want career education programmes in 80% of those schools to promote careers in health care. This could be done in many ways, such as shadowing opportunities or empowering secondary school pupils themselves to come up with their own ideas to boost enrolment into access and degree courses.

ESTABLISHING A PROJECT TEAM

As we discussed in the chapter on teamwork, it is important to create a team with the right skills and abilities to give you the best chance of success. You will also remember from the chapter on change management that the project team's role will be that of a guiding coalition. For a project such as Project Seacole, where commitment is needed from three different sectors (further/higher education, NHS trust and secondary education), it is important to have team members with the expertise and ability to influence in each sector. As a student leader you would try not to choose 'representatives' but rather select people because of their interest and enthusiasm for the task. Additionally you would choose people who will bring diversity of thought as well as skills. Remember that you are aiming for a bit of constructive challenge!

PROJECT SPONSOR'S ROLE

You will also need a project sponsor. This is someone of sufficient seniority in the organisation to champion your project and provide strategic direction. The sponsor also provides support to discuss issues, celebrate achievement and provide access to the various departments that you might need help from, such as human resources (HR), finance, research, communications and IT teams. For this project it is the executive director of human resources, Shanaz Ali, who is acting as project sponsor. She is the one who has commissioned the project from the university, and the project team will report back to her. Project sponsors can be regular project members, attend for 'project milestones' (key achievements marking progress towards the final outcome) or just receive reports and offer advice.

PROJECT MANAGER'S ROLE

It is best to have one project manager who will take overall responsibility for the day-to-day management of the project.

The role usually involves:
- Planning what work needs to be done, including when and who is going to do it
- Assessing and managing risks
- Making sure the work is done to the right standard
- Motivating team members
- Coordinating the work to be done by everyone
- Ensuring that the project is running on time and to budget
- Dealing with changes to the project as and when necessary
- Ensuring that the project delivers the expected outcomes and benefits

Based on the Association for Project Management, www.apm.org.uk.

■ Time Out

Imagine that you are one of the students leading this project. Your university has been commissioned to undertake the project by the local NHS Foundation Trust (FT). You and your fellow students are about to begin by scoping out the project. Look back at the chapter 13 on leading change and what it said about creating a shared purpose—part of the NHS Change Model (Fig. 15.2).

How would you go about creating that shared purpose?

CREATING A SHARED PURPOSE

There are three steps to creating a shared purpose:
1. Listening and communicating with stakeholders
2. Looking for commonalities
3. Designing together

So perhaps you agree as a team to identify your stakeholders. We did this in the leading change chapter (Chapter 13) and discovered that most of the stakeholders are in the three sectors

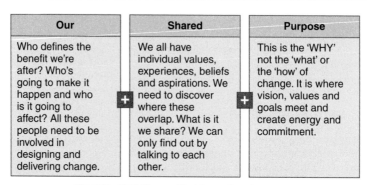

Our		Shared		Purpose
Who defines the benefit we're after? Who's going to make it happen and who is it going to affect? All these people need to be involved in designing and delivering change.	+	We all have individual values, experiences, beliefs and aspirations. We need to discover where these overlap. What is it we share? We can only find out by talking to each other.	+	This is the 'WHY' not the 'what' or the 'how' of change. It is where vision, values and goals meet and create energy and commitment.

Fig. 15.2 NHS Change Model: our shared purpose.

of further/higher education, NHS trust and secondary education. You tell them about the idea and then listen to how the project proposal fits with their values, aspirations, experiences and beliefs.

You invite them to tell you how this project will benefit them—or not—and ask what difficulties there may be and how they might be overcome. You concentrate on the 'why' of the project, but you also listen to their advice on the 'what' and the 'how'.

Let us imagine that Shanaz Ali tells you that the NHS Trust HR department already has a couple of links with local schools because they have been involved in planning careers events with high schools in the past. You get an appointment to meet a teacher, Mr Leonardi, responsible for participation and engagement at a local high school, part of a wider school academy chain in a disadvantaged area.

Mr Leonardi starts to tell you how the project proposal fits with the wider values of the school around aspiration. He tells you that the regulator, Office for Standards in Education (OFSTED) is interested in schools improving their attendance and attainment levels, and that you need to link the project to these two target areas in particular. In addition, OFSTED is interested in the curriculum extending beyond the academic, technical or vocational, enabling learners to develop and discover their interests and talents.

His advice is that schools are under a lot of pressure and that they need to plan events at least 6 weeks in advance. He tells you that careers events should be more geared towards active learning rather than passive information giving, that is, more activities-based. Where possible, he says that activities should build the pupils' soft skills around things like communication, teamwork, problem solving and leadership. He ponders whether the pupils themselves can help shape the project. Finally, he introduces you to the cluster lead for all the local schools in Anytown so you can raise and discuss the project at their next meeting. They confirm Mr Leonardi's advice, offer support, but they query what will happen after the project ends: what are the plans for sustainability and spread?

Anytown NHS Foundation Trust HR and nursing directorate managers tell you that they are concerned about the dropout rate of student nurses and wonder whether this is to do with the way that careers in health care are perceived. They are also very keen to promote certain specialist nursing and allied health professional disciplines such as therapeutic radiography and learning disability nursing, where they have difficulty recruiting. Lastly, they want to create social value (Box 15.1) by encouraging more people from low-income communities in Anytown to gain employment in their trust.

The dean at Anytown University, where you study, tells you that the university has been struggling to compete against nearby Norbrook and DeClancy universities for student enrolments. Like

> **BOX 15.1 ■ Understanding Social Value and the Role of Anchor Organisations**
>
> What came out in these discussions is the desire of these three large public service institutions—further/higher education, NHS trust and secondary education—to see themselves as agents of change to support the wider wellbeing of the community.
>
> 'Social value describes the social benefits achieved from public services and considers more than just the financial transaction. It includes wellbeing, health, inclusion and employment.'
> NHS Confederation (2012).
>
> This means moving away from seeing people and communities as just having needs, but instead seeing their role as identifying the strengths and assets within communities, investing in their education and helping them to develop their skills. Social value is now enshrined in legislation through the Public Services (Social Value) Act 2012, meaning that the public sector must ensure that the money it spends on services creates the greatest economic, social and environmental value for local communities.
>
> Schools, the NHS and universities are often termed 'anchor institutions' because they are unlikely to relocate because of their relationships with the local population. Through their size and scale they can make a positive difference to the lives of local communities by, for example:
> - widening access to quality work—like in Project Seacole;
> - purchasing services and equipment locally and so putting money into the local economy;
> - working to reduce their environmental impact;
> - using their buildings as spaces for the local community to use; and
> - working in partnership with other anchor organisations to learn from each other to spread good ideas and build civic responsibility.
>
> _____
>
> Based on Reed et al. (2019).

the NHS trust, she also wants to create social value and wants to increase the diversity of the students who enrol.

All the stakeholders mention that they want to increase the profile of their organisations and market themselves in as positive a way as possible. Each of their organisations have had negative stories in the press in the last 12 months.

■ Time Out

Make a few notes on what you have learnt from these discussions. How has what you have heard shaped the initial understanding of what you were setting out to do?

You may have noted:
- A desire to move away from careers advice to interactive learning
- A need to help schools do well in OFSTED inspections
- The requirement for schools to have advance notice of activities
- A desire to create a more positive profile of all three sectors by marketing the project well
- A desire to offer local careers in low-income communities
- A concern about how nursing roles are perceived
- Shortages in certain specialties, requiring promotion in schools

You report this back to the project team and project sponsor.

Project Aims and SMART Objectives

The next step is to draft the aims and objectives of the project.

Aims are statements of intent, usually written in broad terms. They set out what you hope to achieve at the end of the project. Objectives, on the other hand, should be specific statements that define measurable outcomes, for example, what steps will be taken to achieve the desired outcome (see Table 15.1).

Although some teams may use these interchangeably, there is a distinct difference between project objectives and project goals. In general, project goals are higher level than project objectives. Project goals should outline what happens once your project is successful, and how your project aligns with overall business objectives.

■ **Time Out**

Draft an aims statement for Project Seacole by completing the sentence:
  Our aim is to...

This might be something like...

PROJECT SEACOLE: AIM

'Our aim is to increase the aspiration of young people aged 12–14 years attending Anytown secondary schools to enter a career in health care locally by enrolling in further and higher education at Anytown College and University.'

The red herrings here are:
■ You might have included how you would go about it, such as improving careers advice or establishing a shadowing project.
■ You may have mentioned the structure—the creation of a student-led project.

Sometimes there is a temptation to add lots of detail to aims statements; for example, we could add in more about students coming from low-income communities or about increasing diversity of enrolments. But then the aim might become complex and difficult to remember. Also, some of this detail belongs in the objectives.

■ **Time Out**

Try drafting three or four SMART objectives for Project Seacole.

TABLE 15.1 ■ SMART Objectives

S	Specific. State what you will do and use action words.
M	Measurable. Make sure your project objectives are clearly measurable things—like percentage change or a specific number of assets.
A	Achievable. Project objectives should be stretching but attainable. Without achievable project goals, your project may suffer from scope creep, delays or overwork.
R	Relevant. Objectives should be relevant to the outcomes you have in mind for the project. Some organisations use 'realistic' for 'R', and this links to the 'A' above of 'achievable'.
T	Timebound. Your project objectives should take into account how long your project timeline is. State when you will get it done and be specific.

Here is my first attempt:

PROJECT SEACOLE: OBJECTIVES

1. Work with volunteer pupils and teachers to create an interactive way for pupils in Anytown schools to learn about health care careers.
2. Engage and deliver interactive careers events, that will help develop pupils' soft skills, in at least 80% of Anytown high schools, including addressing any misconceptions about how health care careers are perceived by pupils.
3. Develop an ongoing student leadership programme within the university faculty for subsequent cohorts of health care undergraduates to continue to raise aspirations in Anytown pupils to have a career in health care.
4. Promote Project Seacole in the local press and on social media to raise the profile of this campaign to increase the aspiration of local pupils, especially from low-income and minority backgrounds, and create a positive image of participating organisations.

■ Time Out

Critique these draft objectives.
- Are they SMART?
- Are they clear?
- What is good about them?

The main details that they are missing is that they are not always specific, measurable and timebound enough. So, for example:

'By the end of month 1, work with a group of up to five volunteer year 8 and 9 Anytown pupils, supported by a teacher, to develop and successfully test an interactive way for pupils in Anytown schools to learn about health care careers.'

The second is that there may be two objectives rolled into one, which makes it complex and confusing. They may be better separated out. For example:

'(By when?) Engage and deliver interactive (how long?) careers events, which will help develop pupils' soft skills (which?), in at least 80% of Anytown secondary schools.'

'During the career events, include identifying and addressing any misconceptions about how health care careers (particularly nursing?) are perceived by pupils.'

Also, we need to check that the objectives are achievable. This is the first time that this initiative has been tried. Do you think the project team will have managed to engage 16 of the 20 schools within 12 months? That is quite a lot for volunteer undergraduates to take on. It may be that you want to target fewer schools (say eight) with a diverse pupil population in low-income communities, where the schools are just as keen as you are to work towards raising aspiration.

What is positive about these draft objectives is that the project team has listened to their stakeholders and tried to include points that they mentioned, such as interactive learning, improving pupils' soft skills and having a plan to sustain the project as a more permanent activity. This will also give future undergraduates a leadership development opportunity.

Project Planning

A project plan (sometimes referred to as a project initiation document, or PID) provides a single source of reference about the project so that everyone involved can easily understand what the project is about. It forms the foundation for a project. It spells out the Rudyard Kipling 5Ws and an H:

- What will be done—aims and objectives
- Why it is needed—link to 'our shared purpose' and the 'system drivers' discussed in the chapter on change
- Who is involved—what they do, specifying key roles, responsibilities and accountabilities
- Where and when—quite often this is put into a chart, listing and allocating all the tasks in order (we will cover this shortly)
- How it will be achieved—resources available, risks, dependencies between one action and another

Three things must always be balanced within a project: the time, quality and cost (or resources) available (Fig. 15.3). Make sure the project team has discussed this before drafting the project plan. More complex and high-quality initiatives, for example, take more time and cost more money. If you only have a short time, you may need more resources to complete projects quickly. Some of the main things to discuss here are the capacity of the undergraduate students involved—who still have study and clinical practice commitments—and the capacity of the schools to accommodate the project.

The NHS Trust in our fictional project has offered a small project budget to the university to cover academic staff time, student volunteer expenses and an allowance to pay the student project manager.

Let us now work through the development of a draft project plan for Project Seacole.

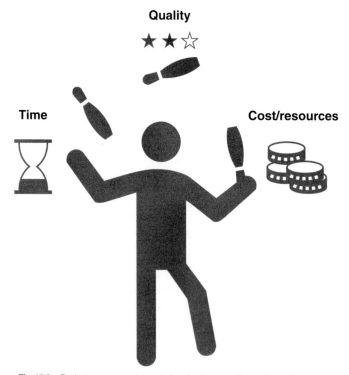

Fig. 15.3 Project managers have to juggle time, quality and cost/resources.

Project Seacole—Draft Project Plan Version 1.0 (Date)

(Version control is important. Always add a version number and date it, so you can make sure everyone is reading the most up-to-date version. Once it is agreed, replace version number with 'FINAL'.)

Aims and Objectives

We have already discussed how to set aims and SMART objectives, and they would be slotted in here.

Background to the Project

Here you would summarise 'our shared purpose': why the project came to be initiated by the NHS Trust, how the NHS Trust approached the university and a summary of discussions with the schools. Link in the system drivers that we discussed in the chapter on change. These may well be around improvements in attainment in education, improving the life chances of low-income and minority communities, workforce development in the NHS Trust, the development of student leadership skills and future student recruitment at the university.

Scope of Project

Scope can be defined in several ways—but here you need to explain how far the project goes and what it excludes. State the geography of the project—you might even name the schools involved if they have confirmed their interest. Spell out both what is 'in scope' and 'out of scope'. State the age groups of the pupils who will be engaged, and be clear about which careers are included and excluded—for example, are social care careers included or not? Will you discuss all health care careers (too big!) or focus on the ones of interest to pupils, where there are shortages, or both?

Benefits

State clearly who will benefit and how. This might include things like tackling inequalities; improving partnership working between the schools, university and the NHS Trust; the development of student leadership skills and how the project may benefit NHS Trust workforce planning in the longer term.

Expected Deliverables

What will you have achieved by the end of 12 months? Be careful what you promise, as you will be expected to deliver it! So, you might for example just say that you will write a project report at the end of 12 months setting out how the project went and what was achieved, plus how you will maintain the initiative if it proves successful.

Timescale

State when the project will start and end and if there are any milestones—a point in the project that indicates that an important phase of the work has been completed. You might, for example, say that getting together a group of pupils to help you develop and testing an interactive way for pupils in the first Anytown school to learn about health care careers (using a PDSA cycle of course!) is a milestone.

Analysis of Risk

A formal risk assessment is completed and added here, listing risks and how they will be mitigated. We shall cover this shortly.

Assumptions

What has been assumed to be in place? The support of key NHS, college, university and school staff? That pupils will be interested and engaged? That the project will be newsworthy? Make this clear.

Resources/Budget

Set out a simple project budget by thinking through how the project would be delivered and what resources are needed to do it. Some commissioners allow a contingency budget and some do not. If they do not, then it is best to be as realistic as possible with costs, getting actual quotes for larger projects, rather than guessing. Do not spend the money in other ways without

Continued

getting permission from the person that commissioned you. Also, be clear how any underspent money is treated—it may be returned to the commissioner or kept.

Item (Inclusive of VAT and Employer Costs)	Cost
20 hours of university staff time @£50/h	£1,000
40 days of student project manager time @£100/day	£4,000
Volunteer travel across Anytown @45p/mile	£200
Refreshments at eight events (pupils bring own packed lunch)	£500
Subtotal	£5,700
University overheads at 10%: stationary, telephone, computing, heating, light	£570
Total	**£6270**

You might also want to list 'in kind' resources—in this case you estimate that five students will each volunteer 30 hours of their time, in total, over a year, giving 150 hours of volunteer time.

Method/Process

In most projects there will be a clear method that can be stated. This project's method, however, is more emergent, because the pupils themselves will be codesigning the interactive career events with you and the NHS Trust, such as shadowing or asking pupils to 'hack' (come up with creative solutions to) real-life NHS problems. It all adds to the pupils' soft skills development and the volunteer students' learning.

Accountability

You might want to set out the accountability in a table or diagram, or just list the roles. Here is a simple example:
- Project sponsor (accountable for delivery)
  - Shanaz Ali, executive director of human resources, Anytown NHS FT
- Project manager (responsible for delivery)
  - Patrick McConnell, student nurse, learning disabilities, Anytown University
- Project team
  - Gino Leonardi, assistant director, Participation and Engagement, Lowville Academy (liaison lead for schools and Anytown College)
  - Sasha Smith, student therapeutic radiographer, Anytown University
  - Helen Maxwell, human resources manager, Anytown University
  - John Pope, Head of Participation, Anytown Local Education Authority
  - Julia Davies, Deputy Director of Nursing, Anytown NHS FT
  - Gina Murray, Senior Communications Officer, Anytown University
- Volunteer team (Sasha Smith links the project team and the volunteer team)
  - Sasha Smith, student therapeutic radiographer, Anytown University (Lead)
  - Melanie Oldroyd, student dietician, Anytown University
  - Chris Fox, student midwife, Anytown University
  - Martin Buchan, student nurse, mental health, Anytown University
  - Aleksandra Kowalska, student occupational therapist, Anytown University
- Academic adviser
  - Duncan Cameron, Senior Lecturer, Child Health, Anytown University

Data and Measures

State what data will be produced and how you will measure success. You might for example:
- Report on the number of schools involved and the number of pupils engaged.
- Get feedback from schools on the process—what worked well and what could be improved.

- Design an evaluation process for pupils to complete reporting on aspiration and how the events helped them to build their soft skills like confidence and communication.
- Design an evaluation for student volunteers measuring change-management skills.
- Get parental permission to film activities and take photographs or interview pupils on camera.

Dependencies (Links Between One Action and Another)

Examples might include coordinating the project between the university and the school annual timetables to consider term dates, assessment dates and key events such as OFSTED inspections.

How the Work Is Going to Be Sustained and Spread

- Spread = actively influencing others to put a change/innovation into their practice
- Adoption = putting a change/improvement into your practice
- Diffusion = occurs naturally
- Dissemination = organised, often 'top down'

One of the project objectives is 'to develop an ongoing student leadership programme within the university faculty for subsequent cohorts of health care undergraduates, to continue to raise aspirations in Anytown pupils to have a career in health care'. You are indicating therefore that this initiative, if it is popular in raising aspiration, could become a permanent initiative between the university, college, local schools and the NHS Trust. You will want to elaborate on this, maybe linking it to leadership development in the undergraduate curriculum as an option for third-year students. You could add that this would create an ongoing win/win relationship between the university, college, NHS trust and the schools.

You might also want to share the idea in a range of ways to facilitate spread and adoption to other universities and NHS trusts. You could for example:

- enter a high-profile national competition;
- publish a project report in a relevant peer-reviewed journal;
- share it through academic networks such as via the Council of Deans of Health;
- share it as an example of good practice through national networks such as the NHS Ambassadors scheme, which encourages people working and/or studying in health care to volunteer 1 hour per year to speak in schools about their roles or participate in careers events and activities; and
- work with Lowville Academy, which is part of an academy chain (a group of schools working together under a shared management structure) to help spread the improvement to other member schools in the academy chain.

GANNT CHARTS: DEPENDENCIES, LEAD AND LAG TIMES

A Gannt chart (named after the inventor Henry Gannt) is a commonly used visual way to spell out the detail of project tasks: how long they will take, in what order and who is responsible.

The ordering of tasks is crucial because some tasks cannot be started before other tasks are complete. For example, you cannot set a date for a careers event before you have recruited the schools. These are called 'dependencies' because one task depends on the other.

Then, the schools tell you that they need 6-weeks' notice for events so they can ensure the teachers are available to supervise, parental consent is gained for videography and the school minibus is booked to take pupils off site. So, the 'lead time' between planning and delivering an event needs to be at least 6 weeks. In addition, it takes an average 3 months for ethical approval to be gained from the university ethics committee to obtain data from 12- to 14-year-olds. For the project manager this means starting tasks 3 months before the project formally begins.

A 'lag time' is the time needed between finishing one task and starting another. So for example some lag time is needed between finishing all eight career events and producing a draft evaluation report.

A simple way for beginners to draft Gannt charts is to invite the project team to help you to brainstorm all the tasks to be done and write each task on small Post-It notes. Then stick the Post-Its to a project timeline drawn on a large flip chart and move them around until they are in the order that they need to be done. Then consider the dependencies, lead and lag times and move them again. Lastly allocate names to tasks. In some projects, the resources needed for each task are also added to the Gannt chart, such as the number of days of key people, or equipment, or portion of the budget.

Template Gannt charts can be downloaded from the internet or can be easily constructed using software such as Excel.

In Fig. 15.4 you can see a black and white version of the project manager's traffic light coloured Gannt chart, dated 6 July, 8 weeks before the project starts but before schools break up for the summer. Duncan, the senior lecturer in child health, has just applied for ethical approval, but approval may not come through before testing out the evaluation with pupils at Lowville Academy. Patrick, the project manager, shows this task as running late (shown as 'R' for red). Sasha is first to volunteer for the project and has been given the role of leading the volunteer team undertaking careers events with schools. She has managed to recruit two schools other than Lowville Academy, who are keen to pilot the project. She has draft dates for their career events (shown as 'Y' for yellow to indicate 'started') but has not recruited the other five—shown as 'B' for blue (not started). Patrick indicates two milestones (via black filled cells): designing and testing the evaluation method with Lowville Academy and presenting the final evaluation. Finally, Patrick has scheduled in project team meetings every 2 months throughout the academic year and circulated them to the project team and project sponsor so they can put them in their diaries well in advance. He has started drafting the agenda and some key documents for the first meeting, such as the risk register, as well as this Gannt chart.

RISK ASSESSMENT AND RISK REGISTERS

A routine part of project management is the assessment, management and mitigation of risk. This is where the project manager would encourage the project team to think about all possible risks associated with the project (Tips Box 15.1).

Risk assessment and planning occur in a series of logical steps, much as you would do in care planning—that is:

1. Identify the risks.
2. Assess the risks.
3. Control the risks.
4. Record your findings in a plan.
5. Review your plan.

Risks can be broken down to include:

- Strategic—is this the right direction that the organisation should be going in?
- Operational—what could go wrong with operational implementation? This includes:
  - Health and safety—and as part of assessing operational risk, looking specifically at the health and safety aspects. The Health and Safety Executive has a range of tools and support focusing on health and safety risks (see Resources section)
  - Data
  - Technology: hardware, software, network
  - Project management: estimates, communication, resources
  - Organisational support: executive support, team support and user or client support

Version 1.0 06/07/20

Task	No	Actions	Who	2020 J	J	A	S	O	N	D	2021 J	F	M	A	M	J	J	A	S	O
Project approval	1	Circulate project outline	SA	G																
	2	Meeting to approve	SA	G																
	3	Recruit project manager	SA	G																
Project structure	4	Seek ethical approval	DC	R																
	5	Recruit project team	PM	G																
	6	Recruit student volunteer team	PM	G																
	7	Recruit schools	SS	Y																
Delivery	8	Project team meetings	PM				Y		B		B		B		B		B		B	B
	9	Design/test evaluation methods with school 1	SS				■													
	10	Careers events with schools 2-3	CC					Y	Y											
	11	Careers events with schools 4-5	SS							B	B									
	12	Careers events with schools 6-8	SS											B	B					
Evaluation	13	Thematic analysis of videos	DC														B	B		
	13	Analysis of Google Forms data	PM																B	
	14	Draft evaluation report	PM																B	
	15	Final evaluation presented to key stakeholders	PM																	■
	16	Agree dissemination	SA																	B

Key

G	Completed	
Y	In progress	
B	Not started	
R	Overdue – state reasons	
■	Milestone	

SA	Shanaz Ali	Project Sponsor
PM	Patrick McConnell	Project manager
SS	Sasha Smith	Lead, volunteer team
DC	Duncan Cameron	Senior lecturer, child health

Fig. 15.4 High-level project Gantt chart for Project Seacole.

The size of the risk is defined by the equation:

$$\text{Risk} = \text{probability} \times \text{impact}$$

Meaning how likely it is that the risk occurs and how much impact it will have.

For example, the probability that an aeroplane will crash into your building whilst you are undertaking your career activities is negligible, but the impact would be massive, so if you score probability as 0 out of 10 and impact as 10 out of 10. The overall risk score would still be zero.

Compare this to the probability that, when handling simulation goggles, a 12-year-old boy might decide to throw them to a friend and they break. You might score the probability of this (helped by the teaching staff) as 6 out of 10 and the impact (based on the cost of replacing them, the fallout from disciplining the boy and the effect on the reputation of the project) as 6 out of 10 too, giving a score of 36.

TIPS BOX 15.1

- Assess risks as a team, bringing in a subject expert if necessary.
- Rather than brainstorming, address risks systematically, either by mentally walking through the project tasks and considering what could go wrong, or thinking about each of strategic risks and operational risks in turn.
- Think about what risks need reporting to others, particularly more senior people like your project sponsor—do not be afraid to ask for advice and guidance.
- At organisational level, risk registers are essential and are usually standing items at board meetings, so risks are reviewed at whatever frequency the board decides. This is good practice for small projects to copy, so project managers usually review risks at an appropriate frequency at project team meetings.

The Project Seacole team has decided to start working with eight high schools, targeted in low-income communities. The eight schools vary in terms of their academic attainment and discipline. Having tested ideas with pupils from Lowville Academy, activities will involve visiting a simulation suite, inviting pupils to 'hack' real-life problems and arranging for pupils to shadow registered health care professions in low-risk activities. The risk register starts with risks, as shown in Table 15.2.

To help readers to quickly identify the problem areas, sometimes the residual risk is colour coded using what is called a RAG rating: a traffic light system to code the risk as red, amber or green, but remember that many people print documents in black and white, so add a letter (H = high, M = medium or L = low) or a number. Also add a key to the names and add their roles if necessary.

■ **Time Out**

Try adding some further risks to the risk register given in Table 15.2.

Communication Planning

The purpose of a communications plan is to get the right message to the right people, in the right way. It sounds simple, but many people fail to plan their communications properly. This can lead to misunderstandings, frustration and missed opportunities. Communication planning is a stepwise process:

> *Step 1*—Agree with the team what the overall communication objectives are. Describe what you want to achieve, when and why. Record your overall objectives in your communications plan (Table 15.3).

TABLE 15.2 ▦ **Example Risk Register, Project Seacole**

Date Added	Review Date	Lead	Description	Probability 0–10	Impact 0–10	Risk Score	Action/ Contingency Planning	Residual Risk
Strategic Risk								
07/04/21	30/04/21	SA	Project fails to attract funding	4	9	36	Link project to system drivers	10
07/04/21	30/04/21	GM	Project attracts criticism from press as 'fluffy', not spending money on health care	2	7	14	Market project internally and externally as an example of creating social value	4
Operational Risk								
15/03/21	30/04/21	PM	Fail to recruit a target of eight schools	4	8	32	Link to attainment Engage cluster lead Make becoming part of the project a desirable, competitive process	25
22/04/21	18/05/21	PM	Evaluation forms ignored by pupils	5	8	40	Design evaluation as interactive game	9
22/04/21	18/05/21	PM	Career events lack pupil discipline, leading to damage/ fights	5	8	40	Two teaching staff at every event and pupil supervision throughout event	30

TABLE 15.3 ▦ **Example of Communication Objectives**

Communications Plan for Project Seacole

Overall Communication Objectives

For example:
1. *Regularly communicate and reinforce the aim of Project Seacole, which is to create interactive careers events for years 7 and 8 in eight Anytown schools in low-income and minority communities, to raise aspiration in health care careers whilst developing pupils' soft skills and undergraduate students' leadership skills.*
2. *Develop two-way communication systems to listen to and learn from our stakeholders, both about the improvement process and about any misconceptions about health care roles.*
3. *Promote Project Seacole in local press and social media to raise the profile of this campaign and the organisations partnering to deliver it (schools, Anytown NHS Foundation Trust and Anytown University).*

TABLE 15.4 ■ **Example of a Communication Plan for Secondary Schools**

Audience	Communication Objective	Message	Channel	Timing
Anytown secondary schools	Keep schools updated on plans, progress and outcomes	Whether project is on track or not Dates, times and venues of specific events Key achievements	Email update with one-page 'flash' report Invite feedback Head teacher cluster meetings	Monthly Quarterly

Step 2—Identify who your 'audiences' are. These are the key stakeholder groups who you want to influence. In the case of Project Seacole they are:
■ Anytown secondary schools
■ Pupils and parents in those schools
■ Anytown College and Anytown University
■ Anytown NHS Foundation Trust
■ Local education authority
■ Press and social media

Step 3—Clarify your communication objectives for each audience. To do this, think about what they need and want to know.

Step 4—List all the communication channels that you can think of that already exist for each of your audiences first. For the schools for example this may include:
■ Email
■ Cluster newsletter to schools
■ Website
■ Notice boards
■ Head teacher briefings from the local education authority
■ Posters
■ Existing regular school meetings
■ Intranet articles
■ School assemblies
■ Parents' evenings or newsletters

It is best to use existing channels if possible because they are familiar; however, you may need to set up new communication channels.

Step 5—For each audience, think through the actual message that they need and want to know:
■ When do we need to communicate this?
■ What is the best communication channel to use?

An example of a communication plan for the eight schools involved in the project has been shown in Table 15.4.

Step 6—Get feedback from your stakeholders on how your communications have been received. Ask them if they understood them, whether you are over- or under-communicating, or about right.

Evaluating Improvement Projects

An evaluation is defined as 'the systematic assessment of the implementation and impact of a project, programme or initiative' (NHS Institute for Innovation and Improvement 2007). The method that you plan to use for evaluating your project should be planned from the start (Tips Box 15.2).

The purpose of doing an evaluation is to:
- Check that you are doing things right.
- Check that you are doing the right things.

Think about who your project evaluation might be for. Is it for:
- Yourself—to give you some feedback
- Leaders in your organisation
- People funding your project
- Partner organisations
- The public, patient groups and the local community

▪ Time Out

Jot down who the target audience or audiences might be for Project Seacole. If there is more than one audience, try to prioritise which is the most important.

There could be multiple audiences for this project, such as the university, the NHS Trust, the local education authority and the schools involved. Consider whether parents and parent governors might be interested too.

The most important audience for any evaluation, however, is generally the one who has commissioned and/or funded the improvement project.

There are many benefits to evaluation, such as:
- Highlight the impact, both intended and unintended.
- Know if the change resulted in improvement or not.
- Know if you set the right goals.
- Know if work practices have changed.
- Know how long improvements take.
- Know if the improvements have been caused by the changes.
- Demonstrate whether the resources put in are value for money.
- Demonstrate if changes are sustainable.

Even small changes can be evaluated to bring attention to what you have done. Evaluations can be small and simple or large and complex. They need not be expensive, especially if you use routinely collected data. Small evaluations can be brought together to show a bigger picture of improvement.

Remember to connect the evaluation of your improvement project to the system drivers that we have been talking about previously.

TIPS BOX 15.2

Develop an Evaluation Plan
1. Develop an outline and explore it with stakeholders.
2. Agree who will undertake the evaluation.
3. Plan when reports will be presented.

DISCOVERING YOUR EVALUATION QUESTIONS

The first step is to draft a plan for discussion with your project team and other stakeholders. In the case of Project Seacole, the schools need to be involved so the teaching staff can help you shape it and are happy with the young people's involvement (Tips Box 15.3).

TIPS BOX 15.3

Ask Yourself
- What question do you want the evaluation to answer?
- What design are you using for your evaluation?
- What data are you collecting, and how will you collect and analyse it?
- What is your timeline, and what are the key stages?
- How will the results be disseminated?

■ **Time Out**

Using Project Seacole as an example, jot down your answers to the questions above.

We need to refer to the aims and objectives of the project:
Will
   ■ delivering interactive careers events,
   ■ addressing misconceptions about health care careers, and
   ■ developing a partnership to do this year on year
increase the aspiration of young people aged 12 to 14 years to become health care profession-als and develop their soft skills to help them achieve it?
Will
   ■ increasing the aspiration of young people aged 12 to 14 years to become health care professionals,
   ■ developing this project as an ongoing student leadership programme within the university faculty, and
   ■ promoting Project Seacole in local press and social media
increase enrolments in health care courses at Anytown College and University, especially from pupils from low-income and minority backgrounds? And subsequently increase employment in health care careers at the local trust?

After 12 months we can answer the first question, but not the second, because it will take several years before any changes show up. So, we want to evaluate pupil aspiration and whether/how much they can develop their soft skills. We also want to evaluate the process to see what happened and what approaches were successful. That learning can then be taken forward into designing subsequent years' activities.

LOGIC MODELS

One of the things that might help here is to understand what is called a logic model (Fig. 15.5). This shows how the inputs can result in outcomes and how you measure change at each stage of the improvement journey.

The logic model starts with inputs, like your time and materials, which turn into activities that you can measure, like learning events, planning meetings and marketing that you might do.

From there you can measure outputs, such as the number of careers events that you have had and the number of pupils who attended. Next come short-term outcomes that you might expect, such as potential improvements in pupils' soft skills, like the confidence they gain from shadow-ing a health professional and being able to ask them questions.

Moving on from this are medium-term outcomes, such as pupils' career aspirations. After several years of running the programme together, the college, university and the NHS trust may start to see more local people enrolling on their health care courses and getting jobs.

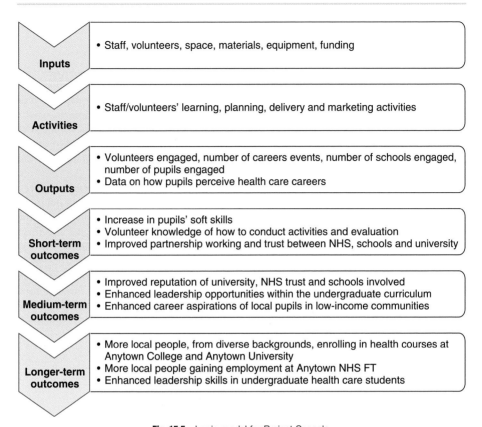

Fig. 15.5 Logic model for Project Seacole.

DECIDING WHO WILL DO THE PROJECT EVALUATION

At the start of a project, you need to think about whether it is best for the evaluation to be done by:

- The project team
- An external team
- An external team alongside your team

Things to consider here are:

- Cost if external and staff time if internal—as a guide, evaluation should cost no more than 5% to 15% of the total cost of the project
- How complex the evaluation is and if your team has the expertise
- Whether an internal team can be objective
- Whether an external team might understand the subject and the culture you are working in
- Whether you might need fresh eyes on a subject
- Whether the project offers staff development opportunities

For Project Seacole, there is no money allocated for an external evaluation, and the method needs to be thought through so that it is valid, reliable and acceptable to schools and doable by student volunteers. The student-led team has access to an academic, Duncan Cameron, who is a senior lecturer in child health, to help them design questionnaires and plan how to conduct the video interviews between pupils. The university has an in-house technical team to help with video interviews. Also, this project is a major development opportunity for the volunteer students and is a key reason why most of them have come forward.

DESIGNING YOUR EVALUATION: QUALITATIVE AND QUANTITATIVE

Evaluation could be qualitative, quantitative or both. Qualitative approaches to evaluation seek to explore a situation and gain understanding of underlying reasons, motivations and opinions.

Some common methods of undertaking qualitative data collection include focus groups or group discussions, individual interviews and observations. The questions that are asked can be structured (you decide in advance what to ask and stick to it), semistructured (you may go on to ask supplementary questions based on replies) or unstructured.

In this picture (Fig. 15.6) you see a university academic interviewing a family who has been involved in one of my asthma-improvement projects. The academic has a number of questions to ask, but she has set the interviews up to be more fun. She asks the children to do the interview in the character of their favourite superhero. She gives them her iPad and asks them to be in charge of the recording of the interview. She also gives them permission to interview her too!

If you plan to use qualitative approaches it may be wise to either commission or seek advice from a local academic organisation to help you decide the best way to do it. You may also need their guidance on whether to seek the permission of an ethics committee, especially if you are interviewing children.

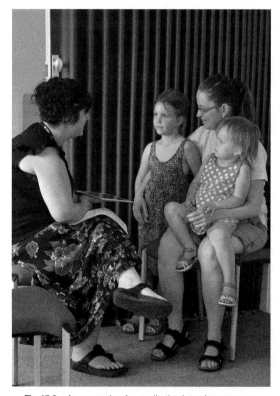

Fig. 15.6 An example of a qualitative interview process.

We know from discussing the risk assessment for Project Seacole with the teachers that pupils may not like completing evaluation forms, so data collection for this project needs to be more participative, and this part of the project is more likely to be qualitative. However, teachers, health care students and health professionals involved in Project Seacole are more comfortable with forms and being asked for written feedback, and ratings of skills and aspirations using something like Likert scales, which can be collated as quantitative data.

DATA COLLECTION AND ANALYSIS

Bearing in mind that you also want to improve soft skills such as communication, confidence and leadership, you agree with the pupils that they can interview each other on camera with a simple smart phone, microphone and tripod borrowed from the university technical team. Their answers to questions on their career perceptions and intentions would be thematically analysed.

You also decide to get written feedback from the two teachers from each school involved in supervising each careers event on how well they think the process works and any changes in soft skills that they observe in their pupils.

The project manager aggregates the data from the feedback questionnaires using Google Forms. He decides to form a subgroup to help plan and analyse the data from the video interviews, involving the academic Duncan, who as a senior lecturer in child health has expertise in working with young people.

The university technical team and communication lead Gina Murray plan to work together to edit the pupils' video interviews into a short report, including commentary from the project sponsor Shanaz Ali and Gino Leonardi, on behalf of the schools.

EVALUATION TIMELINE AND STAGES

A visual timeline is helpful, such as the one shown in Fig. 15.7. The 12-month project coincides with the academic year at both university and secondary school to enable data collection during term time and report writing over the summer break.

DISSEMINATING THE EVALUATION OF THE IMPROVEMENT

You will need to plan how you will disseminate your final report.
Consider:
- Who is the main audience for the evaluation?
- Have you asked them what they want to see and in what format?
- How do you plan to feed back the findings to them?
- Are there learning points from the evaluation to be shared more widely?

For Project Seacole, the project manager (Patrick) meets with the project sponsor (Shanaz), and they agree on a joint presentation in mid-October to senior managers in the trust, the university and the schools first of all. That meeting will then decide on wider dissemination routes.

FORMATIVE AND SUMMATIVE EVALUATION

It is also useful to distinguish between formative evaluation and summative evaluation. Formative evaluation is an ongoing look at how an improvement project is going and suggests ways that it could be improved. A summative evaluation gathers data to make a judgement about the success of an improvement project and whether it met its goals.

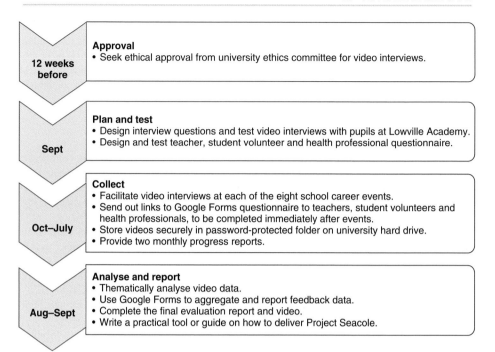

Fig. 15.7 Visual evaluation timeline.

A helpful way to think about the difference is that when a cook tastes a soup, that is a formative evaluation—they will be evaluating the process and why the soup tastes the way it does. When the guest tastes the soup, that is a summative evaluation—they will be evaluating the outcome only (NHS Institute for Innovation and Improvement 2007).

It is up to you to decide whether your evaluation is summative or formative, or whether you want to include both.

Reporting

FLASH REPORTS

Flash reports are one or two-page reports that provide a brief overview of activity over a set period (Fig. 15.8). Because they are short and visual, they are more likely to be read.

These can be set up as a template with the headings agreed with the project sponsor to make sure they get the information they want. A RAG rating of red, amber and green is helpful so people can clearly see if progress is on track at a glance.

FINAL REPORTS

Final reports are more formal (Fig. 15.9).

Template Flash Report

Period/Date/Month:

Resource	Days engaged on project for this period
Project sponsor:	1
Project manager:	1
Project team:	1

Goal

Target, the baseline and progress to date

Actions completed in the last month/quarter
- ✓ Action
- ✓ Action
- ✓ Action
- ✓ Action

What went well and why

What didn't go so well, why, what you've learnt from this and what you might do about it.

Unintended consequences, both positive and negative.

Key actions in the next week/month
- ✓ Action
- ✓ Action
- ✓ Action
- ✓ Action

Issues to be noted by sponsor:
- ✓ Issue

Is the work on track against the project plan and overall aims of the project?

(Use RED/AMBER/GREEN and also supply comments supporting your RAG rating)

Red Amber Green– (insert reasons for your rating here)

Supporting documentation and plans: (These can be embedded as icons)

Fig. 15.8   This is an example of a flash report template.

Template Final Report

1. Executive summary

2. Intorduction and background to the evaluation

3. Outline of any relevant literature

4. Aims and objectives of the evaluation
   The questions you wanted to answer

5. Evaluation method
   Qualitative/quantitative, internal/external, summative, formative

6. Findings, listed and presented as simply as possible

7. Discussion of the findings

8. Implications, especially the impact on stakeholders
   Be sure to have discussed this section with them before writing the report

9. Lessons learned

10. Conclusions

11. Recommendations

12. Appendices

Fig. 15.9   Suggested structure for a final report.

Sustaining Your Improvement

Sustainability occurs when new ways of working and improved outcomes become the norm. Let us assume that your improvement is successful and you want it to be sustained. Some organisations fall into the trap of 'project-itis', where short-term initiatives are completed but there is no longer-term plan around adoption and spread. This can build cynicism and a reluctance for people to commit to future projects (Tips Box 15.4).

TIPS BOX 15.4

For Sustaining Improvement

- *Good enough*—is the improvement good enough or should you improve it further?
- *Measurement*—measuring something indicates that it is a priority, so keep measuring and communicating how you are doing.
- *What is in it for me*—is the improvement considered important to your stakeholders, including your end users (patients, carers, pupils, and so forth)?
- *Win/win*—phrase the improvement according to what others might desire as well as what you want.
- *Redundant*—are there any policy changes or technical solutions that might make this improvement redundant, for example, virtual consultations replacing your improvement based on face-to-face consultations?
- *Mainstream*—ensure the improvement becomes part of your organisation's regular reporting processes and business planning cycle.
- *Set the bar higher*—a new target creates excitement.
  Based on NHS Modernisation Agency (2002).

  Problems with maintaining improvements include:
- The change is seen as an isolated project with a start and end date and fixed, time-limited funding.
- Some stakeholders may not have been involved, do not understand it, are not trained and are not engaged.
- The improvement is not connected to any forward business plans and so no resources are allocated to it.
- The improvement is not linked into the whole system, so the knock-on effects on other departments or teams have not been considered, such as allowing time in the university's schedule for pupil visits to the simulation suite.

  As you go along, consider:
- To which of the related teams affected by your project will you talk? So, for example, if the improvement is about reducing the prescribing of reliever inhalers, go and speak to local pharmacists. If the improvement is about encouraging students from low-income communities to apply to do a course at the university, speak to the admissions team about the barriers that such applicants may face.
- Who else needs to know about positive improvements or lessons learned, such as strategy, training, information and finance teams?
- When might you want to tell them? If there is an annual planning or budgeting cycle then you need to bear this in mind if you want to continue or expand a small idea that seems to be working—speak to the project sponsor early about this.
- What do you specifically want others to do, how much it might cost, how it will be done and what the benefits to them might be?
- What is the best way to keep the wider organisation apprised of what is happening? Discuss this with your sponsor and build this into your communications strategy from the start of the project.

SPREAD AND ADOPTION

Spread is the extent to which learning and change principles have been adopted in other parts of the organisation that could benefit from them. The term spread indicates more of a top-down process, where the organisation uses a strategic approach coupled with tools and techniques.

Adoption meanwhile is more about organisations and teams articulating a need and discovering through conversation and interaction the solution to their needs. This can be facilitated by the opinion leaders who we met in the chapter on power and influence. Such people could be trusted by specific groups but not others, or by a wider group. For example, if a nurse in a popular podcast mentions an improvement idea it may influence nurses but not necessarily doctors. Remember that opinion leaders are often not part of the formal hierarchy, and so it is important to discover who they are and what they think about your improvement.

The wise leader's role in adoption is more of a matchmaker—introducing those who need new ideas to those who have tested them, rather than a commander—someone who just decides that change is required (NHS Modernisation Agency 2002) (See Fig. 15.7).

What improvement leaders across the world have found that it is better to pull people towards you or allow the diffusion of ideas rather than push ideas onto people. Spread is the result of adoption, rather than the other way around (NHS Modernisation Agency 2000).

■ Time Out

Look back at the chapter 9 on power and influence. How does Gladwell describe these opinion leaders?

We may equate the idea of adopting improvement practices to the idea of starting social epidemics. In *Tipping Point* (2000), Gladwell says that it is the mavens who have a significant part to play in the spreading of social epidemics. Mavens are always gaining new information, looking for trends and making links between this information and their knowledge.

Although mavens do not have vast social networks like Gladwell's connectors do, they significantly influence those within that network. Mavens are trusted individuals with insider knowledge. Therefore, people follow their recommendations. What you then do is, via your communication strategy, engage and inform the mavens about the success of your improvement project and openly say that you welcome people who want to copy your successful practices.

Table 15.5 provides the dos and don'ts of spreading ideas developed by Kaiser Permanente, an American integrated care management consortium renown for improving health care.

TABLE 15.5 ■ The Dos and Don'ts of Spreading Ideas

Do	Don't
Make spread a team effort.	Give one person the responsibility to do it all. Depend on local 'heroes'.
Start with small local tests and several PDSA cycles.	Neglect testing—just do a large pilot.
Sustain gains with an infrastructure to support them.	Rely solely on vigilance and hard work.
Allow some customisation as long as it is controlled and elements that are core to the improvement are clear.	Spread the success unchanged.
Choose a spread team strategically and include the scope of the spread as part of your decision.	Require the person and the team who drove the initial improvements to be responsible for spread throughout the organisation.
Check small samples daily or frequently so you can decide how spread practices need adapting.	Check huge amounts of data just once every quarter.
Create a reliable process before you start to spread.	Expect huge improvement quickly Start spreading right away.

PDSA, Plan, do, study, act.
Adapted from: IHI "Seven Spreadly Sins." Institute for Healthcare Improvement. Cambridge, Massachusetts, USA. [Infographic created by Kaiser Permanente Labor Management Partnership]

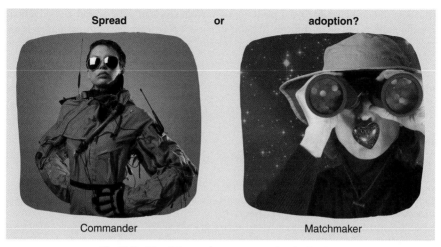

Fig. 15.10   The difference between spread and adoption.

Because each team and organisation may have different contexts and cultures, it is important to enable them to be able to adapt and customise the improvement, rather than blindly copy it. What you are asking people to do is to adopt the change principles—those factors that helped make your project successful—rather than the process as a whole (Fig. 15.10).

Celebrate Success and Learning

Finally, it is always important to engage everyone involved in both celebrating the success of a project and the learning that came from it, even if all did not go to plan (Tips Box 15.5).

TIPS BOX 15.5

Celebrate and Learn

- Review what went well, what did not go so well, what the team has learnt and how the improvement could be made even better.
- Involve the whole team in showcasing what they have achieved directly to their peers. Showcasing can involve presentations, videos, blogs, awards and hosting open events where people are invited to see the work for themselves ('seeing is believing').
- Promote successes through local events, health care awards, media articles, research papers, professional meetings, social media and conferences.
- Express gratitude and thank people for their help.

Summary

Project management is an important part of managing change and making improvements. Projects require good leadership skills from everyone, from the project sponsor to the project manager and the members of the project team. The project team should be carefully selected to combine the right skills as well as the right stakeholders.

The aims and objectives of a project must be carefully written to be specific, measurable, achievable, relevant and timebound. Risks need to be identified and mitigated, communications should be planned and tasks managed according to the three variables of time, quality and cost.

Evaluation and sustainability need planning right from the start. The spread and adoption of successful projects can prove difficult. What is important is to use influencers or opinion leaders, identify principles that can be adapted and customised and 'pull' people towards the improvement rather than 'push' it upon them.

Finally, celebrating what has been achieved is important for 'closure' and recognition of the people involved and the work done.

Resources

Health and Safety Executive. Managing Risks and Risk Assessment at Work. <https://www.hse.gov.uk/simple-health-safety/risk/index.htm>.

Kotter, J., 1995. Leading change: why transformation efforts fail. Harvard Business Review, 73 (2), 59–67.

NHS Improvement, 2018. Seven Steps to Measurement for Improvement. <https://improvement.nhs.uk/resources/seven-steps-measurement-improvement/>.

The Health Foundation, 2015. Communications Approaches to Spread Improvement. London. <https://www.health.org.uk/publications/using-communications-approaches-to-spread-improvement>.

References

Gladwell, M., 2000. The Tipping Point. Abacus, London.

Kaiser Permanente Labor Management Partnership, 2015. The Seven Spreadly Sins. <https://www.lmpartnership.org/tools/seven-spreadly-sins>.

NHS Confederation, 2012. Building Social Value in the NHS. London.

NHS Institute for Innovation and Improvement, 2007. Evaluating Improvement. Coventry.

NHS Institute for Innovation and Improvement, 2002. Improvement Leader's Guide. Sustainability and its Relationship with Spread and Adoption. <https://www.england.nhs.uk/improvement-hub/wp-content/uploads/sites/44/2017/11/ILG-1.7-Sustainability-and-its-Relationship-with-Spread-and-Adoption.pdf>. (accessed 09/01/2022).

Reed, S., Göpfert, A., Wood, S., 2019. Building Healthier Communities: The Role of the NHS as an Anchor Institution. Health Foundation, London.

Leading Through Entrepreneurship

OBJECTIVES

After reading this chapter and completing the activities, you should be able to:
- Differentiate between intrapreneurs and entrepreneurs
- Define social entrepreneurship and how it creates social value
- Describe the basic elements of a business plan using the mnemonic EPOCH
- Explain the differences between inventors, innovators and entrepreneurs, and the roles they play in creating a successful business
- Give an example of closed innovation and open innovation
- Identify those people who are high adaptors and high innovators and describe situations where each would thrive.

Relevance to the Nursing and Midwifery Council (NMC) Code

Promote Professionalism and Trust
Paragraph 21:
Uphold Your Position as a Registered Nurse, Midwife or Nursing Associate
21.1 refuse all but the most trivial gifts, favours or hospitality as accepting them could be interpreted as an attempt to gain preferential treatment
21.2 never ask for or accept loans from anyone in your care or anyone close to them
21.3 act with honesty and integrity in any financial dealings you have with everyone you have a professional relationship with, including people in your care
21.4 make sure that any advertisements, publications or published material you produce or have produced for your professional services are accurate, responsible, ethical, do not mislead or exploit vulnerabilities and accurately reflect your relevant skills, experience and qualifications
21.5 never use your status as a registered professional to promote causes that are not related to health
21.6 cooperate with the media only when it is appropriate to do so, and then always protecting the confidentiality and dignity of people receiving treatment or care

Paragraph 25:
Provide Leadership to Make Sure People's Wellbeing Is Protected and to Improve Their Experiences of the Health and Care System
25.1 identify priorities, manage time, staff and resources effectively and deal with risk to make sure that the quality of care or service you deliver is maintained and improved, putting the needs of those receiving care or services first

The concept of nurse entrepreneurship is still in its infancy and yet it exists, and those who fulfil this description may be so modest that they might not say that this is what they are.

The roots of nursing entrepreneurship can be traced back to the 19th century and to Florence Nightingale and her pioneering work with soldiers in the Crimean War. Following this, she founded the School of Nursing at Saint Thomas Hospital, initiating the scientific foundations of the profession. A more recent example is a district nurse called Ellie Lindsay who founded the Lindsay Leg Club in 1995. There are now leg clubs across the United Kingdom, Germany and Australia, where people with leg ulcers come together in social groups to learn how to self-care and avoid the isolation of being nursed in their own homes (https://www.legclub.org/).

This chapter will define the meaning and characteristics of entrepreneurship and how it differs from intrapreneurship (see Case Study 16.2). It will highlight why nurses might make good entrepreneurs and give some examples. We shall talk about how they lead and influence the nursing community and beyond, and what you might learn from them.

What Is an Entrepreneur?

There are quite a few definitions of what an entrepreneur is. Most say that it is an individual who takes a risk to start a business or businesses to make money. Some say it is about working for yourself and being your own boss. Others say it is a lot to do with innovating to solve a problem and spotting a gap in the market to sell the solution.

The criticism levelled at the idea of nurses as entrepreneurs is that combining caring with business creates conflicting values and therefore many might shy away from the description (Fletcher 2010; Wilson et al. 2003). Certainly, nurse entrepreneurs need to abide by the Nursing and Midwifery Council (NMC) code, described at the start of this chapter, around their financial dealings, marketing their services and working with the media.

However, nursing is about understanding the needs of people and the systems that operate around them and considering how they could be better, more efficient or even reinvented. Therefore, entrepreneurship is a valid option for nurses with courage and vision. Entrepreneurship can be a form of leadership, and therefore it is important to think about how it may be a route for student leaders to make improvements. As we shall see, finding new and better ways to do things this way can happen both in the NHS and outside it, so the 'making money' element might not occur.

Another difficulty that those nurses (or indeed student nurses) with an entrepreneurial flair may face is that nurses are often expected to be 'good employees' and take orders, which goes against their nature (Copelli et al. 2019). Such nurses may be constantly thinking about opportunities and innovation and pushing boundaries. If this is you, look back at the Chapter 8 on assertiveness for ways to rock the boat without falling out (refer to Tips Box 16.1)!

DIFFERENT TYPES OF ENTREPRENEURIAL NURSES

Some examples include:
- Education and training consultancies
- Management consultancies
- Nursing home, home care and care home businesses (see Case Study 16.1)
- Nurses who start social enterprises or charities
- Nurse partners in GP surgeries
- Nurse-led private fostering or adoption agencies
- Aesthetic treatment businesses

The literature on entrepreneurship is sparse, with some differentiating between nurses who set up businesses, those who act entrepreneurially in their workplaces and those who become self-employed (Sæter 2019).

CASE STUDY 16.1   George Coxon, the Fun-Guarding Pioneer and Rebel Leader

'Dear Dementia
I want to put on my wellies not my slippers.'
        IAN DONAGHY, AUTHOR OF *DEAR DEMENTIA: THE LAUGHTER AND THE TEARS* (2014)

George trained as a mental health nurse in the north east of England and now currently lives and works in the south west. He moved on from clinical work to be a commissioner for specialist commissioning and now owns two care homes in Devon and leads a local network of care home providers.

George wonders whether safe has become the enemy of fun in later life and has developed the idea of 'fun guarding', which has taken hold. Writing with colleagues in a series of articles about this for the British Geriatric Society (BGS 2019), he urges care home owners and those who support them to be risk aware rather than be risk averse. He calls for a balance between the two and for care home owners to create a culture where fun can flourish.

He is passionate about care home residents being as fit and well as they can be so that they can do activities that they enjoy. This is personalised care taken to another level, with people encouraged to make 'bucket lists' of things they would like to do, some of which will stretch their capabilities. He enables his staff to lead various types of activities such as wake-up shake-up, singalongs, resistance bands, grip strengthening and post-fall reablement, to name but a few. However, he sees these things as a precursor to having fun and living life to the fullest.

He calls upon NHS professionals such as allied health professionals (AHPs) to cocreate activities and exercises that his staff can learn to do. He wants statutory services to trust that care home owners, who rarely have access to AHPs, can undertake things like breathing exercises without professional support.

The first 'fun-guarding' image that you see on the BGS website is one where two half-scared, half-elated residents are paddling from their wheelchairs at the seaside. His presentations are full of scenes residents tomato planting, weight-lifting and cherishing trophies won in competitions.

He reminds us that leaders are the ones responsible for creating and changing the culture of organisations to enable fun guarding to happen. 'Every day that you're away from the front line as a leader—you lose your credibility inch by inch.' He gets involved personally in ensuring that his residents enjoy themselves safely.

The criteria for success he says are 'excitement, hilarity, competition and exhaustion', and claims that the absence of any two of these criteria suggests room for improvement. The outcomes that he suggests are measured to reflect the concept of social value—such as hearing uproarious laughter or observing sleepy daytime power naps, rather than just using the traditional quality-of-life questionnaires.

FINDING INSPIRATION

George's ideas have been described as inspirational. He says, *'You can't inspire other people until you find people who inspire you...I'm hanging on to their shirt tails because I want to be as good as them.'*

He goes on to list the people who inspire him and gives them credit, such as Nicola Kendall (2020), who wrote about the concept of Namaste care for people living with dementia—the idea of a sensory approach to support people with dementia using loving touch, a tranquil environment, music and, of course, fun.

TRANSFORMATIONAL LEADERSHIP

As an entrepreneur, George's leadership style is visionary and transformational—inspiring positive change in his followers. Like Brian Dolan and the #EndPJParalysis movement, the idea of 'fun guarding' is not owned and the BGS encourages members to take forward fun guarding in their own ways.

TIPS BOX 16.1

George's Tips on Entrepreneurship as a Transformational Leader

- Lead by example: be a role model and be credible.
- Find inspiration and be inspiration.
- Have exposure to different care settings—shadow, mentor or twin so you understand each other.

Continued

- Rewrite your CV every 6 months and add something new.
- Recognise your blind spots and be willing to learn.
- Think about how you will get a return on any investment you make.
- Have several 'fishing lines' (customers) and be patient whilst waiting for a 'bite' (sale).

Intrapreneurs

In contrast to those who build a business from the ground up, intrapreneurs are people who are invited to innovate within an organisation. The term intrapreneur is a portmanteau of the two words 'internal' and 'entrepreneur'. They are often offered protected time and freedom to act, and their role is often to interpret market trends (in our case, the direction that health and care is heading), visualise what could be different and then come up with innovative solutions.

CASE STUDY 16.2   **The Case of an Intrapreneur**

'I am not a hero. I am just a stubborn fighter who does not give up hope of getting a better world for everyone.'

JOAN PONS LAPLANA

A prominent example of an intrapreneur is Joan Pons Laplana (roaringnurse.com), originally from Spain, who is a serial intrapreneur, championing issues such as dementia, dignity and equality, and diversity. He has invented the Flu Bee Game (fluebeegame.com)—a digital game to persuade people to get vaccinated. Joan declares that he is not afraid to change his job, role or location to deliver change.

https://flubeegame.com/

The benefit of working within an established organisation is that the individual has access to all its assets and resources. The downsides are that they do not reap the rewards that may accrue and any successful solutions usually belong to their organisation and not to them personally. Successful intrapreneurs need the support of senior leaders in the organisation, as innovation and change can feel very threatening, and freedom to act can be met with jealousy.

Social Entrepreneurs

Social entrepreneurship in nursing is about mobilising and transforming society via some form of social intervention (Copelli et al. 2019). For many nurses this is about bringing people together in social groups and enabling them to improve their wellbeing by achieving their personal goals (Case Study 16.3).

A social enterprise is a business that has a clearly defined social mission. Its profits are reinvested to pursue this mission. They differ from charities in that most of their income comes via trade, by selling goods and services, rather than being grant funded. They also add 'social value': this is the quantification of the relative importance that people place on the changes they experience in their lives. This includes things like the value that people experience from increasing their confidence, or from being able to see their children if separated or divorced—the things that are important to individuals but not commonly expressed or measured in the same way that financial value is (Social Value UK, online).

CASE STUDY 16.3   **BlueSci Community Interest Company**

An example of social entrepreneurship in mental health services is BlueSci Community Interest Company (https://bluesci.org.uk/), an organisation founded in 2004 in Trafford, Greater Manchester by former mental health nurse Alicia Clare and youth worker and contemporary artist Stuart Webster.

Their fundamental belief is that good mental health and wellbeing are achieved by working closely with local communities, taking its guiding principles from a variety of evidence and best practice. They believe that individuals who have experienced mental health problems and/or services can contribute a wealth of knowledge and experience to its service development. The role of the staff in the journey of recovery for individuals is that of companion or fellow traveller rather than an expert.

Alicia talks about the origins of BlueSci:

'As a matron within the mental health inpatient service at Trafford, I was inspired by Stuart Webster (professional contemporary artist with experience within Forensic and Secure Mental Health Services) and the team of commissioned artists that worked on the inpatient service with service users and staff. They were passionate about their art form and broke down barriers to engagement through this medium. This opened up conversations that removed labels and saw people with skills, interests and more importantly hope and inspirations for the whole ward community (service users, staff, volunteers, carers, friends relatives).'

'The ability for artists to ask curious questions about why things were done in a particular way or not done, created an honest and thoughtful creative learning environment where everyone played a role.'

'The inpatient service was awarded Practice Development Unit Status for its innovative work. Service users wanted to return as volunteers following discharge. Stuart and I thought it would make sense to extend this into the community. We took our "good idea" to commissioners and tendered for what is now the BlueSci Community Mental Health & Wellbeing Service.'

For more information on BlueSci's history, see Clare et al. (2007).

RIGHT TO REQUEST PROGRAMME—NHS SOCIAL ENTREPRENEURSHIP

In the United Kingdom, most primary care contractors (GPs, dentists, opticians and community pharmacists) are contracted to the NHS, and some of them choose to adopt a social enterprise business model and company form. Examples include Salford Health Matters, which provides GP and community services, and Green Light Pharmacy, a group of pharmacies in and around London that provide innovative pharmacy services.

In 2008, social entrepreneurship became part of NHS policy in England when primary care trust staff were enabled to make a 'right to request' to deliver primary and community services through a social enterprise model (Department of Health, 2008). This meant that clinicians, including nurses and AHPs, were able to put proposals to their board and onwards to NHS England to develop social businesses; services would meet local need and maximise the potential to innovate and ultimately improve outcomes for patients, clients and families, whilst remaining part of the NHS family (Case Study 16.4).

By June 2011, 47 such social enterprises had been set up, ranging from microenterprises of six people to those employing over 1,000 people. The Department of Health (2011) produced a report on their progress, finding that many had made cost and service improvements, and some had reduced staff sickness absence rates. However, it also pointed to the fact that, although they had an initial exclusive 2-year contract, when that ended those new social enterprises would have to compete with other, perhaps larger and more established organisations, to continue to provide NHS services. The reliance on one major customer (the NHS) is always a risky business.

Today, some of those early social entrepreneurs have struggled to survive. This might be because the smaller organisations, called microenterprises, do not have the experience or the level of resources to enable them to compete, compared to big NHS organisations. Alternatively, the social enterprise model of trading with, rather than being publicly funded by, the NHS might not be well understood by those who commission or buy its services, and that freedom to act may be interpreted as risky.

CASE STUDY 16.4

Over time, an intrapreneur may become an entrepreneur and start their own venture outside the organisation. Lance Gardner MBE is an example of this.

Aged 16, Lance was inspired to become a nurse after witnessing the nursing care he received when he had his appendix out. He started out as a registered nurse and health visitor in West Yorkshire before moving to Runcorn as a nurse practitioner in a GP surgery. Lance worked alongside innovative GP David Colin-Thomé, who later became the national clinical director for primary care.

He became the general manager of a total purchasing pilot project, where during 1994 to 1998 GPs were given a delegated budget by their local health authority to purchase all of the hospital and community health services for their patients.

Lance moved to Salford in 1996 to become the first owner of a nurse-led GP surgery, which caused upset amongst local GPs because a nurse was in charge and employing GPs. The practice was in a challenging area and, afraid that his surgery would be burgled by local gangs or that his staff may be harmed, Lance went to visit the gang leader (and father to a child on his patient list) at his home to ask for his support. He introduced himself to the gang leader and enquired if he would be safe if he had to visit the house to put a stethoscope on his child's chest. From that day, the surgery and its staff were protected by the gang and a GP was even escorted to a visit on a rival gang's patch for her safety.

In 2011, Lance took advantage of the 'right to request' scheme to start a social enterprise in Grimsby called the Care Plus Group. The social enterprise not only provides personal health and care services, but it operates a charitable trust where local community groups can apply for a grant to purchase equipment.

Lance is now back in Salford as chief executive of Salford Primary Care Together (www.spctogether. co.uk/), a social enterprise operating as a network supporting the GP surgeries across the city.

These are Lance's reflections on entrepreneurship for readers of this book:

'One of the key features of an entrepreneur is their attitude to risk—whether that is personal risk or the risk of attempting something that has possibility of not working. Entrepreneurs don't see trying something and it not working as failure—they see not innovating or trying new things and playing safe as failure.'

'Another feature of a social entrepreneur is their values—these are not negotiable and won't be compromised to achieve a specific outcome.'

■ Time Out

What entrepreneurial characteristics do you observe in the nurses in the case studies given earlier?

The characteristics commonly attributed to entrepreneurs are given here. Many of these are found amongst nurses, and this may be why nurses start their own businesses.

Do a quick self-assessment against these characteristics by marking with an 'x' where you feel you are on a continuum from 'not at all' to 'extremely'. If you tend to be overly self-critical, you might want to do this exercise alongside a colleague who knows you well.

	Not at all	Extremely
Versatile	◄————————————————————►	
Flexible	◄————————————————————►	
Money savvy	◄————————————————————►	
Decisive	◄————————————————————►	
Innovative	◄————————————————————►	
Risk taking	◄————————————————————►	
Ambitious	◄————————————————————►	
Persistent	◄————————————————————►	
Disciplined	◄————————————————————►	
Passionate	◄————————————————————►	
Problem solver	◄————————————————————►	
Able to prioritise	◄————————————————————►	
Resourceful	◄————————————————————►	

There is no 'right' answer here—this exercise is just to get you thinking a little about what entrepreneurship involves. Health and care delivery needs different sorts of people with these sorts of skills. Some are happy to work in existing organisations, services and teams, and others like to strike out in new directions.

Business Skills Are Needed!

Understanding business and having the skills to run a business are essential for entrepreneurs. Nurses interested in taking this path may have a mentor or coach, a background in business or have taken business courses from certificate level right up to a masters in business administration (MBA). There are also MBA courses specifically for health service managers or alternatively you can complete a general MBA and learn alongside people from all sorts of industries so that you can cross-fertilise ideas. Some courses are offered via open learning (such as via the Open University Business School) and can be combined with employment.

There are many sources of information online, but a good place to start is the UK Government website (see Resources section), which contains all the basic information needed, such as how to set up a business, how to choose the right legal form for your company and how to write a business plan, employ people and pay tax.

For companies operating in the voluntary, community and social enterprise sector, such as charities and community interest companies, there are often local voluntary sector support organisations that can offer advice, training and support. Nationally, there are large membership organisations that can help, such as Social Enterprise UK, National Council for Voluntary Organisations and Co-operatives UK (see Resources section).

START-UP IDEAS

To have a successful business you need to have a great idea—one that will differentiate you from the competition. Guy Kawasaki is an entrepreneurial guru. In his book *The Art of Start 2.0* (2015), he claims that great discoveries stem from curiosity and he offers a series of questions as prompts for would-be entrepreneurs which he calls GIST: Great Ideas for Starting Things.

■ **Time Out**

Thinking of your current work or study, which of these questions may be useful to you? Choose one prompt question and jot some ideas down.

Therefore, What? (Slywotzsky 2002)
This technique mirrors the 'five whys' that we ask when understanding problems. This question is helpful when you want to spot or predict a trend. For example: the COVID-19 pandemic allowed scientists to produce, in a couple of months, tests that can be done at home—a process that normally takes 10 years. Therefore, what? This accelerated innovation process can be replicated for other diseases. Therefore, what? The public can be empowered to use tests for other diseases and conditions, such as influenza—self-isolating and thus not infecting vulnerable family members, reducing 'winter pressures' on NHS services.

Isn't This Interesting?
Intellectual curiosity and accidental discoveries lie behind this question. For example, Charles Darwin observed that the finches on the different Galapagos islands had different-shaped beaks. He worked with an ornithologist to discover that each beak shape was adapted to eat different foods such as seeds or insects. From this and other discoveries he put forward the theory of natural selection.

Continued

Is There a Better Way?

This question stems from frustration. Keyhole surgery to reduce recovery times comes to mind. Community care rather than institutionalisation for people with learning disabilities is another.

Why Doesn't Our Organisation Do This?

Many of us may have asked this question out of frustration with our current employers. Nurses understand people's needs better than most and may be thinking of a better way to support them, but no one listens. Finally, you initiate innovations yourself. The case study in Chapter 9 on power and influence, where Joy O'Gorman introduced the MyCOPD app to support patient self-care, is one example here. (Fortunately, in this instance, people listened to Joy!)

It's Possible, So Why Don't We Make It?

This is the 'what the heck, let's go for it' option. Social solutions here include men's sheds to support wellbeing and singing for lung health to improve breath control and wellbeing. Technical solutions include things like ear fold surgery, invented by surgeon Norbert Kang in 2010, for correcting prominent ears. Kang worked with medical technology consultancy Health Enterprise East and formed a spin-out company with West Hertfordshire Hospitals NHS Trust called Northwood Medical Innovation. Following the death of a young patient undergoing otoplasty, Kang pioneered the subcutaneous insertion under local anaesthetic of a shape memory alloy behind the ear. Over time the cartilage reforms around the implant and the ear is permanently bent into new shape.

THE FUNDAMENTALS OF BUSINESS PLANNING

If you are really interested in starting your own business, there is a commonly used list of starting questions, using the acronym EPOCH, to ask yourself (Box 16.1). These questions also form part of a business plan.

Inventors, Innovators and Entrepreneurs

We live in a faced-paced, globalised world, where adapting to change may not be enough. Who would have thought, prior to 2020, that a global pandemic would have shifted the digitalisation of health care quite so quickly? With long-term conditions on the rise as we live longer, health care needs new ways to address the challenges of old age. Health problems are becoming more complex, with a web of interconnectedness between the social circumstances of our lives and the effect on our bodies and our minds. We need creativity and innovation to keep up with changing challenges.

Two of the characteristics often associated with entrepreneurs are that they are creative and innovative. There are many definitions of innovation, but a simple and effective one is that innovations must be both *new* and *useful*. However, not all entrepreneurs are innovative, and it is more likely that they work alongside inventors and innovators to make their ideas into a business, or in the case of intrapreneurs, make changes in their organisations.

The desire for entrepreneurs to introduce innovations often comes from their perception that there is a better way to do something, and for others it is about getting ahead of the competition or a fear that they will be overtaken in the market—say in the pharmaceutical industry, where innovation is constant. In nursing, innovation often comes from a deep desire to literally change the world for the better.

Inventions lead to innovation products such as:

- Discovery of the x-ray → medical x-rays
- Light sensitivity of silver compounds → photography and cameras
- Lasers → CDs and DVDs

BOX 16.1 ■ EPOCH Business Plan

- What are you **E**xcellent at? Focus on excellence, not just what you are good at, because in a competitive business world, others will be better than you! The 'sweet spot' is the overlap between your expertise, your passion and the opportunity (Danner and Coopersmith 2015).
- Which group of **P**eople will benefit from your business? Be specific: people with certain health conditions? In a certain geography? What ages?
- What **O**utcomes do you want for these people? Real outcomes here, not just processes or outputs like training—will it be that you improve their quality of life, or heal their leg ulcers, or reduce asthma attacks?
- Who might your **C**ustomers be? By customers, we mean people or organisations that will buy your services, such as the NHS, local councils, health professionals or patients themselves.
- **H**ow much would they pay you? Work out how much delivering your service will cost. The chances are you will underestimate this at first. Take a look at what others in the same market charge.

And then these innovations become start-up businesses, such as turning photography into a business, like Kodak did.

If you are a student nurse who is interested in innovation and entrepreneurship, it is important to recognise the difference between being an inventor such as Tariq Aslam who invented the Rafi-Tone app (described later), an innovator such Ellie Lindsay, who set up new and more social ways to deliver leg care with the Lindsay Leg Club, and an entrepreneur like Lance Gardner, who has set up several social enterprises.

The roles of innovator, inventor and entrepreneur can combine within the same person, but many times they do not, so it is important that you understand which skill set (inventor, innovator or entrepreneur) applies to you and seek out others to help you (Table 16.1). In general, inventors do not spend time thinking about what comes after the invention has been created—they generally turn it over to the innovator to give purpose to it. The innovator may improve or make some sort of contribution to the invention. The entrepreneur is then thinking about where to place the resulting product or idea into the market.

■ Time Out

Spend some time thinking about which role suits you best. If research ideas, new products or services come into your mind constantly, you may be an inventor or innovator. But if your interest is in introducing a new product or service into the market (or within your organisation), then you could be an entrepreneur or intrapreneur.

Open and Closed Innovation

Originally described by Henry Chesbrough (2003), one thing to look out for as an entrepreneurial student nurse is whether the organisation prefers the process of innovation to be internal (closed innovation) or whether it collaborates with other organisations to innovate (open innovation). This relates back to the chapter on understanding the culture of your organisation.

The philosophy behind closed innovation is around a company being self-reliant and having control over its innovations—and of course getting ahead of the competition. Another phrase frequently used when referring to closed innovation is 'not invented here' (NIH), which suggests

TABLE 16.1 ■ The Difference Between Inventors, Innovators and Entrepreneurs

Characteristics	Inventors	Innovators	Entrepreneurs
Definition	Inventions, research or discoveries are the creation of new products, processes and technologies not previously known to exist	The transformation of new and creative ideas into useful applications Developing proof of concept	Taking a risk to start a new business to make money
Skill sets	Extremely creative Technical expertise Vision	Creative thinking and experimentation Improving inventions Anticipating customer need	Hard working, flexible, forward thinking and passionate
Attitude to risk	Aware of high failure rate and that most ideas do not turn into products	Most are not risk takers	Are risk takers
Interest	Inventing something that has never been made/done before	Once an innovation enters the market, the innovator moves on to develop the idea more or develop a new product	Finds a place in the market for the innovation, makes it into a business venture and works hard to see it become successful
Cause	Solving problems	Make something out of a new thought	Makes a business out of the innovation

Based on DifferenceBetween.net and UniversityLabPartners.org.

that the organisation itself must feel like it owns the idea and may be averse to adopting other organisations' innovations. For example, you may have worked on a ward where they have improved a nursing procedure. When you go to your next ward and tell them about it they reject the idea out of hand, maybe saying 'We've always done it this way and it works fine!' This is NIH in action.

Chesbrough suggests that closed innovation dominated the 20th century but was eroded because of the number and mobility of knowledge workers, meaning that innovation was difficult to control. Workers whose bright ideas were not taken up by the host firm took them elsewhere or formed spin-out companies. Open innovation emerged as companies commercialised their own ideas and those of other firms. The organisation's boundary became porous to allow the flow of ideas and innovations.

The creation of the Academy of Fab NHS Stuff (fabnhsstuff.net), started by NHS commentator Roy Lilley, has enabled anyone to upload and share their open or closed innovations on the website for others to adapt or adopt, thus avoiding 'reinventing the wheel'.

Closed innovations can be quite simple and effective, such as the one uploaded by Kirsty Wood (2021), who is an associate professor at the University of Derby. She held a faith and belief learning event where a student told a story of where she was able to identify and address an Arabic patient in their native language and how this helped to address this patient's anxiety. Together Kirsty and her students developed the idea of adding flags to the students' name badges to identify which language they spoke.

An example of open innovation stemmed from a father and ophthalmologist called Tariq Aslam, whose toddler son was refusing to take his asthma inhaler. He approached Clin-e-cal (clin-e-cal.com), a digital health company spun from the University of Manchester and Manchester Foundation Trust. Working with Clin-e-cal and a company called Clement Clark, they designed a spacer called the Able Spacer. Tariq helped to develop a phone app called Rafi-Tone (named after his son is Rafi). The app, which is now NHS approved, features a game that is played on the phone. When the child has a sufficient inspiratory flow, the spacer makes a whistle. The sound is picked up by the phone, which enables the Rafi-Tone robot in the game to defeat a monster. This encourages young children to enjoy the game whilst they take their medicines.

▪ Time Out

Think of examples of open and then closed innovation that you may have seen. What do you observe to be the main differences, and how successful were the innovations as a result?

One of the things you may have observed is that idea of an asset-based approach that we met in Chapter 7 on cocreation. Innovation requires organisations to engage and harness the strengths and assets of others. Sometimes these assets already exist within the organisation—such as students who speak several languages as in the 'flags on badges' example. At other times they need to look outside their organisations for support. Take the Clin-e-cal example, where a parent with an interest in app design took his ideas forward with a company specialising in digital innovation. However, it required a partner who had the capability of making a spacer that could work with the app and then manufacture and distribute the resulting spacer so that clinicians could prescribe it.

In the modern NHS we see many such collaborations with commercial organisations, universities and scientists. In England, the NHS Innovation Accelerator (NIA, nhsaccelerator.com) is one of the main vehicles for supporting aspiring innovators, including clinicians and academics from industry or from charitable and not-for-profit organisations. Working alongside the 15 Academic Health Science Networks (AHSNs—the innovation arm of the NHS), the NIA offers fellowships to people to help scale up the best innovations. Equivalent organisations work across the UK.

▪ Time Out

Visit nhsaccelerator.com and ahsnnetwork.com (or their equivalent across the four UK nations—see Resources section) to familiarise yourself with what they do. Read some of the case studies on innovations that the NIA has supported and the national programmes currently being run.

Because nurses are ideally placed to spot the potential for innovation, you may want to stoke ambition early on by inviting a member of your local AHSN to speak at your nursing society or student union about how they can support the ambition of nurses to develop innovative solutions.

Innovation Spiral

All innovations have to start somewhere, and it is helpful to have a framework to help to guide you through the journey from finding the challenges to changing the system. One such framework is the innovation spiral (Fig. 16.1), created by the innovation foundation NESTA (online).

Whereas creativity is associated with flashes of inspiration, innovation is actually a planned process. The stages of the innovation spiral involve:

1. Exploring opportunities and challenges: identify the opportunity or challenge, investigate it and understand it (we discussed this in Chapter 12 on problem solving).

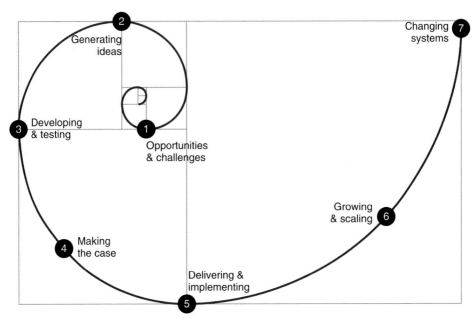

Fig. 16.1   Innovation spiral. (Courtesy Nesta, 2019. A Compendium of Innovation Methods.)

2. Generating (lots of) ideas: then sift out the ones with most potential (Chapter 12).
3. Developing and testing: this is an iterative process often involving prototyping and rapid cycle testing—that plan-do-study-act (PDSA) cycle we looked at earlier is one example of how to develop an innovation (Chapter 14).
4. Making the case: develop the 'proof of concept' demonstrating that the innovation works and is feasible as a solution to the problem. This involves gathering evidence on the impact of your solution.
5. Delivering and implementing: plan and organise for the implementation of your solution, including its ownership and the form and structure you need to create to deliver it. The chapters on managing change and project planning come in here (Chapters 13 and 15).
6. Growing, scaling and spreading: we discussed this at the end of Chapter 15 on project management.
7. Changing systems: we talked about understanding the culture and climate that you are working in and how, with systems leadership, it is important to develop relationships and trust through establishing a common purpose (Chapter 11).

Innovation and Adaptation

Adaptors desire to do things better, whereas innovators want to do things differently—and there is room for both in nursing.

Michael Kirton is a cognitive psychologist and author, who, in 1976 (and further expanded on in 2003) outlined a theory of cognition by which people could identify their favoured approach to problem solving. Kirton (2003) suggested that all individuals can have the capability for being creative, but some may do so by being highly adaptive and others are creative by being highly innovative. Your cognitive style is a mixture of innate preference plus shaping through experiences.

His view is that by understanding each person's preferences, we are better able to understand and embrace each other's diverse styles and thus work together better as a team. In high-pressure, uncertain or unexpected situations, innovators are often more creative. Adaptors will excel in everyday tasks and predictable challenges, improving on the existing methods of the organisation.

The 'KAI test' is a series of questions designed to measure someone's adaptor/innovator score so that they can place themselves along a creativity continuum between high adaptation and high innovation. It is administered by trained KAI practitioners and is used to help organisations with issues such as team building and problem solving (kaicentre.com).

Adaptors prefer well-established organisational structures, systems and processes, whereas innovators like to break the mould, working outside the current restraints to find new and untested solutions.

■ Time Out

In the team that you are currently working or studying in, try to identify:
- Those people who may be highly adaptive, preferring to work within established processes to find solutions
- Those people who may be highly innovative, preferring to push to boundaries and maybe even break the 'rules'

Take a look at how well those people understand and value each other's skills. Would the team benefit if they understood each other's role in the team better?

Unfortunately, Kirton found that innovators and adaptors often clashed because they did not appreciate that they each had different styles and different roles.

STUDENT INNOVATION CASE STUDIES

Case studies 16.5 and 16.6 demonstrate how students can innovate.

CASE STUDY 16.5   Leanne Patrick—Advocacy for Student Mental Health and Wellbeing

In 2019 Leanne Patrick, whom we met in Chapter 2 when we discussed the collaborative leadership style of @WeStudentNurse, was also the instigator of Student Nurse Mental Health Day. The @WeStudentNurse team had observed some of the mental wellbeing issues that students discussed on Twitter. Unlike some of the other WeCommunities groups, they were keen to speak out and advocate for students.

Leanne describes how students want and need to project confidence, but if they struggle with their mental health they may feel that they need to hide what they are experiencing.

'Nursing students often find themselves in a bind; having adjusted to being continually assessed, we fall prey to our own expectations that we must always project competence. We wrongly assume this means we must never be seen to struggle.'

LEANNE PATRICK, WRITING IN *NURSING STANDARD*, 2019

By listening to each other, Leanne thought that they might more readily realise that they were not alone and may come forward to seek help. She was right.

Continued

CASE STUDY 16.5 | **Leanne Patrick—Advocacy for Student Mental Health and Wellbeing—cont'd**

Leanne did a literature search about the mental wellbeing issues of student nurses, but she discovered there was little hard data about the student mental health experience. She put the idea of an annual student nurse mental health day to the team with a view to enabling and empowering students to discuss their struggles with things like anxiety and depression. They agreed.

The @WeStudentNurse team engaged other student nurse Twitter accounts as equal partners in delivery so that they could engage the widest range of students.

The day was launched on 6 May 2019, where the team ran Twitter Polls that revealed that over 94% of 334 students had experienced anxiety or depression over the course of their degree. They signposted students to sources of help in their universities and held Twitter chats to enable students to express their views.

Leanne wrote up the experience in *Nursing Standard* (2019).

Student Mental Health Day was held again in 2020 and looks set to be an annual feature on the student nurse calendar.

CASE STUDY 16.6 | **Brian Webster: Fintry Community Garden**

Whilst many students may think that creativity and innovation end at work or study, Brian Webster, an adult student nurse from Dundee University, thought differently. According to the Scottish Index of Multiple Deprivation, Fintry is a disadvantaged area where fruit and vegetables are not always affordable or accessible, hence the desire to create the Fintry Community Garden. Brian researched organisations like the food bank charity the Trussell Trust and world-renown reports by authors such as Professor Sir Michael Marmot to understand how best to help communities tackle health inequalities and address hunger. He discovered, for example, that Professor Marmot set out six policy objectives to reduce health inequalities, including the creation of healthy and sustainable places and communities (Marmot 2017).

In 2019 he approached his local council to ask if he and eight local people in his community, whom he had reached out to via door knocking and social media, could take over a piece of land and create an allotment and community garden. Fintry Community Garden became a constituted group, meaning that it set out formal roles like chairman and treasurer and had an agreed constitution—the basic rules by which a group operates. Brian himself was elected as secretary. This allowed the group to open a community bank account and apply for small grants. They applied for a grant to the National Lottery Awards For All scheme, receiving £10,000 in funding to progress their work.

The group's purpose is all about tackling the social issues that it sees around it, like poverty, substance misuse and climate change, as well as some of the more traditional lifestyle issues that nurses tackle every day, like obesity, poor nutrition, stress and low levels of exercise. It now provides free, fresh, organic vegetables—and fruit depending upon the Scottish weather—to local people.

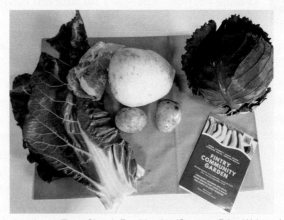

A donation to Fintry Church Food Larder. (Courtesy Brian Webster.)

CASE STUDY 16.6   **Brian Webster: Fintry Community Garden—cont'd**

Both members and volunteers put themselves forward to do tasks in the garden. During the COVID-19 pandemic, some of the food grown was donated to the Fintry Church Food Larder, an initiative to re-distribute food to local people in hard times. Garden workers packed the food into paper bags and included information about the garden and suggested recipes.

The group has formed strong partnerships with immediate neighbours such as the local primary school, library and community centre. They planted 400 tree saplings donated free from the Woodland Trust at local children's nurseries to contribute to the local authority's biodiversity and climate change plan.

The group works hard to communicate what it is doing via its website as well as developing relationships, for example with volunteers at Fintry Church.

Brian adds: 'We have been lucky that the Scottish and UK Governments recognised the importance of food distribution and production, so have been able to continue our work throughout the pandemic and its subsequent lockdowns, which have only exacerbated the disadvantage and struggles of the people of Fintry in the most need.'

In November 2020 Fintry Community Garden received a certificate of recognition from the Royal Horticultural Society.

Find out more on https://fintrycommunitygar.wixsite.com/website.

The Luck of the Entrepreneur?

You may have noticed that the student leaders featured in case studies pushed themselves out of their comfort zone, took opportunities and thought positively. These examples reflect the evidence that luck is not random but can be generated (Wiseman 2003).

There are four basic principles that you can use to take advantage of the scientific principles behind luck:

1. Create, notice and act upon chance opportunities. For example:
   - Apply for that leadership programme rather than think that you will not stand a chance.
   - Widen your network by saying yes to invitations to nursing events. Use this opportunity to meet lots of new people and talk to them rather than just to your friends.
2. Listen to your intuition. For example:
   - Trust your gut feelings—do not apply for a job just because of the proximity to your son's school and if you feel uneasy, do not do it.
   - Practising mindfulness can boost your intuition.
3. Expect good fortune. For example:
   - Practise a daily affirmation 'I am a lucky person and today is going to be another lucky day'.
   - Sit in a chair and visualise yourself achieving—such as doing well in an assessment.
4. Turn bad luck into good luck. For example:
   - Imagine how things could have been worse.
   - Compare yourself to people who are less fortunate than you.
   - Have the mindset that things will work out for the best—many people who are made redundant, for example (myself included), find themselves on a better path.

Adapted from Wiseman (2003).

■ **Time Out**

Using the four principles above, plan for how you will use some of these luck-generating principles in the coming week.

Summary

The nursing community has much to learn from the nurse entrepreneur. They are more likely to think differently and influence the organisation and the system. They may push boundaries or break rules, and that may make peers feel uncomfortable. They can also inspire fellow nurses with their transformational work as well as cause us to question whether a business mentality sits comfortably with nursing values.

Some start off as intrapreneurs before branching out on their own. Past NHS policy via the 'right to request' scheme of 2008 enabled this to happen—but business is business and some organisations fell by the wayside whereas others continue to trade. This reminds us that risk in entrepreneurship is ever-present and the characteristics that are needed include passion, ambition and versatility, as well as strong business skills.

Entrepreneurs are curious and question the status quo to find new ways to solve problems. They may be seen as 'lucky' because they have a positive mindset, listen to their intuition and take up opportunities. They may not recognise the skills of high adaptors and may clash with them—and vice versa—so understanding that both innovation and adaptation have their place is important. Entrepreneurial businesses need a mix of talent, combining invention and innovation with business skills. Innovation itself is a planned process starting with an idea that is tested, then developed and scaled.

Above all, nurses make great entrepreneurs because they understand the needs of their patients, families, communities and organisations, are excellent communicators, are empathic and can find solutions where others cannot.

Resources

Co-operatives UK, <https://www.uk.coop/>.
Digital Health Wales, <https://digitalhealth.wales/>.
Health Innovation Research Alliance Northern Ireland, <https://www.hira-ni.com/>.
Health Technology Wales, <https://www.healthtechnology.wales/>.
HSC Northern Ireland, <http://www.innovations.hscni.net/>.
National Council for Voluntary Organisations, <https://www.ncvo.org.uk/>.
NHS England, Clinical entrepreneur training programme, <https://www.england.nhs.uk/aac/what-we-do/how-can-the-aac-help-me/clinical-entrepreneur-training-programme/>.
Northern Ireland Connected Health Innovation Centre (CHIC), <https://www.ni-chic.org/>.
NurseBuff website, How to become a nurse entrepreneur (without leaving your job) <https://www.nurse-buff.com/how-to-become-a-nurse-entrepreneur/>.
Scottish Health Innovations Ltd, Clinical entrepreneur support, <https://www.shil.co.uk/news-and-events/news/nhs-clinical-entrepreneurs>.
Social Enterprise UK, <https://www.socialenterprise.org.uk/>.
UK Government website for setting up a business <https://www.gov.uk/browse/business/setting-up>.
Welsh Government, 2019. Supporting entrepreneurial women in Wales, <https://gov.wales/sites/default/files/publications/2020-01/supporting-entrepreneurial-women-wales-approach.pdf> (accessed 04/06/2021).

References

British Geriatric Society, Funguarding. Available from: <https://www.bgs.org.uk/resources/resource-series/fun-guarding>. (accessed 04/06/21).
Chesbrough, H.W., 2003. The era of open innovation. Sloan management Review, 44, 3.
Clare, A., Collier, E., Higgin, S., 2007. Enabling mental health through social and cultural inclusion. A Life in the Day, 11 (3), 22–26.

Copelli, F.H., Erdmann, A.L., Santos, J.L.G.D., 2019. Entrepreneurship in nursing: an integrative literature review. Revista Brasileira de Enfermagem, 72 (suppl 1) 289–298.

Danner, M., Coopersmith, J., 2015. The Other F Word. Wiley, Hoboken.

Department of Health, 2008. Social Enterprise – Making a Difference: A Guide to the Right to Request. <https://webarchive.nationalarchives.gov.uk/ukgwa/20081211163243/http://www.dh.gov.uk/en/Publicationsandstatistics/Publications/PublicationsPolicyAndGuidance/DH_090460>. (accessed 10/01/2022).

Department of Health, 2011. Establishing Social Enterprises Under the Right to Request Programme. National Audit Office, London. <https://www.nao.org.uk/report/establishing-social-enterprises-under-the-right-to-request-programme/>. (accessed 10/01/2022).

Fletcher, S.N.E., 2010. Nurse Faculty and Students' Behavioral Intentions and Perceptions Toward Entrepreneurship in Nursing. University of Rochester, Rochester, New York.

Kawasaki, G., 2015. The Art of Start 2.0. Penguin Random House, London.

Kendall, N., 2020. Namaste Care for People Living with Advanced Dementia: A Practical Guide for Carers and Professionals. Jessica Kingsley Publishers, London.

Kirton, M.J., 2003. Adaptation and Innovation in the Context of Diversity and Change. Routledge, London.

Marmot, M., Allen, J., Goldblatt, P., et al., 2017. Fair Society, Healthy Lives. The Marmot Review. <https://www.instituteofhealthequity.org/resources-reports/fair-society-healthy-lives-the-marmot-review>. (accessed 10/01/2022).

Nesta, 2019. A Compendium of Innovation Methods. <https://media.nesta.org.uk/documents/Compendium-of-Innovation-Methods-March-2019.pdf>. (accessed 17/09/2021).

Patrick, L., 2019. Tackling student mental health challenges together. Nursing Standard. RCNi. <https://stg.rcni.com/nursing-standard/opinion/comment/tackling-student-mental-health-challenges-together-151741>. (accessed 10/01/2022).

Sæter, G.B., 2019. Nurses becoming entrepreneurial – exploring learning objectives. International Conference CREE2019. Roanne.

Slywotzsky, A., 2002. The Art of Profitability. Grand Central Publishing, New York.

Social Value UK, What is Social Value? <https://socialvalueuk.org/what-is-social-value/>. (accessed 03/06/2021).

Wilson, A., Averis, A., Walsh, K., 2003. The influences on and experiences of becoming nurse entrepreneurs: a Delphi study. International Journal of Nursing Practice, 9, 236–245.

Wiseman, R., 2003. The Luck Factor. Century, London.

Wood, K., 2021. Creating belonging- flags on student name badges. The Academy of Fab NHS Stuff. <https://fabnhsstuff.net/fab-stuff/creating-belonging-flags-on-student-name-badges-as-part-of-my-role-to-ensure-equity-in-our-programmes-i-joined-our-staff-faith-and-belief-group-this-group-me-the-drive-and-inspiration-to-promote-o>. (accessed 08/06/2021).

This is the just the start of your leadership development, and I hope that these chapters have been useful to you.

Kathryn Perrera at NHS Horizons reminded us in Chapter 4 that we learn through reflecting on experience and not through experience alone. You now have the opportunity to reflect on your own leadership journey with me through this book.

My own reflection on interviewing undergraduate, recently graduated nurses and allied health professionals has been about the power of listening with fascination and without interruption. This in turn has led to those people learning more about themselves as they spoke their thoughts out loud to me.

When I wrote up and sent them the stories that they gave me, this helped them to validate and acknowledge their leadership qualities. There was also an exchange of experience across the generations that helped us both as leaders. A few of the people who I interviewed went on to do something differently. These were the moving and unintended consequences of my book-writing journey.

I mentioned during the introduction that you might:

- Write a letter to yourself to open when you have finished reading this book, or at a later date.
- Write a blog or article on what happened when undertaking the time-out exercises: how did you feel, what did you learn, what did you change, what did you take away? A reflection model will help you organise and systematise your approach to reflection.

I'm hoping that you did keep that diary or notebook with your thoughts and feelings, or maybe you have written notes in the book margins. I do this with most of my management and leadership books, which often include very personal observations as the penny drops when I read—so I can never lend them out!

I still reread the letter that I wrote to myself after completing the Top Manager Programme in 2002! Here's what I wrote:

'To Heather

I learned [on a visualisation exercise during my leadership programme] that my subconscious is a powerful force and that my own self-image is holding me back. It communicated (to my distaste) what I needed to hear. I am not "Barbie", I am an authoritative leader. Only when I believe this will I move on.

I've learnt to:
- Take a risk
- To believe and trust in myself
- To know that I am equal to others'

What will your letter say?

#150Leaders: A 2-year UK-wide student leadership programme targeted at health care students from a variety of disciplines

ABC: An acronym for a model explaining how we can manage adversity by challenging our beliefs and by doing so impact our consequential feelings. ABC also represents, according to the King's Fund think tank, the core needs of nurses and midwives: autonomy, belonging, contribution
ACE: An acronym for leadership that is actionable, connected and extensible
AHP: Allied health professional
APPG: All-Party Parliamentary Group

BAME: Black and minority ethnic
BATNA: A term used during negotiations to mean best alternative to a negotiated agreement
BDA: British Dietetic Association
BSL: British Sign Language

CCG: Clinical Commissioning Group
CIC: Community interest company
CPD: Continuous professional development
CQC: Care Quality Commission
CUS: A safety tool to help people raise concerns; CUS is an acronym for concerned, uncomfortable and safety
CV: Curriculum vitae

DMAIC: Define, measure, analyse, improve and control

EBCD: Experience-based codesign
EI: Emotional intelligence
EPIC: An eco- and e-health academic programme for Cornwall and the Isles of Scilly
EPOCH: The elements of a business plan, standing for what are you excellent at, which people will benefit, what outcomes do you want for those people, who are your customers, how much will they pay you.

FFT: Friends, Families and Travellers (Project)
FT: Foundation Trust

GPN: General practice nurse
GROW: A coaching model using the acronym goal, reality, options, will

HCA: Health care assistant
HEARTS: An acronym used in a leadership workbook devised by Swansea Leadership Academy: honesty, emotional intelligence, authenticity, resilience, true connections
HEE: Health Education England
HIS: Healthcare Improvement Scotland
HLM: Healthcare leadership model

ICS: Integrated care system
ICU: Intensive care unit
IHI: Institute for Healthcare Improvement
IQ: Intelligence quotient

KAI test: Kirton's test for ability to adapt and innovate

Leeds GATE: Leeds Gypsy and Traveller Exchange
LGBT+: An abbreviation that includes people who are lesbian, gay, bisexual and transsexual, but implies with the plus sign that queer, questioning, intersex, asexual people and others who are not specifically identified are included as well
LJMU: Liverpool John Moore's University

MBA: Masters in Business Administration
MBE: Member of the Order of the British Empire
MBTI: Myers Briggs Type Indicator
MOOC: Massive open online course

NASA: National Aeronautics and Space Administration
NHSLA: NHS Leadership Academy
NHSX: A joint unit bringing together teams from the Department of Health and Social Care and NHS England and NHS Improvement to drive the digital transformation of care
NMC: Nursing and Midwifery Council
NQN: newly qualified nurse—today the term newly registered nurse is used in preference

OCEAN: Openness, conscientiousness, extroversion, agreeableness, neuroticism
OFSTED: Office for Standards in Education

PAL: Peer-assisted learning
PbR: Payment by results
PDSA: Plan-do-study-act
plc: Private limited company
PPT: Programme planning team

RBCS: Resilience-based clinical supervision
RCN: Royal College of Nursing
RQIA: Regulation and Quality Improvement Authority

SBAR: Situation, background, assessment and recommendation
SEG: Student empowerment group
SHCR: School for Health and Care Radicals
SMART: Specific, meaningful, achievable, relevant/realistic, timebound
SPC: Statistical process control
STEM: Science, technology, engineering and mathematics
SWANSLA: Swansea Student Leadership Academy

TED: Technology, Entertainment and Design: a nonprofit devoted to spreading ideas, usually in the form of short, powerful talks

WHO: World Health Organisation

INDEX

Page numbers followed by "*f*" indicate figures, "*t*" indicate tables, "*b*" indicate boxes.